THE MENTALLY ILL
IN COMMUNITY-BASED
SHELTERED CARE

HEALTH, MEDICINE, AND SOCIETY:
A WILEY-INTERSCIENCE SERIES
DAVID MECHANIC, Editor

Evaluating Treatment Environments: A Social Ecological Approach
  by **Rudolf H. Moos**

*Human Subjects in Medical Experimentation: A Sociological Study of the
Conduct and Regulation of Clinical Research*
  by **Bradford H. Gray**

Child Health and the Community
  by **Robert J. Haggerty, Klaus J. Roghmann,** and **Ivan B. Pless**

Health Insurance Plans: Promise and Performance
  by **Robert W. Hetherington, Carl E. Hopkins,** and **Milton I. Roemer**

The End of Medicine
  by **Rick L. Carlson**

Humanizing Health Care
  by **Jan Howard** and **Anselm Strauss,** Volume Editors

*The Growth of Bureaucratic Medicine: An Inquiry into the Dynamics of Patient
Behavior and the Organization of Medical Care*
  by **David Mechanic**

The Post-Physician Era: Medicine in the Twenty-First Century
  by **Jerrold S. Maxmen**

A Right to Health: The Problem of Access to Primary Medical Care
  by **Charles E. Lewis, Rashi Fein,** and **David Mechanic**

Gift of Life: The Social and Psychological Impact of Organ Transplantation
  by **Roberta G. Simmons, Susan D. Klein,** and **Richard L. Simmons**

*Mentally Ill in Community-Based Sheltered Care: A Study of Community Care
and Social Integration*
  by **Steven P. Segal** and **Uri Aviram**

THE MENTALLY ILL IN COMMUNITY-BASED SHELTERED CARE

A STUDY OF COMMUNITY CARE AND SOCIAL INTEGRATION

Steven P. Segal
University of California, Berkeley

Uri Aviram
Tel Aviv University, Israel

A WILEY-INTERSCIENCE PUBLICATION

JOHN WILEY & SONS, New York · Chichester · Brisbane · Toronto

Library of Congress Cataloging in Publication Data:

Segal, Steven P   1943–
    The mentally ill in community-based sheltered
care.

   (Health, medicine, and society)
   "A Wiley-Interscience publication."
   Includes bibliographies and index.
   1. Mentally ill—Rehabilitation.   2.   Halfway
houses.   3.   Community mental health services.
4.   Community mental health services—California.
I.   Aviram, Uri, 1936–   joint author.
II.   Title.
RC439.5.S43   362.2'2   77-22474

ISBN 0-471-77400-6

Printed in the United States of America

10 9 8 7 6 5 4 3 2 1

To

Barbara, Ariella, and our families

Preface

In today's world the question of how we will care for our mentally ill, especially for those who are chronically disordered, has become a national and international issue. We face a choice that may, in fact, have already been resolved for us. We question whether it is most efficient, most effective, and in the best interest of mentally ill individuals to have them in mental institutions supported and accredited by the state, and essentially remaining the concern of the state, or whether we should care for our mentally ill in local, privately owned community facilities, perhaps subsidized by local or state government, and certainly licensed or accredited by such governments. Reports of the dismal failure of state hospitals as treatment facilities have led us to reject out of hand the appropriateness of this type of institution. In addition the costs of state hospitals have become so great that we question the wisdom of spending the tax dollar for ineffectual service. We have moved to a system of community care, hoping to provide better treatment, increase recovery, and more adequately insure the civil liberties of people who in the past were sometimes inappropriately confined or deprived of their rights by being placed in mental institutions for long periods of time without due process. We have looked to the community itself to provide the support necessary to maintain its men-

Report says many mentally ill kept in foul cockroach ghettoes

Associated Press

WASHINGTON — A new government report says some mentally ill patients in private nursing homes are living with hunger, cockroaches, leaking roofs, exposed electrical wires and doors made of cardboard and burlap.

The report released today by the Senate subcommittee on long-term care and programs particularly scrutinized New York and Illinois. Senate investigators said private homes were found wanting in both states.

Sen. Frank Moss, D-Utah, chairman of the panel, said the conditions were being fostered by government policy that provides a financial incentive to move patients from public institutions into private-care facilities.

"I have seen hungry people with their faces up against vending machines begging for a quarter," Moss said. "I saw three patients cooking eggs on a hotplate in their room while breakfast was being served in the dining room. I learned that they had bought the eggs with money they had received from begging."

Moss claimed mental patients "are a good investment" in New York and Illinois.

He offered case histories of several private operations, including one in Illinois where the operator housed 180 mental patients who were transferred from public care facilities. The operator received $400,000 a year and managed to keep $185,000 as profit. Moss said the operator spent only 54 cents per patient per day for food.

"He defended this profit, telling us it was below industry expectations," Moss said.

Moss laid part of the blame on Congress and the Social Security Act, including the Supplemental Security Income program.

In 1935, when it approved Social Security, Moss said, Congress barred Social Security funds for residents of public institutions. But if boarded in a private home they could receive the money.

"In short, Congress created the scandal-ridden, for-profit nursing home industry," he said.

In this same way, Moss said, Congress barred receipt of SSI funds by individuals in public institutions and cut SSI funds by a third for individuals living with relatives.

The result, Moss said, was an incentive to leave public institutions for private-care facilities. The same law provided financial incentive for states to move patients into private homes, transferring the cost of caring for a patient to the federal level.

The report says the number of patients in state mental hospitals has dropped 44 per cent from 427,799 to 237,692 between 1969 and 1974.

"The saddest thing is that more often than not patients have been placed in slum housing and forgotten," Moss said. "In some cases, so many discharged patients have been placed in particular areas of our major cities that they have become instant psychiatric ghettos."

Patients in many of these institutions are confronted with poor care and abuse, deliberate physical abuse and unsanitary conditions, he said.

He claimed also they face poor food, high incidence of theft, inadequate control on drugs, fire hazards, reprisal if they complain about conditions, use of restraints and lack of activities and recreation.

"The reason that this scandal has not been discovered up to now is that . . . most states have hidden the problem because of their complicity in moving thousands of patients into such facilities to save money," Moss said.

San Francisco Examiner, Friday, March 19, 1976, p. 1
Reprinted by Permission of *San Francisco Examiner*

tally ill. Yet some mentally ill have no roots in the community, or at least no residence in a community that they call their own or that is willing to accept them. Simply shifting the focus of care from the hospital to the community has in no way changed the issues and problems related to their care. Certainly it has made the policing of quality of care more difficult than it ever was. Yet it may have given the mentally ill a new sense of freedom and a different perspective on life.

The two news articles herein offer a reasonable statement of the issues and dilemmas involved in providing sheltered care to the mentally ill.

During the first 4 months of our project 134 open-ended interviews were conducted with individuals throughout California who were concerned with

Wintonia House

Mentally ill face cash pinch

SEATTLE (UPI) — Nadine considered it a pretty good Thanksgiving even though she may lose her home.

"I don't know what I could do or would do if they closed down," Nadine said as she finished her roast turkey dinner. "There's no comparison between this place and the state hospitals."

Nadine and about 125 other persons live at Wintonia house, which provides transitional care for the mentally ill, mentally retarded and for persons with other disabilities.

The ramshackle, six-story brick building became Wintonia five years ago. It once was a hotel.

"This place is just like a hotel, because you can go out any time you want," she said. "At the state hospital you had to stay on the grounds.

"Last time I was at Western (State Hospital) I was so much out of my head I set fire to myself and they didn't know if I would live.

"They're good to us here. And the food is very good."

The state of Washington pays each resident's room and board fee —just under $9 a day — augmented by counseling and medical service at county facilities.

Despite the aid, the private, profit-making company operating Wintonia — the Danmor Co. — has lost $80,000 this year.

That's even worse than the $50,000 loss in 1974. And, if the residents don't know the specifics, some get the general gist of what's going on.

Independent-Gazette
Friday, November 28, 1975

"We need more money to stay open," said Mike, who looks almost like a Pacific northwest logger with his full beard, broad face and open flannel shirt. "It takes more than it did before to stay open."

The $36,000 deficit for the last four months of this year is being picked up through a onetime demonstration grant, which allows Wintonia to show it provides a unique service to residents.

The staff teaches residents things such as basic as shopping and managing money. But the residents seem to take the most pride in what they do for Wintonia.

"I work on the switchboard three times a week — Monday, Wednesday and Friday," Nadine said. "Lots of times when I was learning I made mistakes and they still didn't fire me. The counselors are very good and I've never seen one get mad."

Despite the help of the residents to keep it going, if someone doesn't come up with more money, Danmor will close Wintonia at the end of the year.

Felix Reisner, chairman of the King County Mental Health Administrative board, said he will personally do what he can to help Wintonia, which he considers unique and valuable. But he says the county can't afford to pay for live-in facilities, only out-patient clinics.

"You have to make choices," he said. "The state needs to provide money for Wintonia."

Dr. Muriel Taylor, in charge of mental health funds for the state, disagreed.

"Felix has the money if he wants to use it that way," she said. "We've got enough in the state budget for 1976 for both out-patient and in-patient facilities."

But Reisner said there is no way the county can appropriate the money by Jan. 1.

the problems of community care for the mentally ill. These interviews often involved walking through neighborhoods with former patients and spending time in service facilities to observe and develop an understanding of the released patient's perception of his world. Also during this first 4-month study period we reviewed the available documents about released patients in California and across the country. It became increasingly apparent as we reviewed the literature and spoke to more people that there was a lack of hard descriptive data on released mental patients and an absence of a clear statement of goals and expectations for helping them. It was also apparent that former mental patients living in sheltered care, whose plight was receiving the most publicity, constituted only a small fraction of the total released-patient population. Yet the distinct needs of this segment of the released-patient population appeared to us to be a justifiable focus of our study. Although general agreement existed during the study's planning phase that changes were needed to better the lives of former hospital patients in sheltered care, there was little knowledge of which services would be most effective and no clear expectation of what different services could achieve.

This book is an attempt to describe what life is like for the mentally ill in community sheltered care and to offer some insight into the factors that may help move the system toward offering better care. The findings offered on community care of the mentally ill reported in this study are taken primarily from the situation in California. These findings and the insights they offer us are not, however, unique to California; they may be used to develop an understanding of the mentally ill in community-based sheltered-care facilities throughout the United States and in other countries, wherever a similar move toward community-based care for the mentally ill is being made.

STEVEN P. SEGAL
URI AVIRAM

Berkeley, California
Tel Aviv, Israel
July 1977

Acknowledgments

We thank most of all those individuals living in sheltered-care faciliti.... who gave their time to help us develop and perform the study, as well as the operators of the facilities we looked at, for their time and cooperation in discussing with us what it was like to run a sheltered-care facility.

We thank the Department of Health of the State of California, and Dr. Earl Brian and Stephen Gibbons of the California Health and Welfare Agency, whose concern and effort helped secure the funding for the initial 2 years of the project; and the National Institute of Mental Health (Grant #5R01-MH25417-03ESR), whose funds enabled us to explore in depth the results we obtained. We thank the Schools of Social Work in California, which provided office space, and Dr. Paul Ekman of Langley Porter Neuropsychiatric Institute, who provided films for training our interviewers. Thanks to George Collins and the Los Angeles Department of Mental Health, and to Richard Gilberg of the Community Care Services Section of the California State Department of Health, for the facility lists. Thanks also to the health, mental health, welfare, and voluntary agencies in California, too numerous to name, whose support made this study possible.

We express appreciation for the expert advice and critical reviews of our efforts given by William Nicholls, Jr., of the University of California, Berkeley, Survey Research Center; Frederick Meyers of the University of California, San Francisco Medical School; Harry Specht of the School of Social Welfare, University of California, Berkeley; and David Mechanic, of the University of Wisconsin, Madison.

We are indebted to Tel-Aviv University of Israel and especially to Joseph Katan and Shimon Spiro for the help extended to Dr. Aviram in funding his travel to California.

We thank all the staff members who have participated in the development and implementation of the project. Particular credit belongs to Reneé Anspach, Lynn Everett-Dille, Kristie Nelson, Peggy Nelson, and Barry Trute. Finally, we thank our families for the time and the support they provided us throughout the project.

                                                                    S.P.S.
                                                                    U.A.

Contents

PART ONE

FROM COMMUNITY TO HOSPITAL AND BACK

A ROUND TRIP SPANNING 150 YEARS

During the past 150 years, ideas about how the mentally ill should be treated or cared for have made a full circle. Public policy on the form and location of care has moved from an emphasis on care of the mentally ill by their local community to one on housing them in state institutions, only to return to a recent reemphasis, beginning with the community mental-health movement in the early 1960s, to move individuals out of institutions back into the community. This may be a result of an idealization of life, an attempt to find a *Gemeinschaft* style of life (one characterized by mutual support based on close personal ties of friendship and kinship) for former patients within the community. It is also founded on the assumptions that one is best cared for by people who care about him and that "caring" people are to be found in local communities.

When the mentally ill were cared for in the community 150 years ago, they were exploited as cheap labor or penned up like animals; in general they were physically and socially excluded from community life. For example,

1

"dumping" was a common practice from the fifteenth to the nineteenth centuries. Mentally ill individuals were taken by coach at night to another town and simply left there. Today we do not do this. But in the return to community care we find old practices translated into new techniques. Some communities now offer financial inducements to leave the area in the form of a one-time general-assistance check.

In Part I, the introduction to our study of the life of the mentally ill in sheltered care, we look at a detailed history of the care of the mentally ill— a history taking them from the community to the hospital and back. In the first chapter—Changing Trends in Sheltering the Mentally Ill—we speak about former community care and the movement to shelter individuals in mental institutions. In our second chapter—Toward a Community-Care System—we look at the movement from the institutions back into the community. Both chapters consider these trends from a national and international perspective. In Chapter 3—Mental Health Reform in California—we consider the policies and practices relating to the development of the community-care movement in California, where our project was conducted.

ONE

Changing Trends in Sheltering the Mentally Ill

Only in the last 150 years has sheltering of the mentally ill as a unique population become an accepted public policy. The behavior and feeling, which is today defined as mental illness, has in the past been described as madness, lunacy, or insanity. Such behavior syndromes today are likely to result in psychiatric hospitalization.

A shelter is "a refuge or defense: a means or place of protection in an area of safety" (*Webster's* Dictionary p. 2093). Synonymous terms are cover, asylum, retreat, or sanctuary.

Public policy relating to the care of the mentally ill has three major functions: (1) the basic humanitarian ideology of protecting the dependent, (2) the social control of a deviant group that poses a threat to the community, and (3) the demonstration of a curative potential that can be realized at a minimum cost.

Until 20 years ago one mode of sheltering the mentally ill predominated throughout the Western world: mental institutions. From their very beginnings these institutions provided a means of sheltering that fulfilled (or often simply claimed to fulfill) the three major functions stated earlier. In the past

3

20 years a new trend has emerged—community care as an approach to sheltering the mentally ill. This trend has emerged largely from the inability of
the large mental institution to carry on (or claim to carry on) its three major
functions.

The three functions of an adequate system of providing care to the mentally ill have not been altered. There is still consensus that shelter is the appropriate solution. What has changed is the means by which shelter is to be
provided. Providing shelter within the community is represented by two approaches. First, there is the approach (anticipated and planned by policymakers and mental-health professionals) whereby the mentally ill are sheltered within an established social network such as the family. In this situation
the family is aided by various community resources that provide treatment
and care, such as short-term hospitalization, psychoactive medication, and
therapy and rehabilitation services.

The second approach, the privately operated sheltered-care facility (which
was unplanned and developed in an *ad hoc* fashion), is a means of providing
shelter to mentally ill individuals who have no access to established social
networks such as families. These people were not given much consideration in
the planning of the thrust to provide community shelter for the mentally ill.
Also not considered were the ability of the family to accept the burden of
sheltering the mentally ill and the possibility that, in response to this burden,
some families would find alternate solutions to in-home care—such as a private sheltered-care facility. Given the need to provide shelter to those without
families and the inability of many families to accept responsibility for their
mentally ill, a new privately operated system of sheltered-care facilities has
developed that acts as a secondary and sometimes primary placement (i.e., in
lieu of the hospital, which has been the major placement resource).

Finding a solution to any social problem depends on concurrent social,
economic, and cultural trends. Public policy reflects people's ideas, theories,
ideologies, social and economic conditions, available treatment technologies,
and knowledge about the issues in question. Thus public policy concerning
the mentally ill, and the provision of sheltered care as a public-policy solution, must be viewed within a broad social context. The focus of this chapter
is on the trends that led to the establishment of public provision of shelter in
large institutions. Further, this chapter considers the roots of the movement
that brought shelter and care out of isolation and back into the community.

RECOGNITION OF MENTAL ILLNESS AS A SOCIAL PROBLEM

Public provision of sheltered care as a solution to the problem of mental
illness cannot occur unless society has recognized mental illness and defined it
as a social problem requiring social intervention. The phenomenon termed
madness, lunacy, insanity, or mental illness in different periods is docu-

mented from prehistoric times (Mora, 1967). In the Bible perhaps the most famous episode of mental disorder is the case of King Saul (1 Sam. 20:18–24), whose behavior might be diagnosed in modern psychiatric terms as manic-depressive. Hippocrates, in his writings about epilepsy ("sacred disease"), was aware of the phenomenon of mental disorder and in fact presented a medical viewpoint, rather than the popular mystical, magic interpretation of the time (Mora, 1967). There are instances throughout history wherein behavior defined today as mental illness was recognized as such.

Until recently, however, the mentally disordered were not classified as a specific group, nor was mental illness viewed as a social problem requiring specific intervention. Rather, the mentally ill were considered members of the marginal groups in the social system and treated as such. Kathleen Jones (1972), in her description of eighteenth-century customs in England, notes that "the problem was a submerged one" (p. 3). If the mentally disordered broke the law, they were judged by the penal law; if their mental condition led to poverty and dependence, they were in the purview of the poor law; if wandering outside their legal place of settlement without means of support, they were dealt with by the vagrancy laws.

Bethlehem Hospital (or "Bedlam," as it is more commonly known) was established in 1377, and private madhouses or "gentlemen's asylums" serviced wealthy people who apparently suffered from mental disorder before the eighteenth century. But the 1744 Act of the British Parliament may be considered one of the first statements of public policy regarding the mentally disturbed. This act, which dealt basically with the problem of vagrancy, had a special clause concerning "lunatics." It excepted "lunatics" from penal clauses applicable to other vagrants, and in addition to provisions for detention, restraint, and maintenance (previously mentioned in the Act of 1714) the Act added the words "and curing" and thus recognized for the first time that people suffering from mental disorders required treatment. The Act did not, however, specify any method by which treatment and care should be carried out.

The situation was not much different in colonial America. Albert Deutsch (1949), in reviewing colonial provisions for the mentally disordered, notes that these provisions consisted mainly of indifference or repressive punishment. The mentally disordered were usually cared for by their families. When they became publicly recognized, they were dealt with as paupers or as criminals (if they broke the law). Incarceration was a common solution. The first institution in American history that received the mentally disordered as patients was Pennsylvania General Hospital, opened by Quakers in 1756. The mentally ill were not, however, the only patients of this institution, nor were they always admitted as "mentally ill." The first American hospital exclusively for the mentally disordered was opened in 1773 in Williamsburg, Virginia, and fully 50 years passed before Virginia opened another institution for the mentally disordered—demonstrating that public provisions specifically for the mentally ill were, as late as mid-eighteenth century, the exception rather than the rule.

INSTITUTIONALIZATION: HUMANE, PROTECTIVE, AND INEXPENSIVE CURE

Although provision of shelter and care for the mentally ill dates as far back as 600 A.D., when the famous Geel Colony was established in Belgium (Henry, 1941) and existed on a small scale in eighteenth-century England and America, it is basically a phenomenon of the latter half of the nineteenth century. At this time the mental institution was "discovered" as a form of shelter for the mentally ill that was humane, guaranteed the protection of the community, and promised "cure" at minimal cost.

A Humanitarian Solution

As a humanitarian solution to providing care for the mentally ill, the institution had demonstrated its utility in the latter half of the eighteenth century and first quarter of the nineteenth century. Moral treatment—as practiced in institutions run by Pinel in France, Tuke in England, and Rush in the United States—broke the pattern of harsh custodialism as practiced in mental institutions. This new approach was based on kindness and warmth toward the patients. Pinel believed that, in addition to heredity, psychological factors were important causes for mental disorders. He was influenced by two movements characteristic of the age of Enlightenment: rationality and social reform. He believed that a patient's faulty education could cause mental disorders and that man could shape his destiny by social action. His program at his asylum was influenced by his zeal for social reform and mental uplift. He asserted that it was impossible to determine whether mental symptoms resulted from mental disease or from the effects of harsh conditions. Treatment of the mentally ill, he believed, was a form of education that could be best achieved in an atmosphere of sympathy and recognition of an individual's worth. The ideas and practices of the moral-treatment approach had a profound influence on psychiatric programs in the United States. Moral treatment appeared to be an effective and humane device for dealing with the mentally ill (Bockoven, 1963).

Social transformation during the French Revolution, the idea of liberating people from bondage, and the "Second Great Awakening" in religion (which increased the philanthropic activities of the wealthy) were essential in bringing about the reform in the care of the mentally ill in the first half of the nineteenth century. Contemporary humanist trends were effectively used by supporters of the mental-hospital movement after the 1830s. Dorothea Dix, a social reformer who almost single-handedly helped initiate the hospital movement, strongly relied on the humanist character of the institution in convincing policymaking bodies of its utility.

A Mechanism of Social Control

As a mechanism of social control, institutionalizing the mentally ill was an attempt to protect the community from dangerous individuals, as well as to reshape these individuals to enable them to make a greater contribution to society. Rothman (1971) points out that, during the Jacksonian period in America, the asylum was seen as an instrument to restore social balance to the new republic. This belief was based on the theory that social problems of the early nineteenth century were a result of faulty organization of the community. The asylum was to fulfill a dual purpose: It would rehabilitate inmates and by virtue of its anticipated success serve as an example for the larger society.

According to Foucault (1965) the asylum was not so much an effort to free the mentally disordered from the harsh conditions of jails or poorhouses as it was a drive to bring madness under the rigid control of reason. The asylum was therefore an attempt at a suitable social mechanism to mold the insane into something more "acceptable" to modern society, using reason as the major tool.

Finally Grob (1966a, b; 1973) attributes the growth of the mental-hospital movement in America to several social, cultural, and economic factors relating to problems of social control. Urbanization caused a breakdown of the traditional informal-care mechanism. Neither socioeconomic conditions nor urban life-styles allowed families and communities to continue to care for the mentally ill as they had in the past. The concentration of the mentally disordered in the city attracted a great deal of attention, bringing awareness of the problems of disturbed behavior in developing urban areas. The waves of immigration and, in particular, the effect of large numbers of lower class immigrants arriving in the United States intensified the problems of dependency and social control for American cities and the public. Alleviating these problems by confining the mentally ill in institutions was a popular solution.

A Curative and Economically Feasible Solution

In the words of Dorothea Dix, "No fact is better established in all hospital annals than this; that it is cheaper to take charge of the insane in the curative institution than to support them elsewhere for life" (Deutsch, 1949, p. 172). What more could a policymaking body ask for than something that is humanitarian, maintains the social order, and does not cost much? The answer as it relates to the mentally ill is the promise that the proposed solution also has curative potential. As Jones (1972) points out, it was cheaper to provide workhouse care than to provide care in a curative asylum. The assessment of cost related to the care of the mentally ill has invariably been bound up in this issue. Without the "curative" component, long-term maintenance is a necessity. The immediate investment of larger amounts of money to avoid future costs has been a primary argument for obtaining public support.

The work of Rush at the Pennsylvania hospital and Pinel at Bicêtre demonstrated the curative as well as the humanistic potential of the institution. Although their work is often placed under the heading of "moral" treatment, along with Tuke's York Retreat in England, Rush and Pinel were physicians and viewed their efforts as curative, whereas Tuke was a Quaker providing his fellow Quakers with a humane environment. But of more importance to the perception of the curative institution was the growth of phrenology in the United States in the first half of the nineteenth century.

During the latter part of the nineteenth century, phrenology became a popular movement in the United States. Today it is colloquially remembered as personality assessment by reading the bumps on one's head. Actually it emphasized the curative aspects of the environment on localized brain functions, and before being discredited it had been used to provide some of the major theoretical justifications for the more humane characteristics of institutional care (Davies, 1955).

Phrenology offered a theoretical rationale for the curative influence exerted by humanistic institutions on the mentally ill. Samuel Woodward, one of the founders of the American Psychiatric Association and first superintendent of Worcester State Hospital in Massachusetts, wrote that:

no man living in charge of a hospital for the insane, and capable of mental analysis and physical observation, reasonably acquainted with phrenology could avoid conviction of its truth (Davies, 1955, p. 94).

Thus institutional shelter, as developed during the last half of the eighteenth and the first half of the nineteenth century, was a solution that was justified as fulfilling all three basic functions of public policy relating to the care of the mentally ill.

CHALLENGES TO THE VIABILITY OF THE HOSPITAL

As soon as a means of sheltering the mentally ill that emphasized humanistic values, social control, and financially feasible cure, had been provided, historical trends began to erode the hospital's ability to justify itself on any of these three accounts. As a financially feasible cure emphasizing the curative aspects of a benign environment, the hospital was threatened by increasing admissions, which reduced or eliminated the ability to provide "moral treatment" at reasonable cost. Overcrowding and bureaucratization played havoc with its humanistic ends. Finally, within the last 20 years social control as a goal has been challenged by proponents of patients' civil rights—that is, civil libertarians and concerned citizens aroused by what they perceive to be an unjustified deprivation of patients' due-process rights in hospital commitment procedures and treatment methods.

The Hospitals' Inability to "Cure" People at a Reasonable Cost

During the second half of the nineteenth century the hospital was transformed to a custodial institution. During this bleak period in American psychiatry the curative aspirations and the optimism of moral treatment were discredited. The hospital became a facility of last resort. Two factors involved in discrediting the "curative potential" of the hospital were (1) the discrediting of phrenology and the practice of moral treatment and (2) the abuse of the notion of cure in promoting the institution as an effective solution to the problems posed by the mentally ill.

First, phrenology fell into disrepute and thus discredited the belief in the curative potential of the practice of moral treatment. The importance of a benign environment in influencing the development of mental illness was given less credence.

Second, in promoting the institution as a public-policy solution to problems presented by the mentally ill, mental hospitals between 1840 and 1850 covered up the effects of overcrowding and poor conditions and reported misleading cure rates as high as 75 and 100%. In 1887, after many years of research, Dr. Pliny Earle published his book *The Curability of Insanity*. Earle found that:

A major factor in the apparently high ratio of cures in institutions for the insane . . . lay in the failure to distinguish properly between the words "case," "patient," and "person." In many instances, the same person was discharged "recovered" from an institution a number of times within a few years, or even in the space of one year. In the statistical report of the time, the reader was given no intimation that the same person might appear as several "recovered cases" in the record. Thus, Earle relates, one woman was discharged recovered six times at Bloomingdale Asylum, and another, seven times at the Worcester Hospital, each within the space of one year. Incidentally, the woman who contributed six "recoveries" to the record of Bloomingdale in one year was reported cured no less than *forty-six times* before her death—which took place in an insane asylum (Deutsch, 1949, p. 156).

The result of these trends, in addition to continued overcrowding and hospital deterioration, was a discrediting of the mental hospital as a curative institution worthy of support. Financing of the mental hospital was reduced or failed to keep up with cost increases and thus at best allowed for custodial care.

The Erosion of the Hospitals' Ability to Meet the Humanistic Goals

From the very outset, pressures on the mental institution to admit large numbers of people compromised its ability to meet its humanistic goals. The expansion of hospitals accelerated the thrust of hospitalizing the mentally ill. This is a trend well known in service delivery: The availability of services increases their use. Grob (1973) contends that families who in the past refused to send their ill relatives to an almshouse or a jail now felt more comfortable sending them to the hospital. The hospital movement increased public awareness of the new alternative, and the "myth of curability" (Deutsch, 1949, p. 132) provided a perfect rationale for sending the mentally disordered to hospitals. With increased use, communities pressured the states to help them with control and custody of indigent and mentally disordered people, and the states responded by assuming greater responsibility.

Larger involvement of the state in the care of the mentally ill was part of a general trend in the United States to centralize public social-welfare services. The fact that the existing apparatus of care did not work caused the state to become more involved, to spend more public money, and to assume greater control over the way this money was spent in an effort to regulate, rationalize, and scrutinize the system. State after state established boards of charities and departments of public charities and corrections. Mental hospitals were included in these centralized systems of bureaucratic control (Grob 1973). During the last quarter of the nineteenth century many states. established central administrations for their hospitals (Deutsch, 1949).

Local communities now had a financial incentive to send their indigent mentally disordered to the state hospital: Doing so, they decreased their local welfare spending. Since the budget of the local community is based on local taxes, the state-hospital alternative became not only an economically sound solution but also a politically preferred one; raising money through local taxes to support the indigent was always a matter of some local dissatisfaction. Local leaders and politicians usually preferred an outside element to pick up the tab. Thus the states' financial responsibility for care of the mentally ill further increased the growth of state hospitals.

State hospitals were filled immediately after they were built. They could never meet the ever-increasing demand to admit more people. Administratively and legally admissions were controlled, not by the state hospital itself, but by elements outside of it. The tendency of judges in commitment proceedings, faced with local pressures and lack of alternatives, was to commit more mentally disordered people to state hospitals. A review of statistics reported by Deutsch (1949, p. 232) reveals that in 1840 about 15% of the total estimated number of mentally disordered people in the United States were in mental hospitals; 50 years later 70% were in mental hospitals. In one decade, 1880 to 1890, the percentage of mentally disordered who were cared for in mental institutions increased from 40 to 70%. While the population in the United States multiplied by 3.7 between 1850 and 1890, the population in mental institutions increased 29 times during this same period.

Grob (1973) points out that the size of a hospital's population, its physical plant, and its manpower distribution led to greater reliance on physical restraint and on strict bureaucratic mechanisms. This in turn led to the development of an environment of a total institution (Goffman, 1961)—an institution where all the life functions of the patients were scheduled and controlled.

Unable to create the humanistic environment that was found essential to the success of the earlier institutions following a moral-treatment ideology, psychiatry turned toward somatic factors within a more traditional medical model. Grob (1973) contends that the trend toward professionalism of psychiatrists isolated them from more humanitarian ideologies that existed in society and further hampered psychiatric care.

Challenging the Hospitals' Social-Control Function

Perhaps the strongest and most enduring function of the mental hospital has been that of social control. The use of the indefinite commitment—incarceration without due process over long periods of time—has enabled the hospital to justify its protective merits for society. Public attitudes toward the mentally ill emphasizing unpredictability and dangerousness have been the foundation of this social-control function. It was not until the mid-twentieth century, with the onset of the Civil Rights movement, that the social-control function of the hospital was challenged strongly enough to cause a major modification in admissions and retention procedures—a modification that threatens the existence of the hospital.

THE SEEDS OF CHANGE

The discrediting of humane care and cure at a feasible cost planted seeds of change that began to bear fruit early in the twentieth century. To remedy the grave overcrowding conditions, farm colonies and custodial institutions were established in the United States. During the economic depression of the 1930s the state hospitals initiated family-care programs—placing mentally ill patients in community foster-care situations to alleviate overcrowded conditions. An attempt was made to distinguish custodial care from acute treatment efforts.

Cultural and scientific changes at the beginning of the twentieth century providing an atmosphere supportive of medical discoveries and the evolution of germ theory, along with the success of the public-health movement in preventing the spread of major diseases, began to replace the prevailing pessimism with optimism. With the hope that mental illness, too, might be prevented, the mental-hygiene movement was established. Psychoanalytic theory provided a new means of understanding human behavior and actually brought about a cultural transformation in the Western world.

Social work developed as a new profession, and its involvement in mental-health services helped create an openness to the importance of environment in the development of community mental-health programs. Psychiatry itself began to look outside the walls of the hospital. Dr. Adolph Meyer insisted at the turn of the century that psychiatry should look at the person in his environment rather than at the disease.

We now turn to how these trends came together to lay the groundwork for a new mode of sheltering the mentally ill, a mode that would meet all three criteria for providing care—humaneness, public protection, and financially feasible curative potential. In reviewing the historical trends of care for the mentally ill, note that a new mode of sheltering could not be a success until it fulfilled all three of the functions that justified the development of the original mode. Thus the mental hospital was not abandoned until a new sheltering solution with components to meet the needs of the mentally ill was found.

REFERENCES

The Bible, *The New Oxford Annotated Bible.* H. G. May and B. M. Metzger (Eds.). New York: Oxford University Press, 1973.

Bockoven, J. S. *Moral Treatment in American Psychiatry.* New York: Springer, 1963.

Davies, J. D. *Phrenology: Fad and Science: A Nineteenth Century American Crusade.* New Haven, Connecticut: Yale University Press, 1955.

Deutsch, A. *The Mentally Ill in America.* New York: Columbia University Press, 1949.

Foucault, M. *Madness and Civilization: A History of Insanity in the Age of Reason.* New York: Pantheon, 1965.

Goffman, E. *Asylums: Essays on the Social Situation of Mental Patients and Other Inmates.* Garden City, New York: Doubleday, 1961.

Grob G. *The State and the Mentally Ill.* Chapel Hill, North Carolina: University of North Carolina Press, 1966a.

Grob, G. "The State Mental Hospital in Mid-Nineteenth Century America." *Am. Psychologist* **21**, 510–523 (1966b).

Grob, G. *Mental Institutions in America: Social Policy to 1875*. New York: Free Press, 1973.

Henry, G. W. "Mental Hospitals," In G. Zilboorg (Ed.). *A History of Medical Psychology*. Glencoe, Illinois: Free Press, 1941.

Jones, K. *A History of the Mental Health Services*. Boston: Routledge and Kegan Paul, 1972.

Mora, G. "History of Psychiatry," in A. M. Freedman and H. I. Kaplan (Eds.). *Comprehensive Textbook of Psychiatry*. Baltimore: The Williams and Wilkins Co., 1967.

Rothman, D. J. *The Discovery of the Asylum: Social Order and Disorder in the New Republic*. Boston: Little, Brown and Co., 1971.

Webster's Third New International Dictionary. P. B. Grove (Ed. in Chief). Springfield, Massachusetts: G. and C. Merriam Co., 1966.

TWO

Toward a Community-Care System

During the last century the mental hospital was the primary resource—often the only resource—for the care and treatment of the mentally ill. Despite some early signs of dissatisfaction with the operations and results of the mental-hospital system voiced in the late nineteenth century, no major change occurred until the middle of the twentieth century. Increasingly large sums of money went for the care of ever-growing masses of people confined in large public custodial institutions. By the early 1950s the number of patients hospitalized in mental institutions in the United States was almost 600,000, 85% in state and county mental hospitals, and the rest in federal or private mental hospitals or in psychiatric departments of general hospitals (Blain et al., 1955).

Statistics on prevalence and incidence of treated mental disorders show that the patterns of care of the mentally ill in the United States changed after the mid-1950s. The number of resident patients in mental hospitals started to decline (Clausen, 1971; Kramer et al., 1961); however, the number of first admissions to mental hospitals continued to grow (Kramer et al., 1972). It is obvious that more people diagnosed as mentally ill were returning to the community than in the past. Care and treatment are provided now in the community by many programs, various facilities, and personnel of different professions who were not part of the mental-health system in the past. Large sums of federal and state money are now provided for various community-care programs (Feldman, 1973)—a key element of which is the new form of sheltered care.

The development of a community-care system required a change of attitudes, new public policy, legal and administrative arrangements, and funds and personnel to execute the new programs in the community. It required the discovery of a new means of sheltering the mentally ill that met contemporary requirements of being humane, providing social control, and being a financially feasible approach to "curing" the mentally ill. How did the change from a hospital-centered care system to a community-care system happen? What caused it? What were its prerequisites?

The development of this new system of care had its catalysts in profound social and political changes of the twentieth century, in the Second World War, and more specifically in the continuing rapid deterioration of the mental-hospital system. Understanding how new public policy regarding the mentally ill emerged and how a community-care system has evolved as a new form of sheltered care is possible only through a consideration of how these factors acted as catalysts.

THE SOCIAL CONTEXT

As we have seen, the mental hospital—the asylum—was the basic societal response to the problem of mental illness at the turn of the century. The exclusion of the mentally ill in large overcrowded custodial institutions cannot be separated from the social context in which these institutions existed. When we view the social context of the time, we are struck by the wide gap perceived between normal and deviant people. Consistent with Social Darwinism, the dominant social theory at the turn of the century (Hofstadter, 1954), mentally ill people were considered biological or hereditary casualties of the natural selection process. Thus the social trend of the time provided a rationale for the meager attempts to improve the lot of the mentally ill: Little should be done for them, to protect future generations from their defective heredity.

During the last 50 years two major social trends have affected the mental health field and brought about changes in it: (1) the psychological revolution (2) democratization and social welfarism.

The Psychological Revolution

The twentieth century can be regarded as the century of the psychological revolution. Freud introduced and made psychological concepts acceptable to the general public. He broke away from the mainstream of clinical neurology and reintroduced emotional factors to an understanding of psychopathologies. He elucidated the relationship between normal and abnormal behavior and emphasized the importance of the individual's early environment in personality development. By placing health and illness on the same continuum, psychiatric theory helped to relax attitudes toward the mentally ill and increased general interest in psychological processes. It provided an optimistic framework for mental-health services, increasing interest in mental illness and renewing hope that cure and prevention were possibilities, and created a demand for increased mental-health services in large urban areas. This demand was crucial in establishing outpatient clinics and creating a cadre of professionals in the community, without which a move away from the hospitals could not have been contemplated.

Since Freud's time, psychological concepts have permeated intellectual and social thought, and psychological interpretations are more readily available than in the past.

Democratization and Social Welfarism

The trend toward community care of the mentally ill has been influenced also by democratization processes that have been taking place in modern society. We are witnessing a trend of inclusion of society's marginal groups into the mainstream of social life. The Civil Rights movement in the United States is both a cause and a consequence of this trend. Recently groups who were considered marginal or deviant have come out in the open, demanding rights and equal treatment. The "Gay Liberation" movement and the decision of the American Psychiatric Association to drop homosexuality from the official manual of mental disorders (*Time,* April 1, 1974) are good examples of this trend. Social Darwinism has given way to more democratic, egalitarian modes of thinking. The liberal attitudes of the 1960s provided the context in which the environment came to be seen as a primary factor in the cause and care of mental illness. The context of democratization was fruitful ground for the development of treatment approaches (such as the therapeutic community and open hospitals), for legal reforms, and for redefinition of social responsibility toward society's indigent members. The economic depression of the 1930s provided an impetus for the change in social philosophy, stimulating a new ideology of social welfarism that promoted federal intervention and the formulation of social planning and public policy at the national level (Marx et al., 1974).

It is inconceivable, without the social-welfare ideology and the large-scale programs it influenced, that the trend toward a community-care system could have taken place. We will see how income-maintenance programs for released mental patients, based on federal policy change, played an important role in facilitating the mass emigration of mental patients from the hospitals to the community (Aviram & Syme, 1974). The large-scale Community

Mental-Health Centers program in the United States was part of this central government acceptance of responsibility and of its intervention. Also, programs such as Medicare and Medicaid, an essential part of the community-care system for the mentally ill, would not have been established without the social-welfarism ideology.

The welfare orientation converged with the psychological revolution. An educated and aggressive middle class created and stimulated the establishment in the community of a human-service industry (Folta & Schatzman, 1968). No community-care system would have been possible without the human-service agencies in the communities and the professionals working in them.

THE EFFECTS OF WORLD WAR II

World War II was a major trauma for the Western world. Military and political victory over Nazi Germany and Japan created a current of optimism. People felt that a better and more just world could be established, and attention was now drawn to the internal conditions of the country. Without this optimism after World War II the subsequent social programs and reform that took place in the West are hard to understand.

The atrocities of the war shocked civilized nations, and to understand the horrible deeds of Nazi Germany, people resorted to psychological theories and their relationships to mass behavior (e.g., Erikson, 1950, Chapter 9). Mental-health problems posed by separation, bereavement, and destruction of homes as a result of the war were a common concern and stimulated interest in mental health and its influences on society. It is not surprising that, following its establishment in 1946, the World Health Organization created a special section on mental health (Roberts, 1967). The community mental-health movement that influenced mental-health policies in the West during the 1950s and 1960s was nourished by the interest of postwar society in mental health. The currents of optimism that followed the war provided the fuel for its achievements.

The war provided psychiatry and other mental-health professions with opportunities to organize and develop large-scale programs involved in selective-service screening. Between the beginning of 1942 and the end of the war in June 1945, about 1,875,000 men were rejected for service because of alleged psychiatric disability (Mechanic, 1969). Despite the hope that psychiatric problems could be prevented by the screening examination, many of the causalties of the U.S. military were related to psychiatric conditions (Felix, 1967; Marx et al., 1974). The conditions created by the war and the fact that soldiers of all social classes were receiving mental-health care helped remove psychiatry from its relative isolation and brought about increased respect and public recognition for mental-health professionals and services.

The psychiatric problems that occurred during the war emphasized the role of the social and physical environment in the onset, process, treatment, and care of psychiatric disabilities (Glass, 1969). Mental-health specialists, no longer able to rely solely on traditional psychodynamic methods, developed new techniques of intervention more suited to dealing with large numbers of people, often in their natural environment rather than in the psychiatric clinic.

Despite fears that wartime anxieties might increase the number of civilian psychiatric patients, the number of patients actually decreased during the war (Jones, 1972). This phenomenon, also apparent during World War I (Roberts, 1967), was attributed to the importance of feelings of group cohesiveness and community in times of war.

The wartime experience stimulated the ideology of community mental health. By the end of the war not only were mental-health services and professionals better known and more respected, but also the number of mental-health workers was much larger than before the war. They were the potential force for many of the new community-care programs that would follow.

THE DETERIORATION OF MENTAL INSTITUTIONS

The deterioration of mental hospitals that continued into this century became another important stimulus for the development of a community-care system. In concluding an analysis of mental institutions in America, Grob (1973, p. 342) stated that the situation "resembles a tragedy in which most participants, to a greater or lesser degree, were well intentioned but their actual behavior gave rise to less than desirable results."

The primary concern of mental hospitals during the first half of this century was safe custody of inmates using a minimum of public funds (Grob, 1973; Wing & Brown, 1970). This resulted in large, overcrowded, and understaffed hospitals, with a high percentage of chronic wards in which long-term patients led a restricted and inactive life. The desire to keep public expenditure down prevented hospital administrators from maintaining the premises in good condition, and patients were constantly exposed to various communicable diseases (Jones, 1972, p. 229). The ineffectiveness of the system in rehabilitating patients, along with the inhumane conditions imposed upon them, caused the hospitals to be known as "The Shame of the States" (Deutsch, 1948).

Public interest in mental-hospital conditions reflected in books and writings led to public inquiries. In Britain, for example, the Prestwich Inquiry was conducted during the 1920s, and the Board of Control undertook several surveys of mental hospitals in the 1930s (Jones, 1972, pp. 232–258). During the 1930s the Rockefeller Foundation financed a mental-hospital inspection project in the United States that illuminated the conditions in mental hospitals and the tremendous need for increased professional manpower and facilities (Rossi, 1969). A study in 1941 revealed that, to raise mental hospitals to an acceptable standard, 74% more social workers were needed (Rossi, 1969, p. 25). It was apparent that mental health could not remain solely a humanitarian concern but would have to become an economic one. In the mid-1950s it was estimated that, to bring existing hospitals up to the American Psychiatric Association standard, $4 billion would be required (Karno & Schwartz, 1974). The prospects were equally sobering in England; a government spokesman called existing mental-hospital buildings an "appalling legacy" and pointed out that replacing them was not a question of a few million pounds but a question of "thousands of millions over many years" (Jones, 1972, p. 291).

In view of the inhumane conditions and financial burden of the mental-hospital system, the steady increase in the numbers of hospitalized mentally ill, and the growing disillusionment with the hospital as a mechanism of treatment and cure, mental-health problems could no longer be ignored and thus became a pressing public policy issue. In 1953 and 1954, after ignoring mental-health problems for 24 years, the British Parliament took up the issue in an intensive debate. The conditions of the mental-health service system were discussed, and the shortages of beds, buildings, staff, and funds were revealed (Jones, 1972, p. 259). At about the same time public concern in the United States over the conditions of mental-health services led Congress to enact the Mental Health Study Act of 1955 (Joint Commission on Mental Illness and Health, 1961), to make recommendations for a national program. Professionals, lay people, and politicians, began a search for alternatives.

ALTERNATIVES TO MENTAL INSTITUTIONS

Alternatives to mental institutions were attempted throughout the period when mental institutions were the major societal response to mental illness. Most alternative programs to hospital care were based on the same principles that had always characterized public policy toward the mentally ill. We are, however, interested here mainly in the alternatives of the twentieth century— alternatives that were to become the building blocks of a community-care system.

Prevention: The Public-Health and Mental-Hygiene Movements

The success of the public-health approach in combating and preventing infectious diseases through environmental and community programs attracted the attention of people interested in problems of mental health. It is beyond the scope of this book to describe in detail the history and concepts of the public-health and mental-hygiene movements (Deutsch, 1944; Felix, 1948; Rosen, 1958). It is of interest to us that these two movements helped provide the ideological impetus for community-care programs aimed at reducing the incidence and prevalence of mental disorders, exposing the public to issues of mental health, increasing the number and quality of mental-health professionals providing care in the community, and stimulating the development of preventive psychiatry (Caplan, 1964) and the community mental-health movement (Felix, 1957; Rosen, 1968).

Outpatient Clinics

The first outpatient clinics were established in the 1880s, as an attempt to improve hospital inpatient programs through an admission service provided by a hospital-connected clinic (Rossi, 1969). These early clinics had little in common with the community clinics that gained momentum after the 1920s (Barhash et al., 1952). The impetus for the community clinics had three sources: the child-welfare movement and child-guidance clinics; the growth of public awareness about mental-health problems, owing to the large number of psychiatric cases during World War I; and the influence of the mental-hygiene movement. With a growing acceptance by local, state, and federal authorities of their responsibility for the welfare of their citizens, and with the aid of increasing tax support, the community clinic became a common institution in most large American cities during the 1940s and 1950s.

Although one may question the effectiveness of the clinics in preventing hospitalization, since the rate of resident patients in mental institutions continued to grow until the mid-1950s, there should be no doubt about their contribution to the establishment of community-care programs. These clinics helped communities to relax their attitudes toward the mentally ill. They offered special training in interdisciplinary approaches for psychiatrists, psychologists, and psychiatric social workers. Further, they developed groups of professional people in urban areas who later became valuable for the development of extensive community-care programs.

Aftercare and the Psychiatric Social-Work Profession

Aftercare programs, like mental-health clinics, resulted from two converging values. On one hand there was the therapeutic function of the aftercare program for released mental patients advocated by Adolf Meyer during the first decade of the twentieth century (Rossi, 1969). On the other hand the hospital not only was a treatment mechanism but also functioned as a social-control mechanism supervising former patients living in the community. Hospitals were reluctant to release patients, especially those who had been committed, because of community pressures. When patients were released for medical, social, or administrative reasons (e.g., overcrowding), hospitals were very self-conscious. Hospitals had to assure the public that patients in the community would be closely supervised by the hospital and that if difficulties developed they would immediately be returned to the hospital. Even the terminology, adopted from the penal system, reveals societal attitudes toward the aftercare program; the term describing the status of patients on conditional leave in the community was "parole."

Regardless of the reasons for the evolution of aftercare programs, they did much to break down the barriers between mental patients and the community. The needs of former psychiatric patients on parole in the community stimulated the development of alternative community sheltered-care programs for them. In California, for example, the aftercare program encouraged the development of family-care homes and brought about the dispatch of psychiatrists from the hospital into the community to provide services for former psychiatric patients (Aviram, 1972). In fact, in some of the community clinics, the first actual activity was parole supervision of former psychiatric patients (Brown, 1969).

Social workers played a central role in the organization and provision of aftercare services, a field where they could use their competence and gain recognition. An emerging profession, social work was provided administrative backing and prestige through cooperation with psychiatry. Thus the incentive to develop aftercare services was based not only on altruistic motives but also on potential organizational gains for the new profession (Aviram, 1972).

The idea of using social workers in conjunction with patients' families to help patients return to their community was developed by Adolf Meyer in 1905 (Rosen, 1968, p. 312). Action to implement Meyer's ideas was taken when Mary C. Jarrett was appointed Director of Social Work at Boston Psychopathic Hospital. During the 1920s, 1930s, and 1940s, psychiatric social workers established numerous child-guidance clinics (*Encyclopedia of Social Work*, 1971, p. 823). In fact social workers were among the leaders in the mental-health movement, and many subsequently assumed administrative or consultative responsibilities in mental-health associations (Rosen, 1968, p. 313). Through their position in child-guidance and aftercare services, social workers stimulated the development of larger programs of community care.

 Family-Care Homes

The family-care program was one of the first attempts to find alternative sheltered care for the mentally ill. Family care is a program that places mental patients in the community with private families other than their own.

The patient is supervised by the caretaker, who is supervised in turn by a professional usually a social worker (Morrissey, 1967). Such programs were conceived as early as 1865 (Grob, 1973) and first introduced in Massachusetts in 1885. But 50 years elapsed before other states introduced the program. The overall growth of the program until the 1950s had not been very impressive, and even though there was some expansion of the program during the 1950s and 1960s, it remained relatively small. Morrissey (1967, p. 14) reports that in 1963 there were 13,000 mentally ill people in family-care homes in the United States, plus about 4000 in similar programs operated by the Veterans Administration. At the same time the resident population in mental institutions in the United States was about one-half million.

Several factors may account for the small size and slow growth of family-care programs. Stycos (1951) suggests that the primary reason for the resistance to the program was "rugged individualism." American cultural patterns were not conducive to care of mental patients in private homes. There were other inhibiting factors, such as the low board rates for providers and public anxiety about the mentally ill. Legislators did not appropriate enough funds for sufficient professional staff and caretakers. Legislative resistance followed from the public's anxiety about the return of mentally ill to the community. Apathy and even resistance on the part of psychiatrists also affected the program. Some psychiatrists—especially those related to the state-hospital system—saw in this type of program a threat to their professional authority. Boarding out patients represented a threat to the psychiatrists' role of authority in the hospital, especially if the process was based on the premise that the family-care home is a therapeutic setting where treatment was offered. This explains why most family-care programs were basically custodial-care programs. In addition mental-hospital administrators were resistant to family-care homes because they were reluctant to take the risk of alienating communities and losing their support because of local placement of mentally ill people.   Historically acceptance of family care has been based on two premises: It was less expensive than hospitalization, and it could free beds for acutely ill patients (Lee, 1963). The early advocates of family care based their arguments primarily on economic grounds. It is not surprising that the growth of the program occurred in the 1930s and 1940s, when the Depression brought both a lack of funds for state mental hospitals and a need for funds for many families in the community. These converging financial conditions resulted in some growth of the family-care programs. During the 1940s a personnel shortage resulting from World War II suggested the family-care program as a relief from the pressures of overcrowded, understaffed wards, since most of the family-care clientele were chronic mental patients who had previously received only custodial care in institutions. Indeed family-care programs were viewed by many as "the one hopeful answer to the perennial problem of overcrowded institutions" (Morrissey, 1967, p. 18).

Despite its relatively small scale the family-care program has made an important contribution to the establishment of a community-care system. It provided the mental-health field with the experience of placement of mentally ill people in sheltered-care arrangements in the community. It showed that custodial care could successfully be provided in the community, and it allowed segments of the public to become accustomed to the treatment and care of mental patients in their communities. The family-care program also brought mental-health personnel into the communities, to conduct the placement and supervision of patients. When additional resources became available during the 1960s and a large placement program was undertaken, the experienced mental-health personnel already in the communities proved very valuable.

 Halfway Houses

Although the formal development of halfway houses is rather recent, many informal parallels have existed for a long time. The halfway house—literally halfway between institution and community—can serve persons who cannot live independently in the community but do not need a complete institutional regimen. In this respect family-care homes can be considered halfway houses.

The early development of halfway houses in Britain consisted of the placement by the British Mental After-Care Association of released psychiatric patients in convalescent or private homes (Apte, 1968). The After-Care Association, founded in 1879, was a voluntary association established to create intermediate forms of care for discharged mental patients (Jones, 1972). In the 1920s the association started to accept residents for placement directly from the community. These individuals have emotional problems to the extent that their ability to function in the community was threatened. It was hoped that, by placing them in "hostels" (actually halfway houses), hospitalization could be prevented. Raush and Raush (1968) state that informal halfway houses are "facilities for mediating between a person with emotional problems and the community with its opportunities and requirements" (p. 4). In view of changing hospitalization patterns, this form of protective residential arrangement will be more frequently used. Glasscote and his associates (1971a) suggest that the recent interest in halfway houses is a "result of an awareness that past practices with the mentally ill have not succeeded as one would like, and an increased concern with the right of every person to participate as fully as possible in the life of the community" (p. 10).

Halfway homes in the United States developed their present form in the 1950s. Rutland Corner House in Boston, opened in 1954, was the first halfway house that operated according to the current concept. When Glasscote and his associates (1971a) completed their survey in 1969, they estimated that there were 128 halfway houses in the United States. These facilities, operating in at least 90 cities and towns, provided homes for about 2500 people who were or had been mentally ill. The houses were relatively small; the average number of beds was 22 (Glasscote et al., 1971a, p. 16). Only 9% of the houses accommodated more than 40 residents. Many definitions of the halfway house emphasize its aim to provide *temporary* residence as a transitional environment immediately following hospitalization and before resumption of normal independent living (Landy & Greenblatt, 1965). Glasscote et al. (1971a, p. 13) contend, however, that halfway houses may also serve as *permanent* facilities for people who are not able to move fully into the community. They define a halfway house as a "nonmedical residential facility specifically intended to enhance the capabilities of people who are mentally ill, or who are impaired by residual deficits from mental illness, to remain in the community, participating to the fullest possible extent in community life" (p. 11).

Another interesting finding of the survey conducted by Glasscote and his associates was that about half of their respondents were intermixing the mentally ill in halfway houses with other categories of people. It appears that halfway houses cater to the needs of variously impaired members of marginal groups, and the trend toward the use of multicategory halfway houses may even increase in the future. The major dilemma of the halfway-house movement will be to find the proper balance between rehabilitative measures and the need to provide a home-like atmosphere. In devising halfway-house rehabilitation programs, the mixing of the mentally ill with other people, as well as the type and number of people from other categories, will have to be dealt with.

Other Alternative-Care Facilities

The development of psychiatric departments in general hospitals has greatly improved the possibility of providing psychiatric services close to the patients' communities without the need to isolate them in remote state hospitals (McKeown, 1965). Day hospitals, which provide mental-health treatment to people during the day who at night use other lodging facilities, are now commonly used in lieu of hospitalization (Kramer, 1962). This arrangement helps the patient maintain contact with family and community, while relieving the patient, as well as his or her family and environment, from much of the burdens that might otherwise have necessitated full hospitalization. Night hospitals were designed for patients capable of maintaining jobs and functioning in the community during the day but still in need of some treatment and support after usual working hours.

Sheltered workshops, psychosocial rehabilitation centers, and former-patient clubs are additional facilities developed in the past two decades for the mentally ill living in the community (Barton, 1962; Palmer, 1966). Only a small number of mentally ill have been involved in these operations, and their effectiveness is yet to be evaluated (Glasscote et al., 1971b). But they represent part of the spectrum of care that can be provided in the community as an alternative to services and treatment formerly available only within the mental institution.

IMPLEMENTING COMMUNITY CARE

Having considered the precursors of community care and the development of some of its components, we turn to its implementation.

The Dual Revolution

The 1950s were very exciting years in the mental-health field. The number of patients in mental institutions started to decline (Kramer et al., 1972), both in the United States and elsewhere. In Britain an article in *Lancet* called the years 1954–1959 "the key years" (Tooth & Brooke, 1961), referring to the decline of the resident population in mental institutions in Britain (Jones, 1972, p. 358). This decline brought a great deal of satisfaction to professional and lay people alike. In particular, state and county mental institutions have been considered the main resource for the treatment and care of the mentally ill (USDHEW, 1969) and have used the major portion of mental-health care expenditure (Clausen, 1971). Thus the decline in the resident population of mental hospitals signaled a savings of public funds.

Two new movements can account for the decline: Policy and administrative changes in the care of the mentally ill began to take place, in hospitals as well as in the communities; and new drugs, first developed in France, were introduced into the mental hospitals for the treatment of patients. Some of these policy changes occurred at the national level and were reflected in increased intervention of the federal government in the mental-health field.

It is difficult to trace the specific course of events leading to the decline in the numbers of mental-hospital patients. In trying to account for the new trend in the United States, researchers have not agreed on the relative effect of psychoactive drugs compared with policy and program changes (Brill & Patton, 1963; Epstein et al., 1962). It is clear, however, that these two movements brought about major changes and can be considered a dual revolution in the mental-health field.

Policy and Administrative Changes.   New treatment and care policies, especially in British hospitals, were introduced before the introduction of psychoactive drugs and have no doubt affected treatment practices, length of stay, and release rates in mental institutions (Wing & Brown, 1970, p. 9). The reform of hospitalization practices in Britain took two main lines: On one hand there was an emphasis on rehabilitation and resettlement through the provision of domestic and industrial roles within an open hospital; on the other hand there was an emphasis on early discharge, or avoidance of admission, to prevent the accumulation of long-stay institutionalized patients. These two lines of reform converged, resulting in various kinds of transitional community facilities, such as hostels.

The "therapeutic community," first used with psychiatric cases in military hospitals during World War II (Jones, 1952), became extremely influential in the mental-health field. The therapeutic-community program involved a total change of the hospital by abandoning formal roles of doctor, nurse, and patient and by restructuring hospital life around four themes: rehabilitation, democratization, permissiveness, and communalism (Jones, 1952). The therapeutic-community concept led to the liberalization of mental hospitals and changed many rigid ones into more flexible and relaxed systems (Jones, 1972).

The therapeutic-community movement was part of the larger "open-door" policy resulting from the changing public climate toward the mentally ill. The use of psychoactive drugs further strengthened this movement. A party of American psychiatrists, visiting British hospitals in 1958 under the auspices of the Milbank Memorial Fund, were deeply impressed with British mental-hospital practices (Jones, 1972). The British mental-health system used industrial therapy (Wing et al., 1962), day hospitals, and "shift systems," where the same facility was used by day patients and night patients. For released mental patients, hostels and patients' social clubs were developed.

Administrative and policy changes in American mental hospitals came somewhat later and were related to federal involvement and legislation. The effect of policy and program changes on the reduction of mental hospitalization cannot be overlooked (Mosher & Feinsilver, 1971). Policy changes that provided federal public assistance to the mentally ill in the community, new release and admission policies, and organizational structures and service agencies in the community (Aviram & Syme, 1974) deserve more credit than they have received for having brought changes in mental-health trends.

Psychoactive Drugs.   The introduction of psychoactive drugs (major tranquilizers, antipsychotics, neuroleptics, etc.) has been considered one of the most important innovations in the mental-health field (Kramer et al., 1961; Mechanic, 1969). These drugs, referred to by many as "wonder drugs" (cf. Jones, 1972, p. 292) and first introduced in 1952, enabled mentally ill patients with disturbing symptoms to relax while remaining fully conscious. The major tranquilizers in particular provided chemical means of control, helping hospital personnel work with mental patients. Many distressing aspects of mental-hospital life—related to the need to control disturbing behavior—disappeared. The hospital atmosphere changed, gave staff greater confidence, and encouraged or facilitated the concurrent "open-door" movement (i.e., the unlocking of hospital wards) and trends toward early release. One of the most significant effects of psychoactive drugs was the new wave of optimism: Feelings of hopelessness and apathy that had prevailed in mental institutions gave way to new hope that patients could be helped and that treatment could be effective.

Although the initial enthusiasm over the potential of wonder drugs has declined (Jones, 1972, p. 292), the drugs continue to be used and have become a major modality in the care of the mentally ill. Patients can go home sooner than in the past, and with the aid of home support or other protective residence and medication prescribed by the community physician, they may remain in the community.

The use of drugs in the treatment of mental patients helped bring psychiatry into the mainstream of medicine. "It promoted psychiatrists to physicians in the eyes of some of their colleagues, and the insane to the status of patients in the eyes of many members of the public" (Roberts, 1967, p. 25). Changes in the status of both psychiatrists and mentally ill people influenced policy and new programs that improved the lot of the mentally ill. The use of psychoactive drugs and the effects on public attitudes helped in justifying the eligibility of the mentally ill for income-maintenance and medical-care programs.

Psychoactive drugs, an important component of community care, met all three requirements previously fulfilled by the hospital. By short-circuiting the psychotic process, they offered an inexpensive solution with "curative potential"; in not interfering with higher level thought processes—that is, not putting the person to sleep—they were humane; and finally, they could effectively control behavior.

The dual revolution of the mid-1950s started a movement that has not stopped. The decline in the number and rate of hospitalizations in mental institutions has been an established trend in the United States for the past 20 years. In 1955, when the patient population in state and county mental hospitals reached its peak, the number of patients was 558,922 (Kramer et al., 1972, p. 31). By 1973 the number had dropped by 55% to 248,518 (US-DHEW, 1975). This trend has changed the mental-health system to such an extent that emphasis has shifted from talk of "aftercare" (which reflects a hospital-centered system) to talk of community care.

The Golden Age of the Community Mental-Health Movement

The passage of the National Mental Health Act in 1946 and the establishment of the National Institute of Mental Health (NIMH) in the same year indicate the beginning of a new era in the mental-health field in the *l*

United States. Mental illness has been recognized as a social problem; since
1946 mental illness and mental health have been a focus and responsibility of
the federal government. The increasing central role of the federal government in mental health has been reflected in policy formulations, in laws, and
in financing many innovative programs in the country. Federal government
involvement, growing public awareness and openness toward mental health,
the interest and focus on interpersonal and community relations, and finally
a strong economy and availability of funds have all brought about the "gold-
en age of community mental health" during the 1950s and 1960s.

The extent of increased federal-government involvement is reflected in the
growth of the NIMH budget: between 1950 and 1967 its budget grew from
less than $10 million to almost $340 million (Mechanic, 1969). Support money provided by various federal agencies and programs for mental-health services increased between 1960 and 1968 by about 120%—from $377 million to
$830 million. During this period the federal government increased its share in
the total public expenditures for mental-health services from 28 to 34% (Harvey, 1973). The whole field of mental health has undergone tremendous
growth during these years. Mental-health centers, nonexistent in the federal
budget before 1963, received $238 million by 1970. The total public expendi-
ture for mental-health services in 1968 was close to $2.5 billion, an increase of
more than 80% over public expenditures in 1960 (Harvey, 1973).

By establishing NIMH, Congress intended to apply the traditional public-
health approach to mental health. Since its creation in 1946 NIMH has
played an important role in formulating and executing federal policy in the
mental-health field. In 1955 Congress passed the Mental Health Study Act,
which directed the formulation of the Joint Commission on Mental Illness
and Health. The mandate of this commission was to analyze and evaluate the
needs and resources of the mentally ill in the United States and make recommendations for a national mental-health program.

The final report of the Commission, entitled *Action For Mental Health* (1961),
was largely an ideological document and was somewhat ambiguous. It emphasized the need for increased mental-health services, substantial federal
support of these programs, and further research. The Commission suggested
the expansion of programs for immediate care of acutely disturbed persons. It
was concerned about the low level of care of chronic mental patients and
strongly criticized the mental-hospital system. It proposed changes in the
programs of care, aftercare, and rehabilitation of mentally ill people and
advocated the establishment of community clinics (Joint Commission on
Mental Illness and Health, 1961). To improve the "mental health of the
mentally ill" and reduce the number of patients in mental hospitals, the
Commission proposed a massive outlay of federal and state funds to increase
state-hospital budgets and improve the quality of service available.

In 1962 President Kennedy appointed a cabinet committee to study the report and to develop alternative courses of action. Political battles developed between those who wished to strengthen mental-health programs according to a traditional medical model and those favoring new approaches based on the public-health point of view (Mechanic, 1969). Those espousing the latter, more radical approach based on prevention and community care prevailed. This resulted in a program proposal by Kennedy that called for the creation of comprehensive community mental-health centers that would make it possible for most of the "mentally ill to be successfully and quickly treated in their own communities and to return to a useful place in society." Congress approved Kennedy's recommendation and, by the enactment of the Community Mental Health Centers Act of 1963, provided funds for the construction of such centers. A 1965 amendment provided funds for staffing them. The centers envisioned by Congress were to include at least five essential services: inpatient, outpatient, partial (day and night) hospitalization, 24-hour emergency service, and community services (consultation and education). Other allowable services were diagnosis, rehabilitation, precare and aftercare, training, and research and evaluation.

The Community Mental Health Centers Act hurled the community mental-health movement from the realm of armchair and academic debates into a national program. The movement still lacked a cohesive theoretical base, and many issues regarding the efficacy of mental-health program alternatives were unresolved. But the movement seized the opportunity provided by federal legislation to establish many new programs. As of June 30, 1971, 452 community mental-health centers were funded and 300 were in operation (Harvey, 1973, p. 93). Although concepts of community mental health seem to vary a great deal (Mechanic, 1969), there is consensus that, no matter how the spectrum of care is defined, community mental-health centers should provide mental-health services to all people on an equal basis, close to where the patient lives, and as soon after diagnosis as possible.

The national mental-health program was compatible with other social-welfare programs such as Medicare, Medicaid, the Poverty Program, and the Model Cities Program. In all of these programs the federal government channeled funds to local authorities and agencies in an effort to solve major social problems of urban America. Although most of the programs of the 1960s were not directly aimed at the mentally ill, they were affected as part of a larger category of indigent people. Increased income-maintenance support, as well as the availability of medical services for the aged and public-welfare recipient in the community, complemented community mental-health centers in establishing a community-care system.

COMMUNITY CARE AS SHELTERED CARE

Today, following the proliferation of community mental-health programs during the 1960s, we have all the ingredients of a community-care system that, in spite of the fact that no one individual oversees its operation (as was the case with the hospital superintendent), is able to justify its existence in terms of all three functions initially fulfilled by the mental hospital. The landmark research of Pasamanick and his associates (1967), *Schizophrenics In the Community,* demonstrated the feasibility of effectively maintaining individuals in the community on psychoactive medications and has been extremely influential in promoting community-care efforts. The individuals in the study of Pasamanick et al. were, however, members of intact families and represent only a small percentage of long-term mental-hospital patients. In addition the middle-class bias of community mental-health centers has led them to offer only minimal service to more marginal patient groups (Chu & Trotter, 1974).

Given these trends, how have the more marginal populations of mental patients fared in today's community-care efforts? Is the community-care system providing shelter for these individuals, and if so, what is life in this new type of sheltered care like for them? Providing answers to these questions is one focus of this book. Yet, before considering them, we must consider the context of community care in California, where our attempt to understand life in community-based sheltered care is focused.

REFERENCES

Apte, R. Z. *Halfway Houses: A New Dilemma in Institutional Care.* Occasional Papers on Social Administration No. 27. London: G. Bell & Sons, 1968.

Aviram, U. "Mental Health Reform and the Aftercare State Service Agency: A Study of the Process of Change in the Mental Health Field." Unpublished doctoral dissertation. Berkeley, California: University of California, 1972.

Aviram, U. and S. L. Syme. "The Effects of Policy Decisions and Administrative Programs on Mental Hospitalization Trends." Paper presented at the Fifth International Congress of Social Psychiatry, Athens, Greece, 1974.

Barhash, A. Z., M. C. Bentley, M. E. Kirkpatrick, and H. A. Sanders. *The Organization and Function of the Community Psychiatric Clinic.* New York: The National Association of Mental Health, 1952.

Barton, W. E. *Administration in Psychiatry.* Springfield, Illinois: Charles C Thomas, 1962.

Blain, D., K. E. Appel, A. E. Scheflen, and R. L. Robinson. "The Current Picture of Mental Health and Psychiatry in the United States." *Am. J. Psychiat.* 112(1), 53 (1955).

Brill, H. and R. Patton. "The Impact of Modern Chemotherapy on Hospital Organization: Psychiatric, Care and Public Health Policies," *Proceedings of Third World Congress of Psychiatry,* Vol. 3. Toronto: University of Toronto Press, 1963, p. 433–437.

Brown, B. S. "Philosophy and Scope of Extended Clinic Activities," in A. J. Bindman and A. D. Spiegal (Eds.). *Perspectives in Community Mental Health.* Chicago: Aldine, 1969.

Caplan, G. *Principles of Preventive Psychiatry.* New York: Basic Books, 1964.

Chu, F. D. and S. Trotter. *The Madness Establishment: The Nader Study Group Report on the National Institute of Mental Health.* New York: Grossman, 1974.

Clausen, J. A. "Mental Disorders," in R. Merton and R. Nisbet (Eds.). *Contemporary Social Problems,* 3rd ed. New York: Harcourt, Brace and Jovanovitch, 1971.

Deutsch, A. *The Shame of the States.* New York: Harcourt, Brace, 1948.

Deutsch, A. *The History of Mental Hygiene—One Hundred Years of American Psychiatry.* New York: Columbia University Press, 1944.

Encyclopedia of Social Work. (16th issue) R. Morris (Ed. in Chief). New York: National Association of Social Workers, 1971.

Epstein, L. J., R. D. Morgan, and L. Reynolds. "An Approach to the Effect of Ataraxic Drugs on Hospital Release Rates." *Am. J. Psychiat.* **119**(1), 36–47 (1962).

Erikson, E. H. *Childhood and Society.* New York: W. W. Morton and Company, 1950.

Feldman, S. (Ed.). *The Administration of Mental Health Services.* Springfield, Illinois: Charles C Thomas, 1973.

Felix, R. H. "Mental Hygiene and Public Health." *Am. J. Orthopsychiat.* **18**, 679–684 (1948).

Felix, R. H. "Evolution of Community Mental Health Concepts." *Am. J. Psychiat.* **113**, 673–679 (1957).

Felix, R. H. *Mental Illness: Progress and Prospects.* New York: Columbia University Press, 1967.

Folta, J. R. and L. Schatzman. "Trends in Public Urban Psychiatry in the United States." *Social Problems* **16**, 60–73 (1968).

Glass, A. J. "Introduction," in P. G. Bourne (Ed.). *The Psychology and Physiology of Stress.* New York: Academic Press, 1969.

Glasscote, R. M., J. E. Gudeman, and J. R. Elpers. *Halfway Houses for the Mentally Ill: A Study of Programs and Problems.* Washington, D.C.: American Psychiatric Association, 1971a.

Glasscote, R. M., E. Cumming, I. D. Rutman, J. N. Sussex, and S. M. Glassman. *Rehabilitating the Mentally Ill in the Community: A Study of Psychosocial Rehabilitation Centers.* Washington, D.C.: American Psychiatric Association, 1971b.

Grob, G. N. *Mental Institutions in America: Social Policy to 1875.* New York: The Free Press, 1973.

Harvey, E. C. "Financing Mental Health Services," in S. Feldman (Ed.). *The Administration of Mental Health Services.* Springfield, Illinois: Charles C Thomas, 1973.

Hofstadter, R. *Social Darwinism in American Thought.* (rev. ed.). New York: Braziller, 1954.

Joint Commission on Mental Illness and Health. *Action for Mental Health: Final Report of the Joint Commission on Mental Illness and Health.* New York: Basic Books, 1961.

Jones, K. *A History of the Mental Health Services.* London: Routledge and Kegan Paul, 1972.

Jones, M. *Social Psychiatry: A Study of Therapeutic Communities.* London: Tavistock, 1952.

Karno, M. and D. A. Schwartz. *Community Mental Health: Reflections and Explorations.* Flushing, New York: Spectrum Publications, Inc., 1974.

Kramer, B. M. *Day Hospital: A Study of Partial Hospitalization in Psychiatry.* New York: Grune and Stratton, 1962.

Kramer, M., E. S. Pollack, and R. W. Redick. "Studies of the Incidence and Prevalence of Hospitalized Mental Disorders in the United States: Current Status and Future Goals," in P. H. Hoch and J. Zubin (Eds.). *Comparative Epidemiology of Mental Disorders.* New York: Grune and Stratton, 1961.

Kramer, M., E. S. Pollack, and R. W. Redick. *Mental Disorders/Suicide.* Cambridge, Massachusetts: Harvard University Press, 1972.

Landy, D. and M. Greenblatt. *Halfway House: A Sociocultural and Clinical Study of Rutland Corner House.* Washington, D.C.: U.S. Department of Health, Education, and Welfare, 1965.

Lee, D. T. "Family Care: Selection and Prediction." *Am. J. Psychiat.* **120**, 561–566 (1963).

McKeown, T. *Medicine in Modern Society.* London: Allen and Unwin, 1965.

Marx, J. H., P. Rieker, and D. L. Ellison. "The Sociology of Community Mental Health: Historical and Methodological Perspectives," in P. M. Roman and H. M. Trice (Eds.). *Sociological Perspectives on Community Mental Health.* Philadelphia: F. A. Davis Company, 1974.

Mechanic, D. *Mental Health and Social Policy.* Englewood Cliffs, New Jersey: Prentice-Hall, 1969.

Morrissey, J. R. *The Case for Family Care of the Mentally Ill.* Community Mental Health Journal Monograph No. 2. New York: Behavioral Publications, 1967.

Mosher, L. and D. Feinsilver. *Special Report: Schizophrenia.* Washington, D.C.: U.S. National Institute of Mental Health, Department of Health, Education, and Welfare, USPHS Publication: (HSM) 72-9007, 1971.

Palmer, M. *The Social Club: A Bridge from Mental Hospital to Community.* New York: National Association for Mental Health, 1966.

Pasamanick, B., F. R. Scarpiti, and S. Dinitz. *Schizophrenics in the Community: An Experimental Study in the Prevention of Hospitalization.* New York: Appleton-Century-Crofts, 1967.

Raush, H. L., and C. L. Raush. *The Halfway House Movement: A Search for Sanity.* New York: Appleton-Century-Crofts, 1968.

Roberts, N. *Mental Health and Mental Illness.* London: Routledge and Kegan Paul, 1967.

Rosen, G. *A History of Public Health.* New York: MD Publications, 1958.

Rosen, G. *Madness in Society.* New York: Harper and Row, 1968.

Rossi, A. M. "Some Pre-World War II Antecedents of Community Mental Health Theory and Practice," in A. J. Bindman and A. D. Spiegel (Eds.). *Perspectives in Community Mental Health.* Chicago: Aldine, 1969.

Stycos, J. M. "Family-Care: A Neglected Area of Research." *Psychiatry* **14**, 301–306 (1951).

Time, April 1, 1974.

Tooth, G. C. and E. M. Brooke. "Needs and Beds: Trends in the Mental Hospital Population and Their Effect on Future Planning." *Lancet,* 1 (7179), 710–713 (1961).

U.S. Department of Health, Education, and Welfare (USDHEW). *Mental Health Facilities Report* (USPHS Publication No. 1921). Washington, D.C.: Public Health Service, 1969.

U.S. Department of Health, Education, and Welfare. *Statistical Note 113: State Trends in Resident Patients—State and County Mental Hospitals Inpatient Services, 1967–1973.* Washington, D.C.: (DHEW Publication No. [ADM] 75-158), 1975.

Wing, J. K., D. H. Bennett, and J. Denham. *The Industrial Rehabilitation of Long-Stay Schizophrenic Patients.* London: Medical Research Council Memorandum No. 42., HMSO, 1962.

Wing, J. K. and G. W. Brown. *Institutionalism and Schizophrenia.* Cambridge, England: Cambridge University Press, 1970.

THREE

Mental-Health Reform in California

California has been one of the leading states in the nation in implementing community-mental-health principles. In 1968 it passed the Community Mental Health Services Law. It created a single system of care based on local responsibility for the treatment and care of mentally ill people. The ideas of community care have been put to the test in California. It is important to review the process of reform before we examine its results.

Comparing California's current system of mental-health care with that of 20 years ago reveals a complete transformation from state-hospital-centered to community-centered service. Before 1957, state hospitals predominated in public mental-health care; today mental-health services exist in all California counties. Community programs now control the use of state hospitals (California State Governor's Budget, 1974).

The state's appropriations for local mental-health care increased tenfold in the decade before 1973 and now far exceed those for state hospitals (California Human Relations Agency, 1972). Residence in state institutions declined from 37,000 in 1955 to less than 7000 in 1973. Three state hospitals have closed recently, with more closures expected in the future (barring any change in the legal-admissions framework). The dramatic decrease in the

33

number of resident patients has been accompanied by an increase in the number of admissions, which have risen from 28,000 to 44,000 between 1961 and 1971. Apparently the incidence of diagnosed mental illness has increased, while the length of inpatient care has declined (Aviram & Segal, 1973).

An increasing number of people residing in California communities have at one time or another been defined as mentally ill. This is reflected in the increased activities of local mental-health programs (California Human Relations Agency, 1972) and in the tremendous increase in the use of so-called protective living environments. Twenty years ago there were fewer than a thousand former mental patients of all ages residing in sheltered-care facilities in California communities (Aviram, 1972, p. 155); by 1973 our sample census indicates there were close to 12,400 between the ages of 18 and 65 in sheltered-care facilities. (This figure does not include persons over 65 living in these facilities.)

Although the shift to community care is occurring throughout the United States, California has pioneered in this area. Many attribute this to the California Community Mental Health Services Act of 1968, which represents a major legal revision of California's mental-health system. Changes in the mental-health system cannot, however, be attributed to a single piece of legislation. Without denying the importance of this law, we contend that it represents only the conclusion of a process that began many years earlier—the result of many converging events. The variety of factors contributing to the dramatic change in California's mental-health system includes policy decisions, administrative programs, new treatment techniques, economic incentives, and an organizational context conducive to change. This historical review describes these factors and analyzes their significance.

THE NEW IDEOLOGY OF COMMUNITY CARE

Community care for the mentally ill, the core of the community mental-health movement's ideology (Roberts et al., 1966), has given a sense of mission to its proponents and provided a rationale for new programs and approaches in California. The idea of community care, based essentially on medical and financial considerations, was first implemented in 1939 with the appointment of Aaron Rosanoff as Director of the Department of Institutions (part of which later became the Department of Mental Hygiene). His attack on the legality of retaining many patients in state hospitals and his belief in community-care programs served as a base for the strong ideological commitment of those who followed him (Aviram, 1972). His ideas and some of his programs (e.g., the "Total Push" program—an all-out effort to return patients to their communities; and "Supervisor for Extramural Care" an aftercare organization independent of the state hospital system) laid the foundation for legislation and programs for the next 20 years, including the Bureau of Social Work (1946), the Short-Doyle Act (1957), and the depopulation policy (1963).

Rosanoff's ideas strongly influenced Portia Bel Hume in directing California's patient-care system away from a state-hospital focus. Hume, whom many regard as the founder of the community mental-health movement in California, was appointed Deputy Director of Community Programs of the Department of Mental Hygiene in 1951. Her most important contribution was to implement the notion of local responsibility. In a recent interview she indicated that it was her firm belief, perhaps one that became prevalent in the early 1950s, that local communities would become more interested in their mentally ill if they were responsible for them (Hume, 1973). Although a state system might be more efficient, Hume considered local interest and responsibility to be the primary factors in successfully meeting the needs of the mentally ill. Toward this end she sponsored the Abshire Act, a noncomprehensive "trial balloon" passed in 1953, which provided a state subsidy for locally operated outpatient mental-health services. Its warm reception ultimately laid the groundwork for the passage of the comprehensive Short-Doyle Bill in 1957.

While Portia Hume and Nathan Sloat (Director of the Bureau of Social Work) were emphasizing the concepts of community care as early as the mid-1950s, the actual community programs operating were few and small. In 1949 Frank Ford Tallman, whose primary focus was on better hospital care, was appointed Director of Mental Hygiene. His appointment illustrates that a strong hospital system was still the major mandate of mental-health policy at that time. Yet a gradual conceptual transformation toward a community-care ideology was taking place in the 1940s and 1950s. By the early 1950s the conceptual shift was adopted by a group of state legislators who would ultimately implement it. Legislative action coincided with advances in the drug and welfare fields.

MAJOR TRENDS IN THE PROCESS OF MENTAL-HEALTH REFORM

Population Trends in Mental Hospitals

The introduction of psychoactive medications and initiation of administrative changes were both important factors in the reduction of the State mental-hospital population in California (Brill & Patton, 1963; Epstein et al., 1962; Kramer et al., 1961; Mosher & Feinsilver, 1971). Without denying the importance of the former, it must be noted that the latter is indeed of major importance. This view is supported by a recent cross-state epidemiologic study that used a time-trend analysis of declines in hospital populations and found marked variation from state to state. These wide discrepancies between states existed in spite of the general availability of modern theories and treatment techniques. The study showed that in California (as in other states) these variations were related to policy decisions and administrative programs undertaken in the 1950s and 1960s (Aviram & Syme, 1974). Taking California as a case in point, our attention is directed to the period starting in 1963; the resident population in California mental institutions reached a plateau in 1955 (when psychoactive drugs were introduced) and declined slightly in 1959; only in 1963 did it start to drop sharply at a rate of six times that of any previous year, the decline rate reaching its maximum in 1966–1967.

Although the percentage of those over 65 in mental institutions in other states grew from 1955 to 1969, the California figures show a decline even more dramatic than that for younger groups. Beginning also in 1963, this decline in the proportion of institutionalized aged between 1966 and 1969 increased by 25% over 1964–1965 (Aviram, 1975). The general decline continued: Between 1969 and 1971 there was about a 20% drop in the number of units providing inpatient services, while outpatient services almost doubled (California Human Relations Agency, 1972).

The number of former mental patients residing in sheltered-care facilities in the community increased only slightly before 1961, rising somewhat faster between 1961 and 1965 and then very rapidly after 1965. Figures of a statewide placement program indicate a 50% increase in the year 1965–1966 (Aviram, 1972). By looking at the relationship between dramatic changes in the mental-hospital population and corresponding community-care figures, we can specify events directly connected with the changes, as well as events that preceded and/or precipitated the change.

Chemical Control, Income Maintenance, and Economic Incentives

In addition to being a treatment center, the state hospital is an agent of social control that provides financial support for its residents. Until recently many patients were kept in hospitals primarily because they lacked other means of support.

We have already seen that psychoactive drugs provided a means of social and emotional control of many mental patients. It has also been shown that the success of community-care programs is considerably dependent on the availability of sufficient funds for released patients to support themselves (Miller, 1965). In 1962 the U.S. Department of Health, Education, and Welfare (DHEW) revised its policy toward mental patients so that persons on conditional release from mental hospitals were no longer barred from eligibility for state public-assistance programs by lack of matching federal funds (DHEW, 1962). The DHEW reinterpretation made categorical-aid funds available to the former mental patients through Aid to the Totally Disabled (ATD) and thus increased their chances of remaining in the community. Seizing this opportunity, California instituted a public-assistance program for the mentally handicapped, and the hospital population began its sharp decline. In addition to medical and humanitarian considerations, there were obvious economic and political advantages to such a program: It was more convenient and economical for the state to transfer responsibility to local communities. Furthermore, the policy change made the forgotten patients in the back wards a transactionable commodity, a source of income to local communities. Thus former mental patients were placed where the economic incentives to accept them were greatest (Aviram, 1972).

In spite of financial support, lack of medical services in the community forced some patients to return to the state hospital for treatment. Since the early 1950s California has had a program of Medical Assistance to the Aged (MAA) for public-assistance recipients. Publicly supported medical services for the non-aged were not, however, available until 1965, when the Social Security Act was amended to introduce Medicaid and Medicare, enabling recipients of public assistance to see local physicians. It is our opinion that the provision of financial support through public-assistance programs was primarily responsible for the mass emigration from state hospitals that began in California in 1962 (California State Department of Mental Hygiene, 1972). The extension of medical services and tranquilizing drugs to local communities in 1965 helped maintain many former mental patients in the community and avoid the lengthy hospitalization of others and thus supported the change in California's mental-health services.

CALIFORNIA'S POLICIES AND PROGRAMS AND THE PROCESS OF MENTAL-HEALTH REFORM

Basically policies are set on two levels: (1) the administrative and (2) the legislative. The ultimate test of policies is achievement of the desired change. In California an interplay of administrative and legislative action led to major change in the mental-health system. Policies and programs most effective in promoting community care included the focus on alternatives to hospitalization, the interest in prevention and the establishment of community psychiatric clinics, the development of placement programs, the "Long Range Plan," the depopulation projects, the Geriatrics Screening Project, the

Bureau of Social Work, and the Community Mental Health and Short-Doyle Acts. We now turn to a more detailed consideration of these important policies and programs in the transition from hospital to community care.

Administrative Efforts

Alternatives to Hospitalization.   In the 1940s and early 1950s, the public mental-health service system was dominated almost exclusively by the state-hospital system. As Karno and Schwartz (1974) stated, this system was primarily designed to house and provide care at a low cost to "the large number of other-than-affluent persons whose behavior had caused others to have them institutionalized as 'insane'" (p. 33). More than 90% of the newly admitted patients in the late 1940s were involuntarily committed (Hume, 1957), and about 80% of state-hospital patients were diagnosed as psychotic (California Department of Mental Hygiene, 1948). The quality of care was low and the conditions in the state hospitals were inhumane. An overcrowding of patients in inadequate facilities was in those days one of the major characteristics of the state-hospital system. In view of California's rate of growth and hospitalization practices the future appeared gloomy. Changing these conditions by building new hospitals and renovating the old ones would have required huge sums of money. Staffing these hospitals with sufficient qualified professionals presented still further problems. The immense investment necessary to improve the system was neither politically nor economically feasible; alternatives to hospitalization seemed more appealing.

California began looking for alternatives in 1939 with the goals of: (1) tightening admission policies, (2) releasing patients not in need of hospital treatment, and (3) developing community-placement and treatment facilities. These three objectives are of course interrelated. For example, unless the state could create a placement program for former and potential patients who could not live alone, admission and release policies could not be changed successfully.

The Development of Community-Placement Programs.   In 1939 legislative and administrative policies first combined to initiate community care for the mentally ill. Through the Family Care Program the state legislature provided funds to support former mental patients in protected living situations in the community. A small "extramural-care" unit was established by Aaron Rosanoff in the Department of Institutions to place mental patients in these community-based family-care homes. In 1946 this unit became the Bureau of Social Work, a major vehicle in the state's placement program. Twenty years after the Bureau's establishment more than 4000 former mental patients were in family-care homes. This represented 20% of the total patient population on conditional release in the community (leave of absence from the hospital)

(Aviram, 1972). Thus, when federal money to support mental patients in the community became available in 1962, California had a well-established administrative mechanism for placing patients—the Bureau of Social Work—and a network of community-placement facilities. We believe that these were instrumental in California's successful exploitation of changes in federal policy.

People involved in the community-placement program claimed that it was preferable to hospitalization for three reasons: It was more humane, it was good politically, it was economical. Removing people from the overcrowded wards was considered humane, especially after the exposés of state hospitals published in the 1940s and 1950s. Politically and economically it was astute because it saved operating costs of the state hospitals, decreased capital outlay for new hospitals, and reduced the number of hospital employees.

The Governor's Conference on Mental Health. One of the necessary conditions for a phenomenon to become an issue of social concern is public awareness of its existence. In this respect the first Governor's Conference on Mental Health, called in 1949 by Earl Warren, then governor of California, is an important event. It was the first time mental-health problems and the mental-health delivery system were discussed at such a level. More than 800 people, professionals as well as laymen, convened to discuss problems and make recommendations. The conference helped make mental-health problems and services a public issue in California and thus contributed to the process of mental-health reform.

The recommendations illuminated the participants' concern with the inadequacy of the mental-health service system and their conviction that improvements could be achieved by establishing programs in preventive mental health, community treatment, and welfare services. Many ideas expressed in this conference became major features of the mental-health service system in California during the 1960s and 1970s. In the final report of the conference we find the following: "With modern methods of treatment, many mentally ill persons . . . need never be sent to a state hospital. An adequate program of mental hygiene must be concerned with both treatment and prevention—with helping people to remain out of hospitals and with promotion of satisfactory living. . . . The goal of treatment is return to community living . . ." (Karno & Schwartz, 1974, p. 36). The conference recognized the importance of welfare services in promoting that goal. Among its recommendations we find one calling for major reorientation of the program of the State Department of Mental Hygiene toward the development and expansion of local community treatment and welfare services. The Bureau of Social Work, which had been in operation for several years, was one of the promoters of the conference (Aviram, 1972) and appeared to receive support for its future operations in the mental-health field in California. Another result of the conference was the establishment of the Division of Community Services in the Department of Mental Hygiene. The Bureau of Social Work and the Division of Community Services became the major proponents of community mental-health programs and contributed a great deal to the development of alternatives to hospitalization and community care.

The statements in the final report of the conference became the ideological rationale for programs in California that tried to establish community-care facilities for the mentally ill. The final report also provided policy goals that were the basis for future legislation, such as the Short-Doyle Act and administrative plans such as the "Long-Range Plan."

The Long-Range Plan. In March 1962 the California Department of Mental Hygiene released its blueprint for future mental-health programs in California, the "Long-Range Plan" (California State Senate, 1963), a document of major interest in the mental-health field. Among its many goals it stipulated that all psychiatric services should be located as near as possible to the people being served and that hospitalization should be used only as long as intensive treatment was necessary. It was implicit in the plan that the goal of the state-hospital system was not necessarily total cure but rather the return of the patient to his former level of functioning or to a level that would allow his stable maintenance in the community. One might argue that the Long-Range Plan's authors believed that the previous presumption of many state hospitals to offer a total cure was one of the factors responsible for the numerical growth of the large back-ward populations in state hospitals.

The Depopulation Projects. At the beginning of the 1960s plans had to be made for two state hospitals with a number of obsolete buildings. Rather than build new wards, it was decided to try to reduce the patient population and eventually vacate the unsuitable quarters. In line with general policy this objective was to be achieved without transferring patients to other hospitals and with no additional budget allocations, taking advantage instead of new federal regulations that would provide many of the potentially released patients with public-assistance funds.

In July 1963 the Department of Mental Hygiene initiated the depopulation project for the two state hospitals. In 5 years their resident population was reduced by 3500, and in 1969 the state closed one of them. Many of those discharged were either senile aged or chronic schizophrenics, who would not improve from continued hospitalization and who could be maintained in the community without danger to themselves or others.

As a result of the depopulation policy the state had to overcome the resistance of hospital employees who feared their jobs were in jeopardy and provide incentives for the project's administrators in addition to relief from over-crowded conditions. The Department of Mental Hygiene dealt with these problems in three ways:

1. The hospital staff was assured that the decline in the hospital's population would not affect their employment.
2. The minimum footage required per hospitalized patient was increased by 40%.
3. The major responsibility for finding alternative care was entrusted to an external organization, the Bureau of Social Work.

The depopulation project encouraged similar efforts by demonstrating viable technical procedures and by providing experience in obtaining community cooperation and in placing released mental patients. The assurance of income maintenance was essential to the success of the depopulation project, especially in the recruitment of community sheltered-care facilities for released patients who could not live independently. As local entrepreneurs—professional as well as nonprofessional—became convinced of the advantages of the new system, the depopulation programs acquired momentum.

Controlling Admission: the Geriatric Screening Project. In spite of the avowed objective of many states to curb unwarranted admissions, the percentage of aged in mental hospitals has increased since 1955. In California, however, the rate of hospitalized aged patients in 1968 was less than half of the corresponding national figure (Aviram, 1975). The reduction of more than 70% of the aged population in mental hospitals from 1963 to 1969 is to a great extent attributable to the Geriatric Screening Program (Aviram, 1975). This project reduced inappropriate commitment of aged persons and promoted the development of community resources for them (Rypins & Clark, 1968).

The Bureau of Social Work: a Major Administrative Mechanism for Change. Policies alone are not sufficient for the achievement of change; administrative instruments are needed as well. Many observers of the California mental-health scene over the past 25 years claim that the Bureau of Social Work was the major instrument in carrying out the state's mental-health reform policies. From the small extramural unit established by Dr. Rosanoff in 1939, by the end of the 1960s the Bureau became an organization of more than 700 employees (400 of them professionals), with a caseload of close to 25,000 (Aviram, 1972). Under the administration of the State Department of Mental Hygiene, the Bureau was primarily responsible for community placements and supervising patients on conditional release (i.e., leave of absence) from the state hospital. A cohesive organization dedicated to developing and strengthening community care for the mentally ill, the Bureau of Social

Work enabled the state to use the opportunities made available by federal funds and psychoactive drugs.

The Bureau established offices throughout California and in some areas was the only professional mental-health unit. New community mental-health programs, especially in nonurban areas, drew heavily on the professional practices, placement networks, and professional manpower pool of the Bureau.

The Bureau of Social Work and its contribution to community care for the mentally ill have been a matter of controversy. Never part of the mainstream of the mental-health service system, the Bureau was first under the state-hospital system, then the Department of Social Welfare, later the Department of Mental Hygiene, and recently local community mental-health programs. The Bureau's position enabled it to be a catalyst in the mental-health system's gradual adaptation to community-care emphasis, allowing new mental-health services to be tested without heavy legal and economic commitments.

Legislative Reform of Mental-Health Services in California

Many attribute California's shift to a community mental-health service system to the Community Mental Health Services Act of 1968 (California Human Relations Agency, 1971), a major legal overhaul of the mental-health system in California (Bardach, 1972; Stone, 1975). This law, comprising two Acts—the Lanterman-Petris-Short Act and a revised version of the Short-Doyle Act of 1957 and 1963—reformed the civil and legal rights of the mentally ill person and revamped funding arrangements of the mental-health service system to create a single system of care and treatment based on county responsibility.

The Short-Doyle Act. The state government realized that, to develop local programs for the care and treatment of the mentally ill, it would have to provide incentives strong enough to counteract the convenience of committing mental patients to state hospitals. Since the mid-1940s, California had directed federal money provided by the National Mental Health Act of 1946 and the Hill-Burton hospital-construction grants to help local communities establish community mental-health centers (while other states, such as New York, used the funds for improving the state-hospital system).

The first state outpatient clinic was established in 1943 in San Francisco. By 1955 there were 57 psychiatric outpatient clinics operating in California; 19 of them were state agencies, 9 were operated by counties and the Veterans Administration, and the rest were supported by private funds (Karno & Schwartz, 1974). The clinics provided some psychiatric services at the local level, strengthened the concept of prevention and local care, added psychiatric manpower to the communities, and increased local interest in providing mental-health care at the local level.

New York State's reform of its Mental Hygiene Law, passed in 1954 (Wiley, 1954), stimulated and encouraged the proponents of community mental health in California to introduce legislation for the provision of "community mental-health services." After 2 years of negotiations within the California legislature and between the proponents of community mental health and some conservative elements (such as the California Medical Association), a bill was introduced by Senator Alan Short and Assemblyman Donald Doyle. The bill was passed and signed into law on July 6, 1957.

The goal of the Short-Doyle Act was to provide early treatment close to the patients' residence. It emphasized the provision of outpatient services and establishment of preventive programs by educating and consulting with care providers in the communities and provided for local administration of community mental-health services. Five services qualified for state reimbursement: outpatient, inpatient, rehabilitation, information and education, and consultation. To qualify for state funds, a local government had to provide two or more of the five services. Once a community qualified, services were jointly funded, half by the local government and half by the state.

It is interesting that the 1957 Short-Doyle Act was passed about 2 years after the first appropriation of funds for new psychoactive drugs for state hospitals. Increased use of these "wonder drugs" helped shorten the patient's length of stay in the state hospital and promote return to the communities. Experience in using the drugs, realization of their potential, and the possibility of maintaining many patients in the community rather than rehospitalizing them lent support for the passage of the Short-Doyle Bill.

Critics of early Short-Doyle programs pointed out that they did not significantly affect inpatient services. The state-hospital system continued to be the main source of these services until the Short-Doyle Amendments of 1968 and 1969. But the original act laid the foundation for community programs for the mentally ill. Local mental-health advisory boards (whose establishment was required by the law) and the Conference of Local Mental Health Directors became forums for discussing local mental-health needs and vehicles for organizing support for community mental-health programs in California.

In 1963 the Short-Doyle Act was amended, and the funding ratio for new programs was increased to 75% state funds:25% local funds. In addition, whereas the Short-Doyle Act of 1957 restricted state reimbursement of community mental-health programs to voluntary patients, the 1963 amendment made services provided to involuntary patients eligible for state reimbursement. This was an important change, because in 1963 more than 80% of the patients in state hospitals were on indefinite involuntary commitment (Assembly Interim Committee on Ways and Means, Subcommittee on Mental Health, 1966). Also in 1963, 95% of state funding was going to state hospitals (California State Department of Mental Hygiene, 1972). Thus it seemed that, unless local community mental-health programs could move into the area of involuntary hospitalization, they would remain at the periphery of mental-health services in California, and the majority of the population needing mental-health services would not receive them close to home.

Even though the 1963 Short-Doyle amendment included involuntary mental patients, a dichotomy emerged in which state-hospital-system funds went primarily to involuntary patients of lower socioeconomic status, while Short-Doyle funds went primarily to voluntary patients of higher socioeconomic status. Proponents of community-based mental-health programs felt, therefore, that the commitment process was the key to changing the mental-health system. The current commitment process determined the flow of patients and funds, perpetuated archaic public sentiment about mental illness as "dangerous," and stood in the way of more modern and humane community mental-health principles (Aviram, 1972). The proponents of community mental-health programs thus joined civil libertarians in an effort to reform the involuntary-commitment process in California. The result was passage of the Lanterman-Petris-Short Act (hereafter LPS) in 1968.

Lanterman-Petris-Short Act.   Many view LPS* as the civil-rights bill of mental patients. However, the perspective and intentions of this law went beyond the civil libertarians' interest in safeguarding the rights of the mental patient. As Alan Stone (1975) states, "it seems designed to implement the concepts of community mental health for those who are and might be committable" (p. 61). The criteria for involuntary hospitalization were made more stringent, providing for screening and local care for those who did not require inpatient care, increasing the legal right of the committed, providing for intensive short-term treatment when needed, and stimulating further localization of mental-health services.

What was the system that LPS reformed? According to the previously existing California law (California Welfare and Institutions Code, 1966, Section 5550), a person could be committed for an indeterminate period of time under one or both of the following conditions:

1. If his/her mental condition warranted supervision, treatment, care, or restraint.
2. If his/her mental condition constituted a danger to himself or to the person or property of others.

---

*See California Human Relations Agency, *California Mental Health Services Act.* Sacramento, California, 1971, for a description of the bill's provisions.

Like many other civil-commitment laws, LPS did not specify how to determine the need for treatment and care, nor did it define dangerousness (Brakel & Rock, 1971). But LPS seemed to advance several social goals, which were (or could be) contradictory. Its aim was to provide treatment and care for those who need it, protect the public from anticipated dangerous acts, and protect allegedly irresponsible people from themselves. In practice there was often a fourth goal—that of relieving society from troublesome and disturbing people.

In *The Dilemma of Mental Commitments in California,* a report issued by the California Legislature in 1966, the possible contradiction between custody of the dangerous person and treatment of the sick was illuminated. The procedures of involuntary mental commitment in California failed to safeguard the civil liberties of the individual and did not comply with good medical practice.

As for the medical examinations and recommendations to the court they tend to presume mental illness, be performed in a perfunctory manner, and are based on vague criteria.

....

As for legal procedures, citizens are often illegally detained in poor facilities for screening, fail to receive adequate legal counsel. . . . (Assembly Interim Committee on Ways and Means, Subcommittee on Mental Health, 1966, p. 177).

This statement was a result of concern in California about the involuntary-commitment process. In 1965 the California Assembly Interim Committee on Ways and Means, Subcommittee on Mental Health, had turned its attention to the California system for handling the mentally ill. The committee thoroughly reviewed California's court commitment process and learned that the average length of a commitment hearing was 4.7 minutes per person. This shocking evidence added strength to the committee's claim that the commitment system was inadequate. In *The Dilemma of Mental Commitment in California,* the legislature viewed the system as inherently defective because it tended to promote long-term custodial care in state hospitals and to discourage short-term noninstitutional care. The report also assailed the involuntary-commitment system because involuntary hospitalization harmed rather than helped many persons, owing to lengthy institutionalization and to the social stigma and legal disabilities involved, even in excess of those experienced by convicted felons. The report pointed out that the trade of "your liberty for your treatment was very often a poor bargain" (Assembly Interim Committee on Ways and Means, Subcommittee on Mental Health, 1966, p. 8).

The subcommittee proposed several changes: (1) elimination of the commitment court, (2) termination of indefinite periods of involuntary placement, and (3) creation of community-service units that would be responsible for helping people reach needed services on a voluntary basis.

The Subcommittee on Mental Health Services and other critics of the mental-health system in California believed that, if the commitment system were abolished, a chain reaction would be started that would, in time, result in fewer involuntary placements, shorter hospitalization periods, a diversion of patients and dollars into a wide variety of community services, a change in attitudes and procedures employed by treatment personnel, and a generally positive change in public attitudes toward the mentally ill.

Basically LPS was a compromise between two major contending groups and was supported by a coalition of various interest groups. The "Dilemma" report illuminated the existing conflict between civil-libertarian interest groups and medical-treatment groups. Civil libertarians objected to the commitment court's lack of due process and to the indefinite deprivation of liberty based on medical judgment. Some treatment-oriented groups led by the medical profession objected to the court's processes as disruptive, untherapeutic, and a serious impediment to treatment.

The legislative compromise entailed in LPS intended to facilitate treatment by giving a great deal of discretion to mental-health professionals to provide services for a specified period of time without mandatory court review. On the other hand the proposed law not only restricted involuntary treatment without court review after this initial period but also eliminated all indefinite-duration commitments. It further responded to concerns of civil libertarians by providing a structured legal process for long-term patients and by protecting patients' civil rights.

The law was supported by what has been called an unholy alliance of liberals and conservatives. The liberals saw in the law an opportunity to guarantee patients' civil liberties and to improve treatment. The conservatives thought it would lead to a reduction of state expenditures in areas that should be the responsibility of local communities. Many mental-health professionals supported the law because they saw in it an opportunity to provide better treatment based on local care for the mentally ill.

The LPS Bill was passed in 1967, with a delayed implementation date of 1 year. The authors of the law were well aware of the need to bolster the law with an adequate funding mechanism that would make it possible for counties to carry out their roles. In 1968 the legislature amended the Short-Doyle Act to finance the new system created by LPS. Both LPS and the 1968 Short-Doyle Amendment went into effect July 1, 1969.

The LPS Bill designed a series of safeguards of patients' legal and civil rights and shifted the responsibility for treatment to the local communities.

The elimination of the commitment court and termination of the indefinite involuntary-treatment status were the foci of LPS. It was primarily concerned with the involuntary treatment of the mentally disordered, alcoholics, and users of illegal narcotic drugs. The old commitment system had been quite simple: Once a person was committed, he was placed in a treatment facility where he remained until the medical director of the facility decided to release him. In contrast the LPS system provided for a series of different procedures applicable to different categories of persons and patients and required severe impairment or danger to justify longer periods of involuntary hospitalization.

The major provisions of LPS are as follows: A person may be involuntarily detained for 72 hours for evaluation and treatment on the request of any private person or police officer and with a written application (following preliminary screening) by a mental-health professional designated by the county. Certification for an additional 14 days of intensive treatment must be recommended by two mental-health professionals (one of whom must be a physician) and filed with the Superior Court. Involuntary detention under the 14-day certificate may occur if the person is found to be dangerous to himself or others, or gravely disabled because of mental disorder, alcohol, or drug abuse, and refuses voluntary treatment. After 17 days any further confinement requires judicial review and decision. If the Superior Court believes the person is suicidal, recertification is authorized for another 14 days of treatment. If the court finds a person imminently dangerous to others, it may allow another 90 days of involuntary hospitalization. If a person is found to be gravely disabled, the court may appoint a conservator. If a continuation of the conservatorship is warranted, a petition is filed with the court, which decides to continue the conservatorship on a yearly basis.

Arthur Bolton, one of the major architects of LPS, states that, in his designing the law, red tape obstacles were deliberately created to discourage involuntary confinement and long periods of involuntary treatment. The system was conceived as a funnel with relatively large and simple entrances, but increasingly narrow and complex procedures for every extended period of involuntary treatment (ENKI, 1972).

One criticism of the mental-health system in California that the Subcommittee on Mental Health mentioned in its "Dilemma" report was that committed persons suffered 16 legal disabilities, 7 more than those imposed on a convicted felon (Assembly Interim Committee on Ways and Means, Subcommittee on Mental Health, 1966, pp. 52, 188–194). One of the objectives of LPS was to reduce the number of legal disabilities and to grant patients various civil rights. Although patients can be certified for 14 days' involuntary treatment, they have a right to judicial review and must be granted a hearing by writ of habeas corpus. This writ may be filed by the patient or by a family member or a friend on his or her behalf. And LPS granted other patients' rights, such as wearing their own clothes, seeing visitors every day, and having reasonable access to telephones, and the right to refuse shock treatment or lobotomy (more recently, 1974, the term *lobotomy* was changed to the more inclusive term: *psychosurgery*). The law further stated that no person might be presumed incompetent because he or she had been evaluated or treated for mental disorder.

The LPS Bill shifted the ultimate responsibility for evaluation of patients' needs, treatment, and planning of mental-health services from the state to the counties, with the goal of creating a single system of care with its locus in the local community. Under the new system each county with a population of 100,000 or more was designated as the local unit of government to provide mental-health services. Except for those services provided for judicially committed patients, services in community and state facilities should be provided under a single system of care under the general supervision of the local community mental-health director, with the advice of a local advisory board. The Department of Mental Health has the responsibility of allocating the funds available to the counties on the basis of approved county mental-health plans. The 1968 Short-Doyle Amendment specified that the net costs of mental-health services are reimbursible on the basis of 90% state and 10% county.

The LPS Bill lists six basic intents:

1. To end inappropriate, indefinite, and involuntary commitment of mentally disordered persons and chronic alcoholics and to eliminate their legal disabilities.
2. To provide prompt evaluation and treatment of persons with serious mental disorders or chronic alcoholism.
3. To guarantee and protect public safety.
4. To safeguard individual rights through judicial review.
5. To provide individualized treatment, supervision, and placement by a conservatorship program for gravely disabled persons.
6. To encourage the full use of all existing agencies, professional personnel, and public funds to accomplish these objectives and to prevent duplication of services and unnecessary expenditures (California Welfare and Institutions Code, 1969: section 5001).

By removing commitment courts, the legislators hoped to achieve the following additional though unstated goals:

1. To reduce involuntary hospitalization and encourage instead voluntary use of mental-health services.
2. To reduce the flow of patients into large state hospitals.
3. To shift the responsibility for mental-health services to the local communities. The law stated that,

after July 1, 1969, no mentally disordered person or persons afflicted with alcoholism shall be admitted to a state hospital prior to screening and referral by an agency designated in the county Short-Doyle plan to provide this service (California Welfare and Institutions Code 1969, section 5655).

With this emphasis on local control, the legislators further hoped:

4. To facilitate the development of a variety of local community mental-health services that would result in individuals' being provided necessary services close to their home.
5. To use better the various services available, both public and private.
6. To reduce the need for inpatient services through the development and better use of alternative facilities and services.

The LPS Act intended, in general, to reform the mental-health service system in California, to create a single comprehensive system of treatment and care for the mentally disordered, and to secure important civil and legal rights for the mentally ill based on the principles of community mental health and continuity of care for mentally ill people.

REFERENCES

Assembly Interim Committee on Ways and Means, Subcommittee on Mental Health. *The Dilemma of Mental Commitments in California: A Background Document.* Sacramento, California: California State Legislature, 1966.

Aviram, U. "Mental Health Reform and the Aftercare State Service Agency: A Study of the Process of Change in the Mental Health Field." Unpublished doctoral dissertation. Berkeley, California: University of California, 1972.

Aviram, U. "The Effects of Policies on the Reduction of Psychogeriatric Hospitalization." Paper presented at the 10th International Congress of Gerontology, Jerusalem, Israel, 1975.

Aviram, U. and S. Segal. "Exclusion of the Mentally Ill: Reflection on an Old Problem in a New Context." *Arch. Gen. Psychiat.* **29,** 120–131 (1973).

Aviram, U. and S. L. Syme. "The Effects of Policy Decisions and Administrative Programs on Mental Hospitalization Trends." Paper presented at the Fifth International Congress of Social Psychiatry, Athens, Greece, 1974.

Bardach, E. *Skill Factor in Politics.* Berkeley, California: University of California Press, 1972.

Brakel, S. and R. Rock (Eds.). *The Mentally Disabled and the Law.* Chicago: University of Chicago Press, 1971.

Brill, H. and R. Patton. "The Impact of Modern Chemotherapy on Hospital Organization: Psychiatric Care and Public Health Policies." *Proceedings of the Third World Congress of Psychiatry,* Vol. 3. Toronto: University of Toronto Press, 1963.

California Department of Mental Hygiene. *Statistical Report 1945–1946.* Sacramento, California, 1948.

California Human Relations Agency. *California Mental Health Services Act.* Sacramento, California, 1971.

California Human Relations Agency. *California Mental Health : A Study of Successful Treatment.* Sacramento, California, 1972.

California State Department of Mental Hygiene. *California's One System Ten Services,* **3,** 8 (1972).

California State Governor's Budget. *Governor's Budget,* 1974–1975. Budget Supplement, Vol. 11. Sacramento, California.

California State Senate. "Final Report on the Long-Range Plan of the Department of Mental Hygiene." Sacramento, California, 1963.

California Welfare and Institutions Code (1966 and 1969).

Department of Health, Education, and Welfare. *Federal Handbook of Public Assistance,* Part IV. Section No. 3533 (1962).

ENKI. *A Study of California's New Mental Health Law (1969–1971).* Los Angeles, California: ENKI Corporation, 1972.

Epstein, L. J., R. B. Morgan, and L. Reynolds. "An Approach to the Effect of Ataraxic Drugs on Hospital Release Rates." *Am. J. Psychiat.* **119**(7), 36–47 (1962).

Hume, P. B. "Mental Health: A Discussion of Various Program Approaches Used in California and the Basic Assumptions Involved." *Calif. Med.* **86**(5), 309–313 (1957).

Hume, P. B. "Portia Bell Hume M.D., Mother of Community Mental Health Services," an interview by Gabrielle Morris, [Earl Warren Era Oral History Project] Regional Oral History Office, The Bancroft Library, University of California, Berkeley, 1973, 126pp. In *Earl Warren and the State Department of Mental Hygiene.*

Karno, M. and D. A. Schwartz. *Community Mental Health: Reflections and Explorations.* Flushing, New York: Spectrum Publications, 1974.

Kramer, M., E. S. Pollack, and K. W. Redick. "Studies of the Incidence and Prevalence of Hospitalized Mental Disorders in the United States: Current Status and Future Goals," in P. H. Hoch and J. Zubin (Eds.). *Comparative Epidemiology of Mental Disorders.* New York: Grune and Stratton, 1961.

Miller, D. *Worlds That Fail: Retrospective Analysis of Mental Patients Careers.* Sacramento, California: Department of Mental Hygiene Research Monograph No. 6, 1965.

Mosher, L. and D. Feinsilver. *Special Report: Schizophrenia.* Washington, D.C.: U.S. National Institute of Mental Health, Department of Health, Education, and Welfare, USPHS Publication (HSM) 72–9007, 1971.

Roberts, L. M., S. L. Halleck, and M. H. Loeb. *Community Psychiatry.* Madison, Wisconsin: The University of Wisconsin Press, 1966.

Rypins, R. and M. L. Clark. "A Screening Project for the Geriatric Mentally Ill." *Calif. Med.* **190,** 273–278 (1968).

Stone, A. *Mental Health and Law: A System in Transition.* Crime and Delinquency Issues. Washington, D.C.: U.S. Department of Health, Education, and Welfare, National Institute of Mental Health, (DHEW Publication No. [ADM] 75–176). 1975.

Wiley, D. E. "Review of Legislation for the Year 1954." *Psychiatric Quart. Supp.* **28**(2), 297–304 1954.

PART TWO
THE STUDY

FOUR

The Study Approach

The study was designed to achieve three specific goals: (1) to provide demographic data on the characteristics of nonretarded, released psychiatric patients between the ages of 18 and 65 currently living in sheltered care; (2) to generate a measure of the level of their social integration; and most importantly (3) to identify factors facilitating or hindering social integration.

We had two reasons for obtaining these demographic data. The first was the tendency of reports to treat all individuals in an area with a high concentration of mental patients the same. This discriminated unduly against the formerly hospitalized group, associating them with several undesirable and often threatening characteristics (e.g., prior criminal offender status) that did not accurately describe the individuals we met while planning the study. Our second reason for gathering data on released psychiatric patients was the problem of reintegrating people into the community without knowing whether they have ever been successfully integrated into society to begin with.

The second and third study goals were based on the observation (made during the study's planning phase) that social reintegratration or integration of the mentally ill was the most frequently stated and common goal of all participants (residents, operators, service personnel, and others) in the sheltered-care situation. Social integration therefore became and remains the central focus of the study.

CONCEPTUAL FRAMEWORK

The major concept in the study is social integration; a second concept, one thought to be an important influence on social integration, is psychopathology. Let us first consider social integration or social reintegration.

Developing a Measure of Social Integration

The reintegration of the mentally ill into their local communities makes assumptions about the status of the mentally ill in society and raises basic questions about the nature of social life in general. Any study of reintegration implies that there are some mentally ill individuals who are not included in the mainstream of social life. This lack of inclusion may be a consequence of mental illness, of failure to "make it" in the first place, or of conscious exclusion by other community members. Moreover "reintegration" and "community" are ambiguous concepts requiring definition and clarification. Therefore two basic questions considered in developing a measure of social integration are (1) What does "community" mean? (2) What do "reintegration" and "integration" into a community mean?

Warren (1963, pp. 9–10) defined a "community" as

that combination of social units and systems which perform the major social functions having locality relevance. This is another way of saying that by "community" we mean the organization of social acitivities to afford people daily access to those broad areas of activity which are necessary in day-to-day living.

Warren views a social system as a community to the extent that it performs five locality-relevant functions: (1) production-distribution-consumption, (2) socialization, (3) social control, (4) social participation, and (5) mutual support. The key to this conception is that living in close proximity necessitates local access to subsystems that carry out these five functions. A theoretical problem arises when we try to distinguish clearly between a system that performs "locality-relevant functions" and its surrounding environment. If, for example, one views "community" in terms of the proliferation of "locality-relevant functions," Goffman's (1961) "total institution" is, in a sense, a community. The problems generated by placing individuals in this kind of "community"—specifically the state mental hospital—have been largely responsible for the concept of returning the mentally ill to the community for care.

To develop a better understanding of the concepts of community and social integration, we included in our planning-phase interviews the question, "What does 'reintegration into the community' mean?" Whereas answers varied, they generally related to Warren's description of community as involvement in "locality-relevant functions." Five levels of involvement were identified: (1) presence, (2) access, (3) participation, (4) production, (5) consumption.

These levels of involvement are not expressed as part of a continuum of increasing community integration, but each was described usually as in itself a necessary and sufficient condition for being integrated into the community. For example, some thought that when an individual had access to supermarkets, jobs, parks, movie-houses, and so forth, he was integrated into the community whether or not he chose to make use of these facilities or opportunities. (For purposes of analysis, however, we have given these concepts equal weight and added the scores relating to each to determine an individual's level or degree of integration.)

Many owners and operators of sheltered-care facilities believed that the facility was the only community available to residents. Some, if not all, involvement in locality-relevant functions could be achieved within the facility, and it was usually considered unnecessary, and sometimes undesirable, to attempt integration in the outside community. In this view the community was synonymous with the facility.

We conceptualized community integration of the mentally ill within a two-by-five matrix, the vertical dimension representing level of involvement in locality-relevant functions and the horizontal representing internal versus external community focus. Figure 4.1 illustrates this framework for assessing integration.

Levels of Involvement in Local Life	Community Focus	
	Internal: Toward the Facility	External: Toward the Local Area
Presence		
Access		
Participation		
Production		
Consumption		

Figure 4.1. Multiple conceptions of the reintegration of the mentally ill into the community.

Presence refers to the amount of time spent at a given place—the amount of time a resident spends inside versus outside his sheltered-care placement. This level of involvement is reflected in the comments of residents and social workers, who expressed the need to "get out" of the facility and to "get out in the community."

Access refers to the availability to residents of places, services, and social contacts open to other community members. This level of community involvement is best reflected in the response of a Mental Health Association member to the question about integration into the community:

What people do, the organizations they join, vary according to the personal needs of different individuals. I couldn't stay home by myself but others prefer this type of existence. What is important is that individuals not be denied the opportunity to do what they want and live where they want simply because they are former mental patients (F.N.).*

Ruesch (1969, p. 663) states that "an impairment becomes a disability if it leads to a person's permanent exclusion from work, play or family life, thus precluding access to the material and emotional rewards that society has to offer."

The internal/external dimension of "access" refers to whether the facilities, services, and other opportunities for interaction are under the sponsorship of the sheltered-care placement or of channels followed by other community members.

Participation is a concept of integration into the community shared by many sheltered-care operators and mental-health professionals. It refers to a resident's degree of behavioral involvement in social activity and is reflected in the desire to provide activities for residents. One social worker stated, "It's not just having these things available but doing and becoming involved in them that tells you a person is integrated into the community." The internal/external dimension of participation refers to whether these activities are organized inside or outside the residence.

Production relates to a type of participation frequently identified as a key factor in reintegration, especially by professionals involved with rehabilitation services, and refers to income-producing work. (Because of the considerable emphasis placed on this activity as a reintegration criterion, we treat it separately from participation, which is not income-producing activity.) The internal/external dimension of production refers to whether the income-producing activity is performed, or its prerequisites pursued, inside or outside the confines of the sheltered-care placement.

*F.N. refers to field notes taken at the time of a structured or open-ended interview.

Consumption, another distinct type of participation, refers to the control of finances and purchase of goods and services. This aspect of integration has been underemphasized in the literature. Consumption is one of the key factors in social interdependence and is therefore uniquely important in community integration. Whether purchases and finances are handled through the sheltered-care placement or independently of it determines the internal/external dimension of consumption.

The operational definition of integration into the community used in the study was the extent to which a person was involved in his internal and external environments. Two broad criteria were developed for the study. The first, an external-integration scale, describes the totality of an individual's involvement in the external community—the extent to which his life was focused outside the facility. The second, an internal-integration scale, describes an inward focus—involvement in the sheltered-care facility in which an individual lives and the mediation by the facility of his contacts with the broader outside world. The statistical procedures used to develop these scales are described in Appendix A.

Assessing Psychopathology

To assess levels of psychological disturbance, multiple measures were included in the resident interview. The first measure was the Langner Scale, a paper-and-pencil test involving resident self-report of psychophysiological symptomatology. These items were most predictive of psychiatrists' ratings of psychological disorder in the Mid-Town Manhattan Survey (Srole et al., 1962) and distinguished between a hospitalized and nonhospitalized population (Manis et al., 1963). We thought, however, that they were more reflective of neurotic symptomatology and psychophysiologic disability than of psychotic behavior.

Because we could not find an adequate self-report measure of psychosis, we hired interviewers with at least 1 year of experience with hospitalized mental patients and had them rate resident symptomatology on the Overall and Gorham Brief Psychiatric Rating Scale (BPRS). This scale requires estimates of the severity of 16 symptom categories. The rationale for using this rating scale—previously used only by psychiatrists—was that the interviewer's prior exposure to psychotic symptomatology would give them an understanding of the range of behavior, and their ratings would closely approximate those of psychiatrists.

During the interviewer-training session, four interview films of patients admitted to and released from a California mental hospital were shown. Each interviewer viewed a film and independently rated the patient on the BPRS. The completed ratings were handed in and put up on a blackboard. Differences in ratings and the rationale for such differences were discussed, and an effort was made to reach agreement on the correct score. The project psychiatrist participated in these discussions, which included symptom categories from two psychiatric dictionaries, using observed content as opposed to inference and assessing the seriousness of a given symptom and the time frame that behavior reports were to cover. It was agreed that all ratings should be confined to behavior during the week before and including the interview and that ratings were to be based on actual reported or observed content (i.e., content observed during the interview), not on inference.

STUDY DESIGN AND METHODOLOGY

Our study design was to describe the influence of individual characteristics and the social environment on the internal and external integration of formerly hospitalized mental patients living in community-based sheltered-care facilities. The sheltered-care facility was defined as any residence, excluding licensed hospitals and nursing homes, offering at least a minimally supervised living arrangement (e.g., a halfway house, family-care home, or board-and-care home).

Data Sources and Study Samples

Two data-gathering methods were employed: (1) open-ended interviews and (2) structured interviews. The open-ended interviews, in addition to helping in the conceptualization of the study, related primarily to our goal of determining those factors facilitating or hindering social integration. Open-ended interviews with key people in the system—that is, residents, facility operators, mental-health professionals, administrators, and policymakers—enabled us to review trends in sheltered care and to become familiar with patterns of service delivery and community reaction. Most importantly these interviews, now numbering more than 200, added a depth of understanding to our analysis of the life situation of residents that facilitated our efforts to interpret the results of the structured-interview survey.

The major component of our research was a structured-interview survey that was designed to be a sample census and involved sampling every 36th bed in California sheltered-care facilities. A description of the survey methodology (sampling plan, data-gathering procedures, and data analysis procedures) is included in Appendix A. Interviews were conducted with a sample of 499 nonretarded sheltered-care residents between the ages of 18 and 65 with a history of psychiatric hospitalization, and with the operators of the 234 facilities in which they lived. The samples of interviewed residents and operators are representative of their respective California sheltered-care populations. Each resident (with the characteristics just mentioned) and operator in California had an equal chance of being interviewed. Formal interview data were supplemented with the interviewer's observations and commentary following the completion of each structured interview.

Structured Interviews and Data Analysis

Two structured-interview schedules were designed: one for residents and the other for operators.

Using our conceptual framework of social integration to deal with the second and third objectives of the study, we included items in the resident interview to measure the degree of an individual's integration into the facility and the external community. Included in the resident interview were factors we thought would affect the social-integration measures, such as the community's reaction to former patients in the neighborhood, the resident's level of psychopathology, and the resident's degree of satisfaction with the living environment. Items were also added to both the resident and the operator interview that related to the social nature of the environment.

Operators and residents were asked many of the same questions. In addition operators were asked about their role as an operator and about their reception in this role by the neighborhood. The operator interview included questions about the relationship between the operator and his residents and about the social and medical services available in the community.

Throughout the project we have combined a conservative approach to design, measurement, and data gathering (doing whatever was possible to ensure the reliability and validity of our findings) with an unorthodox approach to data analysis (using the most powerful statistical procedures known to us to obtain the maximum amount of information from our data).

REFERENCES

Goffman, E. *Asylums: Essays on the Social Situation of Mental Patients and other Inmates.* Garden City, New York: Doubleday, 1961.

Manis, J. G., M. J. Bruner, C. L. Hunter, and L. C. Kercher. "Validating A Mental Health Scale." *Am. Sociological Rev.* **28,** 108–116 (1963).

Ruesch, J. "The Assessment of Social Disability." *Arch. Gen. Psychiat.* **25,** 655–664 (1969).

Srole, L., T. S. Langner, S. T. Michael, P. Kirkpatrick, M. K. Opler, and T. A. C. Rennie. *Mental Health in the Metropolis: The Midtown Manhattan Study.* New York: Harper Torchbooks, 1962.

Warren, R. *The Community in America.* Chicago: Rand McNally, 1963.

PART THREE

THE CURRENT STATUS OF COMMUNITY CARE

Our sample census indicates that, as of September 1973, there were approximately 12,430 formerly mentally ill people between the ages of 18 and 65 in sheltered-care facilities in California. This figure represents approximately 1 out of every 1000 in the general population. If we compare the number of individuals between 18 and 65 living in community-based sheltered care and state mental hospitals in 1973 with the corresponding 1953 figures, we see that there has been a major shift in the pattern of care offered to the mentally ill (Department of Health, Education, and Welfare, 1953 and 1973; U.S. Census, 1952 and 1973). The community is less likely to be a provider of bed-and-board service to this group, as shown by the following facts:

1. Relative to the general population the number of individuals housed in community-based sheltered-care facilities and mental hospitals in 1973 (14 in 10,000) is only a little more than one-third of what it was in 1953 (37 in 10,000).
2. If we accept the 1953 rate of 37 in 10,000 as the true number of mentally ill in need of care in a protected environment in 1973, we would expect to

find approximately two-thirds of this population—who in 1953 would have been housed in state mental hospitals—now living in a community with family or relatives or alone.

3. Since the number of individuals in state mental hospitals in 1973 was 4 per 10,000, we conclude that, compared with the number of patients retained in hospitals in 1953, only 11% are retained in 1973.

Despite the smaller number of mentally ill now given sheltered care outside established social networks (i.e., the family), the population now in community-based sheltered-care facilities represents a significant and growing segment of today's mentally ill. The population in these facilities in 1973 was 10 times greater than it was 20 years earlier. Comparing this with the 1953 estimate of 37 per 10,000 in community-based sheltered care and state hospitals, we assume that the population living in sheltered-care facilities in 1973 represents approximately one-fourth of those currently at risk of hospitalization (i.e., those individuals whose chances of being hospitalized are high by virtue of their life situations). Given these statistics, it is crucial to gain an understanding of what the new system of community-based sheltered care is like—that is, how communities accepted it, what its organizational arrangements are for delivering services, how services are delivered, and what types of facilities are available to the residents.

Chapter 5—Community Reaction to the Development of a Sheltered-Care System—discusses community response as a major unanticipated consequence of the move to community care.

Chapter 6—Placement and Services in Sheltered Care—compares past and current approaches to service delivery for community-based sheltered-care residents. Finally, in Chapter 7—The Community-Based Sheltered-Care Facility—we describe the facilities themselves, the neighborhoods in which they are situated, and the relationship between these facilities and their neighborhoods.

REFERENCES

U.S. Bureau of the Census. *Census of Population: 1970*, Vol. 1, Characteristics of the Population, Part 6, California—Section 2, Part 1. Washington, D.C.: U.S. Government Printing Office, 1973.

U.S. Bureau of the Census. *Census of Population: 1950*, Vol. 2, Characteristics of the Population, Part 5, California. Washington, D.C.: U.S. Government Printing Office, 1952.

U.S. Department of Health, Education, and Welfare, Public Health Service Publication, Part II. *Public Mental Hospitals for the Mentally Ill*. Washington, D.C.: U.S. Government Printing Office, 1953 and 1973.

FIVE

Community Reaction to the Development of a Sheltered-Care System

In the past 13 years a new and largely ungoverned system of community residential care for former mental-hospital patients has evolved in California. The evolution and public visibility of this new system are major unanticipated consequences of the trend toward community care for the mentally ill. Other unanticipated consequences are extensive public reaction to the presence of former mental patients in the local community and the development of policies to exclude them from the community. As a result of these consequences and of the political activity of interest groups involved in the community-care controversy, there is a move toward a statewide regulation of the mental-health system.

Institutional care for the mentally ill excluded them from their local communities, and one of the primary goals of the community mental-health movement has been to combat this exclusion, based on the assumption that treatment and care outside of an institution would help maintain one's social integration or facilitate reintegration into the community.

The mental-health reform acts in California were designed to implement the concepts of community mental health. The designers of the Lanterman-Petris-Short Act (LPS) believed that elimination of the commitment court and termination of indefinite commitment would drastically change patterns of mental-health care. They further believed that LPS would start a chain reaction ultimately leading to fewer involuntary placements, shorter hospitalization periods, diversion of patients and funds to a wide variety of community services, development of more and better community mental-health services, a change in attitudes and procedures employed by treatment personnel, a positive change in public attitudes toward the mentally ill, and a higher level of social integration of the mentally ill in the community.

To the extent, however, that the placement of individuals in mental institutions has been the major vehicle of exclusion from the local community and has been functional in the community social system—a possibility often alluded to by deviance theorists (Cumming & Cumming, 1957; Scheff, 1966)—one would expect that the closing of these institutions would lead to a new system of exclusion. Did the proponents of the mental-health reform in California consider that their proposals might result in a new system of exclusion? Even if they did, no plans were made before the reform went into effect to combat new patterns of exclusion.

The LPS Act did intensify the trend of deinstitutionalization of many chronic patients. It also resulted in shorter hospitalization time and in an increased number of mentally ill residing in the community (Aviram & Segal, 1973; ENKI, 1972). Many people from state hospitals did not, however, return to their homes or did not have homes to return to. The system of care that developed to meet the needs of these people, and the community's reaction to them, are the new focus of community mental health.

THE DEVELOPMENT OF A HIGHLY VISIBLE SYSTEM OF RESIDENTIAL CARE FOR THE SOCIALLY DEPENDENT

The antecedents of community care for the mentally ill have already been discussed. A new system of residential care developed not only to meet the needs of the released mental-hospital patient but also to meet those of a broader category—the socially dependent. Thus, to some extent, the community-care system represents a step back to the "poorhouse" concept by providing care under the same roof for all types of individuals who are unable to "make it" in our society.

The availability of Aid to the Totally Disabled (and later Supplemental Security Income—SSI) funds created a business opportunity for the small entrepreneur to provide residential care for the mentally ill and other disabled groups. The additional funds have opened a new avenue of upward social mobility for attendants, nurses, aides, and other service personnel. They have offered supplemental income to families who open their homes to the mentally ill, while also providing a new market for established providers of residential services—for example, owners of boarding homes for students in university areas or owners of old hotels in deteriorating areas catering to the aged or a largely transient population. All of these facilities joined the small number of professionally operated halfway houses and certified family-care homes to form the large number of residential-care units currently serving the mentally ill and other socially dependent groups in local communities.

The involvement of established providers of residential services is especially important. In California and throughout the country (Chase, 1973; *New York Times,* 1974; *Washington Post,* 1974), the socially dependent (and specifically the mentally ill) have become concentrated in residential facilities previously used for other purposes but no longer competitive in these other markets. The tendency for hotels, boarding houses, and so forth to locate in a single geographic area is common. Resort areas have large numbers of beds to serve the tourist population; areas near universities have many boarding houses to serve a transient student population; and older hotels located in deteriorating urban sections now provide another source of beds for people who require community care.

These types of facilities provide quick and, in many cases, easy placement for an individual leaving a mental hospital (Segal, Baumohl, & Johnson, 1977). Their proliferation has, however, created visible and sometimes problematic concentrations of former mental patients in communities throughout the country.

A major example in California of such a development is the concentration of socially dependent persons around the San Jose State University campus. During the late 1960s cultural and economic changes in the local student population made living in campus-area boarding houses less appealing than renting an apartment. Boarding-house operators, finding it difficult to get student boarders, were more willing to take in patients released from Agnews State Hospital. These released patients constituted a more stable and possibly more profitable residential group. In Long Beach, New York, primarily a tourist community for well-to-do people, deteriorating hotels no longer able to compete in the tourist market also willingly provided services for former mental patient and other socially dependent groups (notably the aged).

To date, it is difficult to determine the exact number of residents in sheltered care. The rapid growth of this population was discussed in Chapter 3, but there is a paucity of information about who these people are and what sort of facilities they live in.

COMMUNITY REACTION

The rapid influx of released state-hospital patients was described by *The San Jose Mercury* as a "mass invasion of mental patients" (1971). The following KNTV editorial was aired on October 2, 1972:

Saturday night a resident of one of San Jose's halfway houses was stabbed to death during an argument. If you are a citizen of San Jose and have not visited the areas between Santa Clara and Williams and First and Twenty-fourth streets, you should do so, but only in a locked car during the daylight hours and never alone.

The halfway houses are in the greatest numbers between South Tenth and Thirteenth streets. The situation is pathetic. It is difficult to believe that some of these people, many of whom are out-patients from Agnews, are allowed to wander the streets. We doubt that anyone can give us an exact number, but we have been told that there are as many as 15,000 residents of the halfway houses in San Jose. Many of them within a few blocks from SanJose State University. A co-ed walking home at night is taking a chance with her life.

The rhetoric of fear in this editorial is further enhanced by distortions. The total population of the area is 15,000, with only 1790 beds available in sheltered care. Not all sheltered-care beds are filled by the mentally ill—who in fact are *released* patients, not state-hospital outpatients.

Communities have also reacted negatively to the threat of moving of mental patients to areas where they have not previously lived. An example is the vocal protestations of homeowners at Los Angeles City Council hearings on board-and-care zoning regulations. When such vocal protestations occur, the question of what leads to such community reaction cannot remain unanswered.

The Bases of Community Reaction

Community reactions seem to be based on five factors: (1) a stereotypical fear response to the mentally ill; (2) an actual threat to the community posed by the total former-patient group (as opposed to only those former patients living in sheltered care); (3) the housing of individuals who represent a real threat to the community in the same facilities or the same local area as the mentally ill; (4) norm-violating behavior—for example, loitering, odd or bizarre behavior; and (5) a concern that the value of property will decline in those areas of the community where the mentally ill reside.

Stereotypical Responses to the Mentally Ill. The fear expressed by community members is largely the result of a stereotypical concept of mental disorder— that is, unpredictable behavior manifested by a totally irrational and often harmful individual (Starr, 1955). Studies of public attitudes toward the mentally ill have indicated that inability to explain a person's action in the context of one's life experience leads to interpreting behavior as mentally disordered (Cumming & Cumming, 1957). The behavior of the mentally ill is seen as unpredictable and therefore as posing a personal threat. With the "raving maniac" in mind even the most liberal groups are reluctant to engage in close interpersonal relationships with the former patient (Aviram & Segal, 1973).

Actual Threats Posed by the Total Former-Patient Group.   Stereotypes do not exist in a vacuum; they usually have some basis in fact, though the facts may themselves be unperceived. Rappeport and Lassen (1965) made one of the most thorough studies of the threat that discharged patients represent to the public. In reviewing previous studies of this question, they observed a consensus that released hospital patients were found to have lower arrest rates than the general population (from data gathered before 1947). Rappeport and Lassen questioned whether the recent trend to earlier discharge would result in comparable results with a present-day population. Their study of arrest rates for individuals released in 1957 is, in fact, more ambigious. When they compared these figures with those for the general population, they found that the arrest rates for robbery for released hospital patients were significantly higher and about the same for aggravated assault. (The results for murder and manslaughter were ambiguous.) Recent studies in California and New York add evidence suggesting a trend. These studies report high arrest and conviction rates among discharged patients for murder (California State Department of Health, 1973; Sosowsky, 1974; Zitrin et al., 1976). But even the highest crime rate reported indicates that only 31 in 10,000 former patients represent a real physical threat to others (California State Department of Health, 1973). There are no data to support a conclusion that "would suggest any accuracy in the distorted view of the average mental patient as an unusually and predominantly dangerous person" (Giovannoni & Gurel, 1967, p. 152).

Miller (1964) reports that approximately 9% of the former-patient population she studied in the San Francisco Bay Area were released to a sheltered-living environment. The majority return to family, relatives, or more transient life-styles. Those released to sheltered-care situations were, and have traditionally been, older long-term hospital patients rather than younger and perhaps more transient people. One finding consistent in all studies is that older people (in both the general and the mentally ill populations) have the lowest rates of violent crime. Even the California findings, indicating increased violent crime among released patients, report a lower crime rate in the older than in the younger group (Sosowsky, 1974). Whereas the incidence of violent crime among older former patients was lower compared with the younger group, the rate was significantly higher than the comparable age-specific rate for the general population. In the high-incidence group (ages 20 to 29) the rate for former male patients was 5.2 times that of the general population, and in the low-incidence group (ages 50+) it was 9 times that of the general population. These findings are consistent with the statewide report of the State of California Department of Health, November 28, 1973 (Sosowsky, 1974). Yet these figures represent the total released-patient group. Current evidence provides little understanding of the extent to which the small percentage of released patients who go to sheltered care contribute to the higher crime rate. Information cited here and in Chapter 8 gives the impression that the involvement of released patients in sheltered care in violent crime is minimal and is overestimated by the public, owing to the publicity given such crimes.

Responses to More Real Threats. The third factor contributing to negative public reaction is the housing of former mental-hospital patients in the same facilities and the same areas as former convicts and drug addicts, who present a more real threat to the community. In one community, former-offender and former-addict halfway houses and a Job Corps Training Center have been established along with many boarding houses serving former mental patients.

Since the incidence of violent crime is highest in the age group 20–29 (Sosowsky, 1974), the crime rate is likely to be higher among the former-convict and drug-abuser residents, since many of them are of this age group, than among the older former patients living in sheltered care. When, however, all of these groups live in the same area, they are not differentiated. Reports from San Jose refer to 1790 mentally ill residents who are impacted in the downtown area (Garr, 1973; Garr & Linebarger, 1974; Thornton, 1974). This figure refers to the total number of beds available in residential facilities, not just those filled by former mental patients (Housing Office, San Jose State University, 1973). The crux of the issue is that total crime statistics are perceived by the general population and governmental planners without reference to subgroups within the sheltered-care population, and frequently these crime statistics are attributed only to former mental patients.

Norm-Violating Behavior. Observing a stranger standing outside a house or in a public place such as the local bank for an extended period of time is a violation of social expectations sufficient to justify a public response. Police are likely to encounter "walkaway" patients or receive calls from storekeepers and homeowners complaining about "odd-looking" individuals "disturbing" their customers or standing in the street. These situations are common among the less capable mentally ill in downtown areas. Police involvement with mentally ill sheltered-care residents requires special skills and time commitments, and the police believe this requirement lessens the amount of protection they would otherwise be able to offer the community (ENKI, 1973; Garr, 1973). Whether this latter perception is true or not, it affects the public's willingness to welcome the mentally ill in the community.

Effects on Property Values.   Given the stereotypical fear response and the evidence (real or imagined) of rule breaking and higher crime rates, homeowners become concerned that the value of their property will decline because of sheltered-care facilities serving the mentally ill. This concern is not solely related to the mentally ill; homeowners resist the intrusion of other marginal groups as well. This resistance and concern over property value is implicit rather than explicit because of civil-rights issues; nevertheless, these concerns are present and contribute to the negative reaction of the community.

Evidence regarding the actual impact of sheltered-care facilities on property values is scarce but indicates little if any effect (Dear, 1977). Neighborhoods likely to attract sufficient numbers of facilities to show such an impact are usually on the decline. The influx of sheltered-care residents, often revitalizing the economic situation in an area, may, in fact slow the decline of the neighborhood. Garr (1973), referring to figures obtained from the county assessor's office, demonstrates a steady increase over a 5-year period in property values in an area with many sheltered-care facilities. Whether this increase is consistent with surrounding areas and in line with inflation is not considered, but in a declining neighborhood any positive price evaluation is welcomed.

Patterns of Community Reaction to the Presence of the Mentally Ill

Perhaps the best illustration of public reaction to community care for the mentally ill is the development of measures to keep residential-care facilities out of local areas. No community has gone as far as Long Beach, New York, in passing an explicit exclusionary ordinance. Its provisions relating to registration in local hotels state that

any person requiring continuous psychiatric or medical or continuous nursing services shall not be registered. Residents requiring medication for a mental illness or requiring out-patient medical or psychiatric care shall not continue to be registered if without said medication the resident may be a danger to himself or others or may not know the nature or quality of his acts or where the resident's actions may become so disturbing as to interfere with the comfort and safety of the other residents. (Long Beach, New York, City Ordinance #1195/73, p.3)

We observed various exclusionary measures in California communities that were directed primarily against sheltered-care facilities for the mentally ill.

These include the use of zoning ordinances, city ordinances and regulations, neighborhood pressures, and bureaucratic obstacles.

Formal Mechanisms of Exclusion

Formal mechanisms of exclusion are those rules, regulations and legal administrative procedures which are used in order to accomplish exclusion.

Use of Alternative Legal Routes. California's mental-health reform blocked the routes of exclusion through the use of indefinite civil commitment. However, the penal mental-health system operates as a reciprocal system for the control of deviance (Stone, 1975, p. 63).

A person in California can be committed under the penal code if (1) he is charged with a criminal offense and is found not mentally competent to stand trial and/or (2) he is convicted of crimes but found not responsible because of insanity (California State Penal Code, 1976). Several studies have found an increase in the use of penal-code commitments to mental institutions since the enactment of LPS in 1969 (Abramson, 1972; California State Senate, 1974; ENKI, 1972). Referrals of mentally ill people to the Los Angeles Police Department, for example, increased about 80% in the first 2 years following the enactment of LPS (ENKI, 1972). A California Department of Mental Hygiene study (1970) concluded that the annual admission rates under the penal code for the whole state, as well as for the four specific counties studied, were higher after the new mental-health law went into effect. The results support the conclusion that "the superior courts of at least some counties began to use commitment by the penal code as an effective admissions procedure for securing long-term care for patients" (California Department of Mental Hygiene, 1970, p. 1).

The increase of about 15% of the governor's budget for 1972–1973 over the 1970–1971 allocation for care of people committed by the penal code also indicates the increase in the use of the penal code for committing people to mental institutions. Neither inflation nor the increase of California's population can serve as a sufficient explanation for the 15% increase of anticipated expenditures for committed people under the penal code in these 2 years (California Department of Finance, 1971).

The use of alternative legal routes to commit people may be evidence of the system's adaptation to the closure of civil commitment resulting from the enactment of LPS. Many who in the past might have been committed indefinitely now return to the community much faster—some because they refuse to accept voluntary treatment and some because there was nothing in their behavior to persuade the court to extend their involuntary treatment beyond the certified 14 days. There is also some evidence that local mental-health services may not admit as easily for inpatient service as the state hospital used to. There are now incentives for discouraging local mental-health services from using state hospitals. At times there are people in the community who may become a local nuisance, but there is no way to exclude them in the mental institution. Law enforcement officers, under pressure to deal with a community's undesirable elements, often report their frustration. Some resorted to an alternative solution—they arrest the mentally ill and charge them with a minor crime they have committed! Indeed one study reported a dramatic increase in the number of arrests followed by rulings of incompetency to stand trial. In many cases the court commits those arrested to a mental institution via the penal code (ENKI, 1972).

Blocking Entrance Through the Use of City Ordinances and Regulations. Many local communities base their resistance to the upsurge of sheltered-care facilities for the mentally ill on the facts that the present level of care in the homes is not satisfactory and that the local community has not been given sufficient time and money to develop appropriate alternatives. We have no dispute with many of these claims. The fact remains, however, that in the past when the number of former patients in the community was low and alternative routes were open, the communities did not object so vehemently to the low level of care. It is only now, with diminished access to the state-hospital system and the unavailability of arrangements with other counties and neighborhoods, that we see the furor in some communities over the quality of care given the mentally ill within the community. The lack of alternatives for routing the mentally ill "out" suddenly revealed the low quality of care.

Local communities use legal measures, some justified as safety needs, to block the entrance of the mentally ill into the community. Although California law requires the community to provide care and treatment for the mentally ill, it cannot prevent communities from exercising their local responsibilities. One example is a California city's demand that every new board-and-care home operator obtain a permit from the fire marshal. A week later the city announced a moratorium suspending the authority of the fire marshal to issue permits for a period of time (*San Jose News,* December 14, 1971), effectively blocking new boarding homes in that community.

Another restrictive mechanism has been the use of strict definitions of what should be considered a "family" for zoning purposes, definitions that restrict the mentally ill from certain residential zones. There is accumulating evidence of other types of ordinances, such as fire-safety requirements and building codes, that support exclusion trends now operating in the communities.

Exclusion by Informal Mechanisms

Informal mechanisms are the various group pressures reflected in neighbors' attitudes and various bureaucratic obstacles that exclude. Bureaucratic obstacles are efforts taken through legal action or by the bureaucracy that manipulate the system so as to create a preferred (but unofficial) goal. The example of the fire-permit requirement, which was rendered impossible to fulfill, is an example of such maneuvering. High fees for use permits for sheltered-care homes is another example of manipulating the system. The fee can be instituted to discourage potential local operators of facilities for the mentally ill from going into business. In addition to the fee one city can also demand expensive structural repairs in accordance with current building codes. Executing the repairs does not ensure the permit, but once a person applies, he risks having his house condemned for noncompliance with code standards! The influence of this risk on the decision to apply for a permit should not be minimized; many potential sheltered-care operators live in old homes and are in a low-income bracket.

Stalling, red tape, and threats of legal action are also used in bureaucratic manipulation. Bureaucracies may send forms back and forth for minor technical problems. Counties have been known to withhold approval of public-assistance grants (although it is illegal), causing difficulties and delay in placement programs in the communities for released mental patients. A request for a legal opinion, in the hope that the issue would not be resolved for some time, probably served the same purpose of manipulating the system in such a way as to block the mentally ill from the community (*San Jose News*, December 14, 1971, and June 1, 1972).

The process of ghettoization of the mentally ill, that is, their restriction to certain neighborhoods, may be in part a result of economic conditions. The current amount of public assistance provided allows them only to subsist in rundown neighborhoods like the ones so often found in the downtown area of many American cities.

Economic reasons are not, however, a sufficient explanation of ghettoization of the mentally ill. Many move or drift to certain areas because their previous efforts to live in other neighborhoods failed. Facilities also fail to open in nonghetto areas. There is evidence of neighborhood pressures upon citizens who wanted to open and operate sheltered-care facilities for the mentally ill outside a former-patient ghetto. In one case a man wanted to buy a house for his family and four former patients and was threatened by other people in the neighborhood. He gave up the idea and said: "I know I am entitled to live there but that is not the issue. My wife and kids, that's what's most important" (*The Press*, December 1, 1971).

Since the road back to the state hospital for these former patients has been made extremely difficult, many drift into ghetto areas. The recent increase in the number of former mental patients in some California neighborhoods has been observed and reported by professionals as well as lay people. If future study substantiates this phenomenon, it would define one type of physical exclusion of the mentally ill that takes place within the boundaries of the geographically and administratively defined community.

Incentives, Risks, and Social Exclusion

Physical inclusion is a necessary but not a sufficient condition for the integration of the mentally ill in the community. Earlier we mentioned the economic incentives that operate in the development of sheltered-care facilities in communities. These economic incentives, positive in the sense of creating numerous facilities, had some unintended consequences that might have contributed in part to a process of social exclusion. Some economic risks are involved in caring for the mentally ill in the community. Steps taken to deal with these risks are at times contrary to programs and goals of integrating the mentally ill in the community. Payment according to the number of filled beds, and awareness of community sensitivity to and low tolerance of former mental patients, have led many operators to keep their residents at home. The less contact residents have with the outside community, the less likely it is that the operation of the house will be disturbed. The goals of avoiding conflicts with the community and of developing a stable population in the home to ensure constant income may intensify social exclusion (i.e., lead to a reduction in individual levels of social integration).

Overuse of psychoactive drugs contributes to social-exclusion trends. It is not surprising to find a quite docile population in many sheltered-care homes in the community. Lamb and Goertzel (1971), in a study of discharged mental patients, note that some of these homes resemble long-term hospital wards isolated from the community. One wonders whether a change in the economic incentive system would be sufficient to change this trend. It may be that community fears and uneasiness in relation to the mentally ill are an even more significant factor than the lack of economic incentives in the seclusion of the mentally ill within the community.

QUALITY OF CARE AND INTEREST GROUPS

Up to this point we have referred to the community at large and its reaction to the rapid growth of a residential-care system for the socially dependent. However, along with community resistance to sheltered-care homes, there has also developed a number of distinct, politically active interest groups whose concerns center on board and care. Homeowners, mental-health professionals, sheltered-care operators, and advocates for the residential-care population agree that "quality of care" is the most important issue, but each faction has defined resident need in terms of its interest or at least of its own perspective.

For example, Los Angeles homeowners' groups have defined quality of care in terms of supervision and medical services. Speaking derisively about "mamma-papa operations," they maintain that only a large facility is capable of providing quality care, bringing them into an uneasy alliance with the operators of large board-and-care facilities located outside single-family residential zones. This alliance is consistent with the homeowners' stated desire to exclude sheltered-care facilities from single-family residential areas.

Mental-Health Professionals

Mental-health professionals have defined quality of care largely in terms of the delivery of services. This group argues for open zoning, supporting the small "home-type" environment under professional supervision as the key to high-quality care. Such a facility, one administrator noted, is the most amenable to professional control and sanctions. Mental-health professionals also support the halfway house when it is sponsored by the professionals and imbued with a liberal dose of psychiatric ideology. An interesting consequence of this is that several more astute sheltered-care operators, to gain professional backing and, more importantly, referrals, have learned the jargon of professionals and can now give the "right" answers to questions about quality of care. A few have even hired public-relations people to articulate their efforts in appropriate professional language. This is not to imply that professionals do not support development of a responsible, high-quality system. In fact, professionals exert pressure on operators to maintain standards (e.g., they stop referrals to low-quality homes). But, a professionally controlled system may have some drawbacks if residents' independence is a primary and realistic goal. Moving out from under the protective umbrella of the mental-health profession may be a necessary step toward independence.

Sheltered-Care Operators

Sheltered-care operators have defined quality of care in terms of their own self-betterment: to become better care givers through training. Training satisfies the operators' need for accreditation and legitimacy in what is now a highly competitive market in several areas of California and seems to be a productive approach to upgrading care. A recent report issued by the State Department of Health (Hazleton et al., 1975) on the situation in Santa Clara County (including the controversial San Jose area) emphasized that highly trained operators were less likely to receive "inadequate" ratings by survey interviewers in providing needed services to their residents. The continued training and licensing of operators may, however, create a new professional cadre, simply extending the principles and prejudices of hospital care into the community and losing the benefits of the more natural, though perhaps not as intellectually elegant, environment.

Resident Advocates

Resident-advocate groups have defined quality of care in terms of residents' civil rights. More particularly they argue for quality of care as freedom from substandard living conditions and for the right of the resident not to be excluded from community resources open to the general public. Advocates view themselves as representing the resident population; however, we found only one small consumer-oriented group in Los Angeles with resident membership.

Interest-Group Politics: The Zoning Controversy

These viewpoints of quality of care all have merit and potential, but they are by no means congruent. The interests they represent, as well as the community-fear reaction discussed earlier, have come to the forefront in zoning controversies throughout California.

An example is a controversy that has taken place over a 3-year period in Los Angeles. Proposed zoning ordinances would have restricted residential-care facilities to certain zones and limited their development in others. Recently homeowners and operators considered a compromise that would mean the end of future facilities in single-family residential zones and would therefore obviously discourage the future development of small facilities that tend to locate themselves in these areas. Another proposed solution in Los Angeles would permit small facilities in single-family residential zones while drastically limiting the zones in which larger facilities would be allowed to operate. This solution threatened the existence of currently operating larger facilities in residential areas and would have severely limited the neighborhoods in which these facilities could operate. All of the proposed compromises considered in Los Angeles were more restrictive than state legislation, which allows a home with up to six individuals to operate in a single-family residential zone. Finally operators of residential-care homes in Los Angeles seemed primarily interested in ensuring their continued existence without regard to future facilities. This status quo has been temporarily maintained by default, in that the Los Angeles City Council has failed to pass a compromise.

STATE REGULATIONS

The problem facing the state is that, by taking decisive action on any of the quality-of-care issues and on the zoning questions, it will be opting for one solution and encouraging the growth of a particular type of residential-care facility to the exclusion of others. For example, the continuation of restrictive zoning in small residential areas in some parts of the state would probably lead to a reduction in the growth of small facilities with a "home-type" atmosphere. In the past several years the combination of community fear of released mental patients, increased media coverage, and the assertions of the several vocal interest groups has made the sheltered-care population much more visible to the general public. This situation has pressured the state toward regulating the board-and-care system. Pressures based on community resistance to the sheltered-care industry and criticism of quality of care endangered the very stability of the new system established by LPS. Reservations were expressed about the pattern and pace of change (California Senate, 1974).

In July 1971 the Braithwaite Bill (AB344), which requires licensure of sheltered-care facilities, was passed. The bill initiated a detailed exploration of the requirements the state could legitimately impose on sheltered-care facilities and of the modifications needed to promote the best interests of residents. These explorations were not mandated by the bill but resulted from the general confusion it raised regarding the future of existing sheltered-care facilities and the requirements necessary to develop high-quality and new facilities.

In October 1973 the Community Care Facilities Act (AB2262) was passed under the sponsorship of Frank Lanterman. This legislation established a citizens' advisory group on community care and allowed for the levying of fines against violators of regulatory standards, which were to be specified before July 1, 1975.

Although the move toward regulation seems to be improving the quality of care in sheltered-care homes, one should not overlook the dangers of this trend. One intention of the legislators of mental-health reform was to guard the civil rights of the mentally ill. It was hoped that those not requiring hospitalization would be able to live in the community, allowing their buying power and market conditions to determine their life-style. Regulating sheltered-care homes emphasizes that former psychiatric patients are still considered a special class of people—a class requiring the state to interfere to assure them shelter and care of proper quality. Regulation may eventually create little state hospitals in the community. Our hope is that the state will find a way to use minimum regulation to ensure quality of care while protecting the civil liberties of residents.

Although minimal regulation is desirable, it would not be fair to leave the mentally ill without protection from negative community reaction, completely exposed to changing market conditions and to trends of social exclusion. Recent changes in the LPS Act (California State AB1228 & 1229, 1975) following the completion of our study have modified the commitment laws to allow for a 90-day certification when a person is *considered an imminent danger*. Previously, to get a 90-day certification, there had to be *direct evidence* (such as an observed physical attack) that the individual was dangerous.

We have gone from community to hospital care and back in 150 years. Is the pendulum starting back the other way again, and on what basis is this move being made (California State Senate, 1974)? This is the dilemma we attempt to solve in our report on the lives of the mentally ill in sheltered care and on the factors that facilitate and hinder their social integration.

REFERENCES

Abramson, M. F. "The Criminalization of Mentally Disordered Behavior." *Hosp. Community Psychiat.* **23**, 101–105 (1972).

Aviram, U. and S. Segal. "Exclusion of the Mentally Ill: Reflection of an Old Problem in a New Context." *Arch. Gen. Psychiat.* **29**, 120–131 (1973).

Dear, M. "Impact of Mental Health Facilities on Property Values." *Comm. Mental Health J.* **13**(2), 150–157 (1977).

The Braithwaite Bill, California, AB344, July 1971.

California Department of Finance. "Population Estimates for California Counties." Sacramento, August 16, 1971.

California Department of Mental Hygiene, Bureau of Biostatistics. "The Impact of the Lanterman-Petris-Short Act on the Number of Admissions by Penal Code Commitment to State Hospitals for the Mentally Ill." *Statistical Bull.* 3(12). Sacramento, June 8, 1970.

California State Assembly Bills AB1228 and AB1229, October 1, 1975.

California State Department of Health. "Special Study on Community Care in Santa Clara County." Sacramento, December 20, 1973.

California State Penal Code, Sections No. 1370; No. 1026, 1976.

California State Senate, "Select Committee on the Proposed Phase-out of State Hospital Services, Final Report." Senator Alfred E. Alquist, Chairman, California Legislature, Sacramento, March 5, 1974.

Chase, J. "Where Have All the Patients Gone?" *Human Behavior,* October, 14–21, 1973.

Community Care Facilities Act, California, AB2262, October, 1973.

Cumming, E. and J. Cumming. *Closed Ranks: An Experiment in Mental Health Education.* Cambridge, Massachusetts: Harvard University Press, 1957.

ENKI Research Institute. *A Study of California's New Mental Health Law* (1969–1971). Los Angeles, California: ENKI Corporation, 1972.

ENKI Research Institute. *The Burden of the Mentally Disordered On Law Enforcement.* Chatsworth, California: ENKI Corporation, 1973.

Garr, D. "Mental Health and the Community: San Jose, A Preliminary Assessment." Unpublished paper, San Jose State University, San Jose, 1973.

Garr, D and D. Linebarger (Eds.). "The Residential Care Environment: San Jose, A Case Study." Department of Urban and Regional Planning, Studies in Urban and Regional Development No. 3, San Jose: San Jose State University, July 1974.

Giovannoni, J. M. and L. Gurel. "Socially Disruptive Behavior of Ex-Mental Patients. *Arch. Gen. Psychiat.* **17**, 146–153 (1967).

Hazleton, N., D. Mandell, and S. Stern. *A Survey and Education Plan Around the Issue of Community Care for the Mentally Ill: The Santa Clara County Experience.* Sacramento, California: State Department of Health, 1975.

Housing Office, San Jose State University. "Statistical Breakdown of Area Board and Care Facilities." Unpublished Memo, 1973.

KNTV, Editorial Statement, October 2, 1972. San Jose, California.

Lamb, H. R. and V. Goertzel. "Discharged Mental Patients: Are They Really in the Community?" *Arch. Gen. Psychiat.* **24**(1), 29–34 (1971).

Long Beach, New York, City Ordinance #1195/73.

Miller, D. "Who Are the Family Caretakers?" *Calif. Mental Health Res. Digest.* Sacramento: Department of Mental Hygiene **2**(2), 5 (1964).

New York Times, 1974 (see articles: January 10; February 8, 15, and 20; March 10, 12, 18, and 30).

The Press, December 1, 1971, Vista, California.

Rappeport, J. R. and G. Lassen. "Dangerousness-Arrest Rate: Comparisons of Discharged Patients and the General Population." *Am. J. Psychiat.* **121,** 776–781 (1965).

The San Jose Mercury, November 16, 1971.

San Jose News, June 1, 1972.

San Jose News, December 14, 1971.

Scheff, T. J. *Being Mentally Ill: A Sociological Theory.* Chicago: Aldine, 1966.

Segal, S., J. Baumohl, and E. Johnson. "Falling Through the Cracks: Mental Disorder and Social Margin in a Young Vagrant Population." *Social Problems,* **24**(3), 387-400 (1977).

Sosowsky, L. "Putting State Mental Hospitals out of Business—The Community Approach to Treating Mental Illness in San Mateo County." Unpublished Paper. University of California, Graduate School of Public Policy, Berkeley, 1974.

Starr, S. "The Public's Ideas About Mental Illness," Paper presented at the Annual Meeting of the National Association for Mental Health. Indianapolis, November 1955.

Stone, A. *Mental Health and Law: A System in Transition.* Crime and Delinquency Issues, U.S. Department of Health, Education, and Welfare, National Institute of Mental Health, DHEW. Publication No. (ADM), 75-176. Washington, D.C. 1975.

Thornton, P. H. "Board and Care Homes: Society's Rejection of Community Mental Health." Unpublished Master's Thesis, San Jose State University, Department of Sociology, San Jose, June 1974.

Washington Post, February 17, 1974.

Zitrin, A., A. S. Hardesty, E. I. Burdock, and A. K. Drossman. "Crime and Violence Among Mental Patients." *Am. J. Psychiat.* **133**(2), 142–149 (1976).

SIX

Placement and Services in
Sheltered Care

Placement in sheltered care involves fitting potential residents to facilities that will best meet their needs. Traditionally services to sheltered-care residents were organized to meet the requirement of providing continuous care—that is, a progression of services emanating from the state mental hospital to the community, leading to different levels of care coordinated to meet patients' needs. The conductor or orchestrator of community sheltered-care services was the placement worker, for the nature of the placement itself was a statement of the client's needs. This latter fact is illustrated by the observation that community-based sheltered care serves three functions:

1. A temporary-transitional facility for people released from the mental hospital who are not able to live independently in the community.
2. A permanent home for chronic mentally ill people.
3. A placement alternative to hospitalization. A temporary arrangement to avoid mental hospitalization.

The major goal of the transitional community-based sheltered care facility is to provide the mentally ill person with help necessary to "bridge the gap" between hospital and community. In an attempt to do this, the halfway house has been the primary placement facility. Apte (1968) indicates that the preponderant social situation "that makes the halfway house necessary is the failure of the family, for a variety of reasons, to provide meaningful help for the mental patient during the critical period of transition from hospital to community" (p. 9).

For some mentally ill people, community-based sheltered care provides a newfound home, one that will be permanent and one in which they would probably spend the rest of their lives. In most cases intensive mental-hospital treatment would not change their condition, and they can be maintained in the community in a supportive, protected living environment. The use of this type of community-based sheltered care as a long-term placement for the chronically mentally ill has been a part of mental-hospital policy since the mid 1930s (Morrissey, 1967).

The third function of community sheltered care is relatively new. The placement alternative to hospitalization is used by mentally ill individuals living in their own homes as a place to go to avoid mental hospitalization during periods of excessive stress or emotional crises (Apte, 1968).

Placement in a facility emphasizing any of these three functions to a large extent determined the orientation of services a resident received. Given this perspective, we look first at the knowledge base of sheltered-care service, then at the placement system as the fulcrum of service, and finally, at who gets what service how and why.

THE KNOWLEDGE BASE OF SHELTERED CARE

The knowledge base supporting policy and program for the care and treatment of the mentally ill in sheltered care in the community is composed of those findings related to the detrimental effects of long-term confinement in mental institutions and of empirical findings on the effects of the use of alternatives to mental hospitals. This knowledge base, especially in regard to the goal of promoting an individual's involvement in the community, is rather small. The results of previous research can be summarized under three headings:

1. Long-term hospitalization with total confinement in a desocialized environment.
2. Short-term hospital care with supportive outpatient services.
3. Sheltered care in community-based facilities.

Long-Term Hospitalization with Total Confinement in a Desocialized Environment

The detrimental nature of this type of care can be attributed to three factors: (1) extended hospitalization, (2) the degree of confinement (locked wards or facilities), and (3) a desocialized environment. Looking at duration of hospitalization, Kramer (1969) found that the chance of a patient's ever leaving a mental hospital after 1 year of continuous residence approaches zero. The consequences of long-term hospitalization have been described by Barton (1959) and Wing (1962) in the concept of "institutional neurosis," defined as increasing dependence on the institutional environment. External social roles break down and the patient's place in society is lost.

The degree of confinement seems to have the most detrimental iatrogenic effects on people in long-term hospital care. This is evident in the miraculous cures reported by Pinel in the unlocking of wards in two Paris asylums in 1792 and is continually rediscovered by individuals responsible for the care of the mentally ill. In the early 1950s, before the introduction of psychoactive drugs, Dr. T. P. Rees initiated the modern-day open-hospital movement in England (Gruenberg, 1966). Rees's concept of the open hospital involved not the extensive release of patients to the community, but simply the unlocking of wards. This change in itself significantly reduced the amount of bizarre social behavior exhibited in these hospitals.

The French psychiatrist Henri Ellenberger (1960) compares a state mental hospital with a zoological park, pointing out that animals confined in zoos are likely to experience the "trauma of captivity," including prolonged stupor, hunger strikes, severe agitation, and the manifestation of violent symptoms. He also reports the phenomenon of "nestling behavior" among animals in zoos, whereby they "take root" in their environment after being there for some time. This latter behavior phenomenon lends support to Wing's (1962) observations on institutional neurosis: that the key factor in institutional dependency is time itself rather than degree of confinement.

The works of Goffman (1961) and Zusman (1966) have illuminated another factor in the negative impact of long-term hospitalization; the necessity of the patient to be perceived as an individual in his own right if his identity as an individual (and therefore his social responses to others) are not to deteriorate. Gruenberg (1966) has appropriately termed patients' deterioration the "social-breakdown syndrome," stressing the importance of the patient's continuing to conduct himself as a human being. In the past, institutions created a desocialized environment—taking symbols of individuality and identity away from the patient: his own clothing, grooming aids, and a place to keep personal items with which to prepare himself for the everyday world.

The interaction of these three factors—confinement, protracted duration of hospital stay, and a desocialized environment resulted in the negative experiences of mental-hospital patients during the past 100 years. Thus future hospital care or community-based sheltered care should strongly discourage long confinement in a desocializing environment. Whether long-term care in a pro-social environment should be encouraged is a question we explore further in the latter sections of this book.

Short-Term Hospital Care with Supportive Outpatient Services

The definition of short-term care has varied a great deal over the years. Five years ago hospitalization of from 6 months to a year was defined as "short term"; today, the phrase suggests a stay of a few days. Today's approach to care of the mentally ill is exemplified by the current "revolving-door policy" with respect to the use of inpatient hospital facilities, whereby patients experience an increasing number of brief admissions.

Basic problems in understanding short-term hospitalization and outpatient services are the difficulty of determining the optimum pattern of care and the lack of controlled research to illuminate the relation between the hospital and the community-based sheltered-care facility. Retrospective studies of outcomes of differing terms of hospitalization have generally shown a benefit associated with shortened care.

Controlled studies of hospital care have shown that little difference in improvements in social functioning can be attributed to duration of patient stay (Caffey et al., 1968, 1971; Glick et al., 1974). (This is consistent with the observation that duration itself leads to settling-in behavior but not to more bizarre symptomatology.) Caffey et al. (1968, 1971), for example, in a study of 201 Veteran's Administration hospital patients found that:

The brief treatment group showed as much sustained improvement as those who stayed longer. The longest-stay groups tended to be more symptomatic at their discharge. The short-stay group did not demonstrate a greater incidence of readmission or a shorter mean time out of hospital prior to their first readmission . . . (1971 p. 81).

Studies comparing provision of partial hospitalization with outpatient supportive service (i.e., no inpatient care) have also found little difference between treatment groups. Langsley et al. (1971), in their study of 300 patients requiring immediate hospitalization, randomly assigned 150 to outpatient family-crisis therapy and 150 to treatment at the university hospital inpatient unit. Measures were taken at 3, 6, and 18 months following admission. While both groups showed a significant remission trend at 3 months, they did not differ significantly from each other.

Finally, evaluative efforts comparing day-hospital care with inpatient care

(Craft, 1959; Herz et al., 1971; Smith & Cross, 1957) and outpatient care with long-term hospitalization (see Pasamanick et al., 1967) have also found little difference in patient-behavior outcomes. Of interest in these studies is that a great amount of behavioral remission occurs within 3 months following patient admission regardless of the type of care received. Thus rapid remission of behavioral symptoms may itself account for the lack of treatment difference.

None of the studies contend that care is useless and should not be given. Rather, the results of these studies indicate that our understanding of inpatient care for the mentally ill consists primarily of knowing what not to do: Do not ignore minimal social necessities, do not allow long-term confinement, and do not aggregate individuals in long-term facilities by neglect rather than by plan. If long-term care is provided, we can expect that individuals will want to stay in such arrangements indefinitely.

Sheltered Care in Community-Based Facilities

In this section we refer to all protected living situations that serve primarily as alternatives to prolonged hospitalization. Foster care or family care for the mentally ill has been under study since the early 1930s (see Crockett, 1934; Crutcher, 1944). The use of community-care facilities as placements of first resort was legitimated in the study of Pasamanick et al. (1967). This study established the ability of schizophrenic patients to be maintained in the community without prior hospitalization and with the help of antipsychotic medication.

The initial emphasis in family-care homes was on providing a nice place for the individual to spend the rest of his life. The concept of moving back into the community—both in the halfway house and family care—did not become prevalent until the mid-1950s and has received serious and well-founded criticism because of what in the past was found to be the limited ability of the population to reintegrate themselves (Olshansky, 1969).

In the development of the halfway house and other sheltered-care living arrangements, the work of Fairweather et al. (1969) has been most influential. Fairweather, in his attempt to design an alternative living arrangement for released mental patients, created a facility that had its own economic functions and could supply employment for its members. To a certain extent the facility encouraged the member to focus life internally, in an attempt to develop a mutual-support system among the residents that would ultimately enable them to become independent of any professional support or supervision (though not necessarily independent of this mutual-support system). This system tended to increase the length of stay in the community as opposed to the usual aftercare services. In addition, although the system enabled residents to participate in full-time employment sponsored by the facility, when the facility closed, their employment potential quickly approached zero, the normal experience of patients who leave a Veterans Administration Mental Hospital. Fairweather also noted that social interaction in the facility was quite limited. The results of this study raise questions about the realistic possibility of "total" rehabilitation, at least from within the facility. Given a concentration solely on the internal-facility environment, former patients may need to continue in such a supportive environment.

The "high-expectation" environment, which reinforces normalcy by requiring the individual to be responsible for his own actions, was codified in the work of Wilder et al. (1968). Lamb et al. (1969), in their work at El Camino House in San Mateo County, have extended the "high-expectation" environment to include "satellite housing," which enables the resident to move out of sheltered care into an apartment subsidized by the facility. Facilities throughout the country have instituted "high-expectation environments" and satellite-housing programs.

Other sheltered-care facilities are more therapy oriented. Although characteristics of these facilities are not entirely agreed upon (though an attempt at definition is made by Cumming & Cumming, 1967), it has been assumed that they promote transition back into the external community. It is not known, however, whether the therapeutic milieu actually has this effect or in fact promotes the involvement of individuals in the facility at the expense of their involvement in the outside community.

Current knowledge of sheltered care and its relation to social integration leaves many questions unanswered. Sheltered care comprises highly diverse environmental settings with the common goal of reintegrating the individual into the internal activities of the facility and the external activities of the broader community. We understand that long-term care will promote a wish to stay in care and an asocial setting will produce asocial behavior. We do not know how to optimize the use of the hospital in relation to the facility, though we have begun to identify the type of social environment that should be encouraged in sheltered care. What is not well understood is the relationship between the environment (i.e., both the facility and the community that surrounds it) and the individual's level of social integration in the facility and in the community; our study is an attempt to deal with this question.

PLACEMENT AND SERVICE PRIOR TO MENTAL-HEALTH REFORM

Although the knowledge based on empirical studies on community sheltered care is rather limited, there is a wealth of information on subjects related to the placement process and services to the mentally ill in sheltered care. This information is based on practice experience of agencies and professionals involved in establishing and developing the system. Let us review the main features of this practical experience in California.

Sheltered-care services and placement were provided in California primarily by two organizations: the state hospitals and the Bureau of Social Work. The state hospitals were the major (if not the only) source of clientele for the sheltered-care facilities. The Bureau of Social Work (now Community Care Services Section of the Department of Health, henceforth: CCSS) was the major aftercare organization with the public mandate to place patients in the community and provide services to them. Patients in sheltered-care facilities were under the jurisdiction of the state hospital, most of them on indefinite commitment and, when placed, on conditional convalescent leave or "parole." The community held the state hospital responsible for the supervision and medical care, both physical and mental, of the mentally ill placed in sheltered care. In the beginning, funds for board and care also came from state-hospitals budgets; community resources were hardly used at all. After 1963, public-assistance funds became available, and local welfare departments became involved in allocating them. However, until the 1969 mental-health reform (LPS) most of the services to the mentally ill were provided by the Bureau of Social Work, a centrally administered state aftercare agency, and by the state-hospital system rather than by community agencies.

Before 1963 the major resource for placement in the community was the family-care home. The Family Care program entailed the placement of up to six state-hospital patients in private homes. Since the patients were on indefinite commitment, they were under the legal authority of the state hospital and received all their medical care (physical and mental) from it. The Bureau of Social Work performed the role of brokerage between the hospital and community facilities. The Bureau of Social Work was the facilities' referral source or supplier of clients and was also a regulatory agency with authority to certify family-care homes for the placement program. Certification is the property of the certifying organization, unlike a license, which is the property of the facility. Certification can, therefore, be withdrawn more easily than a license. If a home was decertified by the Bureau of Social Work, the clients were simply moved out of that home—either returning to the hospital or moving to another facility.

Until the mid-1960s the Bureau of Social Work was the sole provider of services to the mentally ill in sheltered care in the community. By the time the Community Mental Health Services Act went into effect in 1969, this organization provided services from 39 offices in various communities throughout California with a total budget for services and program support of more than 8 million (Aviram, 1972).

The Bureau of Social Work provided both direct and indirect services to sheltered-care residents. Its program had four foci: the residents of the sheltered-care facilities, the operators of these facilities, the general community, and the state hospital. The Bureau was considered the "community arm" of the state hospital. By placing hospital patients in sheltered care and by providing supervision and social support to former mental-hospital patients in the community, the Bureau helped the hospital maintain its leave and sheltered-care programs and even strengthened the state-hospital system.

Dorothy Miller (1965), in her study of former mental-hospital patients on leave of absence in the community, lists two services provided within the "supervision" function: (1) reports to the mental hospital regarding the condition of the former patients and (2) referral of former patients for medical care and social services. Bureau workers in the community were responsible for returning to the hospital any former mental patient in the community who caused problems because of behavioral or medical conditions. Unless communities had been given this assurance by the Bureau, the large community-care programs developed in California would not have been possible. Indirectly the Bureau helped the state regulate the size of the resident population by supervising and serving large groups of patients in the community who otherwise would have been in the hospital.

The assurance that the road to the state hospital would be kept open by the Bureau's workers was an important service provided also to the sheltered-care operators. The social workers also provided information about case management to these operators and were essential in facilitating medical services and payments for board and care.

Six basic types of social services were provided by the Bureau of Social Work to former mental-hospital patients in sheltered-care facilities: (1) mediating, (2) facilitating, (3) protecting, (4) supervising, (5) advocating, and (6) counseling.

Social workers from the Bureau mediated between the state hospital, the patient, the public-assistance agency, and the operators in the placement and maintenance of the person in the facility. Through mediation, the social worker acted as a "social broker" on behalf of the person placed in the facility.

The social worker facilitated many services necessary for placement and continuous maintenance in the community, including: (1) prerelease services in the hospital; (2) acquisition of board-and-care funds, public-assistance grants, and medical care funds; and (3) acquisition of medical care from hospitals or general practitioners in the community.

Between 1955 and 1966 the state hospitals assigned Convalescent Leave Psychiatrists who operated through the offices of the Bureau of Social Work and provided drug maintenance programs. After the Medicare and Medicaid

legislation in 1965 the Bureau of Social Work helped obtain drug maintenance programs from community general practitioners. When necessary, the
Bureau workers helped establish eligibility for various medical programs
(such as Medicaid) for people in sheltered-care facilities.

In providing supervision the social workers indirectly helped the former
mental-hospital patient. Without supervision the community, the hospital,
and the operators would have been reluctant to continue with the program.
Most of the protective services entailed facilitation of services and referring
the former mental patients to another state, local, or private agency for specialized medical and financial support and, at times, for vocational and social
rehabilitation in former mental patients' social clubs. When the placement
did not work out, the social workers helped relocate the resident in another
facility.

Because of the civil commitment procedure of institutionalization, former
mental-hospital patients were often in need of advocacy services. Social workers served as advocates for the patients in their dealings with the state hospital. For example, state-hospital authorities resisted discharging a patient from
leave of absence less than a year after his hospital release. When early discharge and restoration of rights might facilitate inheritance, social workers
sometimes negotiated an early discharge.

Social workers also provided counseling to the resident, his family, and the
facility operator. Although most of the social workers at the time were trained
in the psychodynamic tradition of casework (Miller, 1965), intensive psychotherapy was not a major service, because (1) the population in these
facilities was mainly chronic schizophrenics, and psychotherapy based on
psychodynamic concepts did not seem to work with this type of patient; (2)
even if it did work, the heavy caseload (an average of 78 patients per worker)
did not allow time for intensive treatment (Miller, 1965). Rather, services
were supportive and included advice, encouragement, suggestion, reassurance, ventilation, education, and direct help to modify external conditions
(Farber, 1958; Hollis, 1964; Kaplan, 1956).

Although various community clinics existed from the early 1950s, they did
not cater to the needs of the former state-hospital patients in sheltered care.
Even after the establishment of the Short-Doyle program, and its expansion
in the 1960s, local mental-health outpatient clinics were not a source of services for the sheltered-care population (Aviram, 1972; Bardach, 1972). With
the availability of public-welfare assistance after 1963 and Medicaid and
Medicare programs after 1965, community resources started to replace state-
hospital resources in providing social and clinical supports. Usually a general
practitioner provided antipsychotic drugs and physical medical care. The
Bureau of Social Work continued to be the major provider of social services to
residents until the early 1970s. Although county mental-health departments

were made responsible to this population in the late 1960s, they were reluctant to accept this responsibility (Aviram, 1972). It took several exposés (California State Employees Association, 1972; Lamb & Goertzel, 1971), public concern, and legislative action (California Legislature, 1970) to draw county mental-health departments into service provision. Only recently, and still with great reluctance, have the counties begun to accept responsibility for serving residents, relieving the Bureau of Social Work somewhat and setting the stage for the development of a service system provided by local service organizations.

The Negotiated Process of Placement

By the time the mental-health reform (LPS) went into effect in California in 1969, the Bureau of Social Work provided services to 20,000 people with more than 600 workers throughout the state (Aviram, 1972). One of its major functions was placement services. The district office of the Bureau was responsible for finding facilities for the placement of former mental hospital patients in the community. Each office had a worker or workers who served as liaisons with the state hospital in the area. The hospital made referrals for placements. These referrals contained "a summary of the clinical chart, a psychosocial evaluation of the patient, and recommendations to assist the patient's community adjustment" (Lee, 1963, p. 562).

The hospital usually referred a patient to the area he or she chose or to the area where he or she had previously lived. In practice a great many of the placement referrals were made on the basis of personal acquaintance between the hospital worker and the Bureau worker. Each worker developed close contacts with family-care homes and used these homes as a pool for placements. If one Bureau worker could not find a facility, the patient would be referred to another Bureau worker. At times this was quite a lengthy process that kept patients in a state hospital longer than they needed to be there. The Bureau of Social Work did not use any well-developed, rational criteria for matching patients with homes but left placement to the discretion of the social worker. Social workers felt a commitment to family-care home operators with whom they were acquainted and continued to use the homes as placement resources. (Operators wanted always to have their beds full; they were not paid for available empty beds.) Because of this commitment it was possible for a patient to be placed in a home without regard for his needs or the suitability of the home. This paternalistic approach did, however, often function to ensure at least minimum quality of care; that is, a worker often had personal knowledge of a resident's and an operator's needs and attempted to find the best available "fit." In addition to this relationship to the operator the social worker had another reason for maximizing the "fit" between the client and facility: Failure to maximize this "fit" usually resulted in the return of the client to the hospital within 3 months (Lee, 1963).

One may criticize the parties involved for not developing a more rational system of placement; it is questionable, however, whether a highly systematic rational system was possible in the early stages of community placement of the mentally ill. The placement of the mentally ill in communities not accustomed to their presence, within a legal system that did not encourage discharge of patients from hospitals, required delicate negotiations between parties involved—the state hospital, the Bureau of Social Work, the placement facilities, operators, and the communities. The development of personal commitments and some abuses of patients' true needs are inevitable by-products of the compromises required in such negotiations. No binding policy required communities to accept patients who originally came from their area. Thus social workers had to make placement arrangements in areas that were least resistant and among population segments that were more accepting of such a program for either altruistic or economic reasons.

Some communities preferred their former patients to be placed in other areas. Los Angeles County, for example, was only too glad that some patients who had lived there before their hospitalization and who needed sheltered care would be placed in Placer County (500 miles northeast of Los Angeles), where former patients became the basis of a whole industry of sheltered-care placement facilities. The Bureau's statewide program allowed its social workers to ignore the previous residence of a person in their placement decision. Their negotiations and sensitivity to local pressures and desires resulted in a concentration of placement facilities in certain communities close to state hospitals, such as East Palo Alto and Vallejo, and in poor and lower middle-class neighborhoods such as Oakland and San Jose.

The Effect of Changing Federal Welfare Regulations on Placement

Because of the far-reaching effect of changes in federal regulations making patients on conditional leave eligible for public assistance, the need for placement facilities and their availability increased a great deal. At the same time the county welfare departments became involved in placement. Since state-hospital social workers had to establish contact with the county to apply for public-assistance grants for patients, they also discussed with county public-assistance workers their placement plans for patients on leave. As a result of the new opportunities and demands county welfare departments developed their own placement programs for former mental patients in the community. No formal criteria were ever developed to determine which patients were placed by the Bureau of Social Work and which by county welfare departments. Rather, it was a result of informal processes and local conditions, in which interpersonal relationships played an important role. The availability of homes at any specific time and place was also a factor affecting the placement process and case distribution.

The Bureau of Social Work continued to be the major public agency dealing with the placement of the mentally ill in the communities throughout the tremendous increase in community facilities in the 1960s. Whereas in 1960 fewer than a thousand former psychiatric patients were placed in California communities, mainly in family-care homes, by 1968 the number of patients on the Bureau of Social Work caseload had increased to more than 7500, 75% of whom were placed in unlicensed board-and-care facilities (Aviram, 1972).

The Placement Role of Local Mental-Health Programs

The mental-health reform in California at the end of the 1960s further accelerated placement activities and brought drastic changes in the system, introducing Short-Doyle mental-health programs as an important element in the placement process. We have already mentioned the fact that until 1963 the Short-Doyle legislation did not allow county mental-health programs to claim reimbursement for involuntary patients. Since most of the potential clientele for placement in the communities were state-hospital patients who had been committed, the county mental-health programs had nothing to do with placement. Even after 1963, when the counties could claim reimbursement for involuntary patients receiving this service, very few clients did receive services from local programs. The mental-health reform that went into effect in 1969 forced the county mental-health centers to become involved in the placement arena, giving responsibility and authority over services to the counties. Placement of former mental patients was part of these services.

PLACEMENT AFTER MENTAL-HEALTH REFORM

The LPS Act created shock waves in the whole placement system, changing both the status of the client and that of the Bureau of Social Work. The client was no longer legally the commodity, the subject of barter within the system, but was granted the rights and responsibilities of a consumer. The dominance of the Bureau of Social Work in the placement business was challenged and the importance of its certification procedure minimized.

The Diminished Role of the Bureau of Social Work

By creating a system based on county rather than state mental-health services, the California mental-health reform in effect eliminated the need for the Bureau of Social Work. The Bureau had, however, several assets to offer in its attempt to regain legitimacy: its experience in placement services, its state-wide connections, and its ability to obtain federal money and thus save state expenditures on mental health.

According to the mental-health reform, the county mental-health services should have accepted responsibility for all services in the county, including placements. County services were, however, somewhat reluctant to enter the placement arena. The Bureau of Social Work remained the main placement agency, and the private sector remained the major resource of facilities.

This situation, viewed by some as an anomaly not in concordance with the mental-health reform, was basically the result of the mutual interests of the parties involved. Most community programs were unprepared to handle the increasing number of released patients who needed placement services because of the reform; they had neither the experience nor the staff to move into that area. The law did not, moreover, initially give priority to aftercare and placement services. The emphasis in the state's policy was on reduction of inpatient services. The state even offered incentives to counties to reduce their inpatient services by allowing them to use part of the savings in the development of new services.

It soon became obvious that placement services might become the bottleneck of the system. The placement services of the now-experienced Bureau of Social Work were provided free to the county mental-health departments. (If the county provided the services, it had to pay 10% of the cost under the state reimbursement schedule.) Also, the Bureau was a statewide agency that could operate across county lines. At a time when many counties did not have sufficient facilities within their boundaries, the ability of the Bureau to place people outside county boundaries was helpful.

The state, especially the Department of Finance and the governor's office, preferred the continued use of Bureau apparatus for placement services because they believed it saved the state money. The Bureau, at that time part of the State Department of Social Welfare, was able to claim from the federal government 75% reimbursement of the cost of services provided to welfare recipients. Since many of the patients needing placement referrals were welfare recipients, the services provided by the Bureau were less expensive to the state than if the county mental-health programs had provided placement services. (In this latter situation the services would have not been considered welfare services and would not have been reimbursable.)

For a time all the organizations concerned agreed to the Bureau's central position in the placement arena. The Bureau of Social Work expanded its placement program a great deal and in 1970 was viewed in the mental-health system as primarily a placement agency. Patients were referred to the social workers of the Bureau by the social workers of the state hospitals. The relationship between the Bureau of Social Work and the county programs was more complicated. Many counties, some reluctantly, signed a contract with the Bureau for services. The continuous existence and operation of the Bureau became a threat to the counties' authority in the provision of services. The Bureau also became a symbol of the counties' failure to perform their duty. Some counties decided to stop using the Bureau's services and to provide placement services by their own staff or through contracts with other agencies (such as the county welfare department).

What in the past had been a homogeneous system now became heterogeneous, with an increased network of interdependencies. The number of agencies providing placement grew, the number of facilities increased, and the new legal status of residents—many were actually free to come and go—introduced a dynamic element into the system. Because sheltered-care facilities could open with a simple business license, they diminished the effectiveness of the Bureau's certification program. There is now no established pattern of placement for the entire state. The process is based on local arrangements, on the organizations involved, and on the market conditions of supply and demand of facilities.

Major Placement Agencies

Before discussing the current placement process, let us review the five major agencies involved at present in placements of mentally ill in sheltered care in California. They are the following:

1. State mental hospitals.
2. County mental hospitals.
3. County-community mental health services.
4. The county social-service departments.
5. The Continuing Care Services Section (formerly The Bureau of Social Work) of the California Department of Health.

Since placement arrangements in California vary from place to place, it is important to remember that the agencies just mentioned are not involved always at the same time and at the same rate in placement.

In some of the state hospitals patients are placed directly by staff members who assume that responsibility. At times a hospital staff member links a voluntary patient, who plans to leave the hospital, to a placement facility in the community. Most of the state hospital's direct placements are those related to people who need convalescent care.

Some of the county hospitals have placement personnel on their staff. For example, in Contra Costa County, hospital social workers of the inpatient medical social services staff place their patients. These social workers are not under the supervision of the head social worker of the county mental-health services. In some counties, however, the county mental-health services are active in placement either in a coordinative capacity or in a direct way through an assignment of this task to their workers.

County social-service departments may be involved in placements under the "out-of-home" care provisions for adults in Title XX of the Social Security Act. Generally some element of physical disability would have to be involved for them to place an individual in out-of-home care. A mental disability may be part of the condition of the person placed. In some counties the Board of Supervisors designates the county social-service departments to act as conservators of the gravely disabled mentally ill. In such cases the county social-service agency may be involved directly in placements and supervision of the conservatees in sheltered care.

The former Bureau of Social Work has now become the Community Care Services Section of the Department of Health (CCSS). Under a variety of arrangements, formal and informal, it has continued to be the major agency involved in placement in sheltered care. In the local CCSS unit each placement worker has a group of homes she/he is familiar with. There are placement specialists who place and follow the client for about a month and then refer him for follow-up services by another social worker in charge of the area.

We find that 53% of the state-hospital referrals are placed by CCSS; thus CCSS is still the major broker between the state hospital and the facility. It also places 20% of the county-hospital residents and thus assumes a dominant role in all placements from large institutions. Other major participants in making institutional placements are mental-health services, which place about 15% of the state-hospital referrals, and the public-welfare department placing 36% of the county-hospital referrals; 9% of the facilities who get most of their residents directly from the state or county hospitals do so by informal arrangements.

The Variety of Local Placement Procedures

The emerging system of community care in California is characterized by a variety of placement agencies and procedures of placement. Placement arrangements—the placement agency, the referral procedures, and so forth— vary from one place to another. The procedures are related to historical conditions, organizational relations, existing manpower in the specific area, and even personal relationships. In areas where a strong community mental-health program has developed, the county mental-health service was usually the major placing agency. In areas with a strong CCSS and a relatively weak county mental-health program the chances are that the former would be the primary placement agency. Common features of placement procedures are the haste with which they are done, the limited choice given to residents, and the lack of established criteria to match residents with facilities.

Difference in placement exists between and within counties. In one county we studied, several subdistricts have different procedures and responsibilities. For example, in one subdistrict, the placement agency is the CCSS, and follow-up services are provided by liaison workers from the county program; thus no continuity of care is maintained. In other subdistricts the hospital takes major responsibility for discharge planning, or it is done by social-service workers in the community.

In Los Angeles County, Departure Centers were developed in state hospitals in 1972 with Federal Social Rehabilitation Service Funds; the CCSS has been servicing these facilities. Although discharge and placement plans in these centers have been required for some time, few have been developed. As part of the Departure Center placement program, preplacement visits are planned to the proposed facility; in practice, however, many patients were placed without first visiting the facility. As already noted, this problem was due to a lack of financial support and staff to facilitate such visits.

Recently the State has attempted to get facility operators to recruit their own residents. *The General Licensing Information for California Community-Care Facilities Handbook* prepared for facility operators by the State Department of Health stated:

You can get clients through being listed with social agency registries, pastors of churches, placement agencies, advertisements in newspapers, a listing in the yellow pages of the telephone book and through senior citizen centers (p. 16).

Although the placement system can be characterized by its variety, we attempted to reconstruct what may be considered as a typical placement procedure.

The Typical Placement Procedure

A local CCSS or county mental-health social worker, called a liaison worker, is responsible for following up on people after they are placed in the state or county hospital. The worker is supposed to visit the patient in the hospital. Shortly before the patient is to be released, the worker discusses with her/him a continuing-care plan. This is not always possible, however, because this liaison worker may get to the hospital only 1 day a week. This continuing-care plan is arranged by a committee composed of County Mental Health (CMH) staff. The patient's history and particular care and program needs are considered in the creation of the continuing-care plan. If several homes would meet the patient's needs, the patient may visit all or a subset of them and decide which he or she prefers (though CMH makes the final choice). The liaison worker is responsible for explaining details of placement to a patient and for arranging a visit before placement. Given limitations on staff time, funding, and transportation, however, preplacement visits are often limited to the one facility selected by the placement worker, and sometimes even this preplacement visit is not possible. If possible, the placement is made in the district in which the person lived before hospitalization.

The patient is not obligated to agree to a continuing-care plan (on the assumption that the patient is not a conservatee). Clients often believe, however, that failure to agree on this plan will result in the county's getting a conservatorship for them and carrying it out anyway. The hospital may dismiss the person without making arrangements for further treatment. Patients will often, moreover, leave the hospital at the completion of their 72-hour detention period without ever seeing a liaison worker (who, as already noted may get to the hospital only once a week). Sometimes people are placed in certain board-and-care homes because a staff member at the hospital is a friend of a particular operator. The liaison worker is supposed to follow up on a person even if she or he does not agree to a continuing-care plan. People (who are not conservatees) may leave board-and-care homes or move to another home if they so desire; these alternatives are not frequently chosen, however, because of the residents' perceived threat of involuntary detention under a conservatorship.

Major System Problems Affecting Placement

There are at least four major system problems affecting placement: (1) finances, (2) county and within-region jurisdictions, (3) lack of outreach, (4) needs assessment.

Aside from the shortage of funds needed to cover preplacement efforts, there is need for funds to cover placement costs for those not already eligible for Supplemental Security Income (SSI). Processing SSI may take from 6 weeks to 18 months and does not have presumptive eligibility (i.e., they will not pay until the qualification process is completed). To allow patients to leave the hospital and have a place to live, the state advances family-care funds appropriated annually. When retroactive SSI checks are received by the client, he is asked to repay the fund. Unfortunately, to get family-care money, the prospective resident has to be considered a "good risk" for getting on SSI. Often the most disturbed clients cannot get such funding, because they are not considered stable enough to qualify for SSI. Some problems concern jurisdiction. A liaison worker has responsibility for only the homes and residents of his own region; thus if a patient wants to move to some other region, it is possible that neither the liaison from the old nor the liaison from the desired region can help him. It may be up to the patient to contact the new liaison worker. The difficulty is compounded if the patient does not know where he wants to go.

The jurisdiction problem is further magnified for intercounty placements. With county workers responsible for services for their own county residents, and the county responsible for paying for their residents' care, barriers are raised to prevent patient movement across county lines. Not only are there problems with the number of persons involved at the provider end and the different rules for each region, but also there is the major hurdle of whether the receiving county will accept the person considering the questions of follow-up services—who will provide them and who will be responsible if the client needs to be rehospitalized.

This jurisdictional barrier contrasts with the ease of intercounty transfer under the former Family Care system operated by the state, whereby cases were accepted for service around the state when referred by one office in the system. This system was dissolved, and no substitute has yet been implemented for out-of-county placement.

Lack of outreach has been described as another problem. If a discharged client not previously oriented regarding placement does not respond to a letter from a mental-health facility offering follow-up services, he is often listed as not requiring them. We observed at times that this situation occurred even though the only address the client listed was the police station from which he was initially hospitalized.

The lack of outreach might have left many patients needing placement services unserved. This problem, coupled with other difficulties related to the placement system, brought about the enactment of the "Need Assessment Act".‡ This act became effective in California on August 31, 1975. It specified various problematic areas in the placement system. The law requires evidence of needs assessment, evaluation of progress, and guarding of the civil rights of the patient. It also requires that the person participate in and consent to the selection of the facility and have a medical examination no later than 30 days after entry. A large variety of "needs assessment" plans has developed since the act became effective, indicating the lack in the regulations of a clear directive of responsibility.

Regulations say that the assessment should be done by the person's physician, by the local mental-health program or its designee, or by some other appropriate community agency in the case of the mentally disordered. The state has not appointed an agency to make the assessment, and there is a question of whether it will be done uniformly in all cases or in all homes.

‡California Administration Code (Title 22 Division 6 #80329).

Market Conditions

The need assessment requirement is one approach to improve the quality of the placement system. Another approach, and by no means exclusive of the first one, is the use of market conditions as a means of bringing about quality of care. Level of payments for care and other incentives that could be given to operators may create market conditions of competition for clients and consequently lead to improvement of services and care in the community-based sheltered-care system. Our findings indicate that currently there is a good deal of competition in the market. Approximately 30% of the facilities in California report a vacancy rate above 25% of their available beds; 20% report a 1 to 24% vacancy rate, and 50% report no vacancies. This is particularly important in view of the competitive structure of quality service; what is necessary is more considered planning in the placement arena so as to maximize the benefits that can accrue from such a competitive market.

When facility operators were asked to state the source of most of their residents, 10% indicated that they obtain residents from other sheltered-care facilities; another 5% said that residents come primarily from families and relatives. Thus at least 15% of the facilities claim that most of their residents come from nontraditional sources of placement; 65% of the facilities report that they receive most of their patients from the state and county hospitals, the traditional mode of entry; another 20% report multiple sources.

Given these findings, it appears that a full third of the population may enter the system through nontraditional means. Any attempt to maximize the use of competition and regulation in this arena must be dealt with in this light. Focusing programs on the hospital or the social-work follow-up agency to rationalize the placement system may be inappropriate owing to the large number of residents moving into the facilities through other sources.

SERVICE PRECIPITANTS: WHO GETS WHAT, HOW, AND WHY

The question of who receives services is best answered by the saying "It's the squeaky wheel that gets the grease." The data we now discuss demonstrate that the residents likely to cause the most trouble and be the most demanding are more likely to get services.

Support for the "squeaky-wheel" hypothesis is offered by the significant difference in the amount of treatment offered to groups with different problems. Only 28% of the residents in our sample were receiving therapeutic treatment at the time of the survey. Young residents and those more likely to be involved in social disturbances—that is, in loud arguments as opposed to contemplating suicide—were more likely to receive treatment and to be treated more frequently.

Moving from a focus on therapeutic treatment services to an analysis of the total range of services, we developed a composite score relating to the reported frequency with which operators said they used 11 different types of services—that is, day care, socialization centers, psychiatric inpatient care, general medical care from a private physician, general medical care from public facilities, volunteers, paid helpers, public-health nurses, social workers, vocational rehabilitation, and sheltered workshops. Looking at who receives the total range of services adds further support to the squeaky-wheel hypothesis.

With regard to facility operators, we found a positive correlation between the number of complaints received about residents' behavior and the amount of services an operator used. Several aspects of residents' problems explain this correlation. First we found that facilities with a high percentage of residents who had been hospitalized in the past year were more likely to receive complaints. This finding would seem to indicate that the residents' illness-related behavior tends to precipitate complaints. Yet aggregate ratings of psychiatric symptomatology on the Brief Psychiatric Rating Scale (BPRS) indicate that facilities with a large percentage of "well" or "not severely disturbed" residents were the ones that received complaints. It seems, therefore, that complaints, the hospitalization, and the services were not precipitated by the severity of the illness, but by the reaching-out behavior of the resident. This observation is consistent with the findings reported in Chapter 10, "Involvement in The Outside World." Reaching-out behavior precipitates complaints, which in turn precipitate the delivery of services. This phenomenon is also consistent with the squeaky-wheel hypothesis.

Our findings show that frequent use of service is related more strongly to the characteristics of the operator and the facility itself than to the characteristics of the area and the facility's residents. The length of time the operator has been in the sheltered-care business being controlled for, operators who use services frequently have a treatment orientation and a more "professional" facility. They see themselves more as a friend than as a parent or caretaker and will have entered the business for reasons of past professional experience with this resident group. This professional or business-oriented attitude toward sheltered care is reflected in the characteristics of the facility. Those facilities identified by the operator as having a hotel, boarding-house, or commune atmosphere (versus a family or home atmosphere) are more likely to be service users. Larger facilities are also more likely to be service users.

In addition to a businesslike approach, service use is predicted by operator's experience or contact with services (especially where such service has a clear social-control function involved with it): Operators who have contact with other operators, whose residents have been in the hospital within the last year, or whose residents have been picked up by the police are more likely to use services. In addition, operators who have more education and see services as helpful will be more likely to use services.

Operators' Use of Services

Social workers are the most consulted helpers in the sheltered-care environment. Only contact with general practitioners approached the frequency with which social workers were consulted. Table 6.1 is an analysis of the type of problems presented by residents and the helper operators selected to help deal with these problems.

Social workers were selected 42% of the time, general practioners 26%, and psychiatrists 15%. Table 6.1 breaks down problems into three types: intrapsychic (i.e., made no sense talking, talked to himself, attempted suicide, seeing and/or hearing things), psychosocial (i.e., avoided people, felt persecuted, constantly needed coaxing, felt people were talking about him, misbehaved sexually, hostile to staff, hostile to other residents, exposed him/herself), and social (i.e., came in drunk, disobeyed house rules, refused to take medications, bought foolishly, did not pay rent, hit someone, stayed in bed). The table shows that social workers are called upon to deal with social problems 56% of the time, but only 27% of the time for intrapsychic problems. On the other hand general practitioners are called upon almost twice as frequently as psychiatrists to deal with intrapsychic problems. Although the efforts of psychiatrists generally parallel those of general practitioners, they are much less involved with the population than general practitioners are.

Table 6.2 is a more detailed account of the problems with which different helpers are asked to deal, with varying frequency. A task division emerges between the general practitioner, who is called upon for intrapsychic problems (which might be most amenable to the use of psychoactive medication), and the social worker, who is called upon to deal with difficult social situations.

Operators were asked how frequently they would seek help for the 19 specific problems listed in Table 6.2. Half responded that they would seek no outside help for nine of the problems. Only 6% indicated that they would seek help for all 19 problems, while less than 1% of the operators reported that

Table 6.1   Operator's Choice of Help for Various Resident Problems[a]

Resident Problems	Operator's Chosen Helper				
	Social Worker	General Practitioner	Psychiatrist	Other	Total
Intrapsychic	27%	33%	19%	20%	100%
Psychosocial	42%	25%	18%	15%	100%
Social	56%	19%	7%	18%	100%
All problems	42%	26%	15%	17%	100%

[a] Total number of possibilities for selecting help is the number of problems times the number of operators responding to each question, or 19 x 1155.

Table 6.2 Type of Helper and Frequency of their Selection in 19 Problem Situations

Problem Situation	Social Worker	General Practitioner (M.D.)	Psychiatrist	Welfare Worker	Owner	Police	Hospital	Other	Number of Operators Requesting Help
1. Disobeyed house rules	85%	8%	2%	1%	0%	0%	1%	3%	425
2. Bought foolishly	78%	4%	6%	1%	1%	0%	3%	7%	330
3. Did not pay rent	71%	1%	0%	20%	1%	0%	0%	7%	982
4. Hostile to other residents	62%	9%	9%	1%	0%	10%	4%	5%	593
5. Came in drunk	61%	6%	5%	5%	0%	10%	5%	8%	440
6. Hostile to staff	54%	12%	10%	1%	1%	10%	8%	4%	661
7. Hit someone	44%	17%	9%	1%	0%	21%	6%	2%	640
8. Constantly needed coaxing	42%	26%	17%	5%	0%	1%	6%	3%	532
9. Avoided people	40%	34%	21%	1%	0%	0%	1%	3%	527
10. Talked to him/herself	39%	35%	22%	0%	0%	0%	2%	2%	411
11. Felt people were talking about him/her	39%	28%	21%	2%	0%	2%	6%	2%	410
12. Exposed him/herself	39%	23%	20%	1%	0%	2%	12%	3%	654
13. Made no sense talking	34%	31%	26%	1%	0%	0%	6%	2%	912
14. Misbehaved sexually	33%	37%	14%	1%	0%	5%	9%	1%	892
15. Felt persecuted	30%	29%	34%	1%	0%	0%	4%	2%	745
16. Refused to take medication	30%	41%	18%	1%	0%	3%	4%	3%	855
17. Stayed in bed	27%	55%	7%	1%	0%	0%	10%	0%	376
18. Seeing or hearing things	26%	40%	25%	1%	0%	0%	7%	1%	798
19. Attempted Suicide	10%	24%	7%	1%	0%	26%	25%	7%	1137

they would seek help for none of the problems. There was a distinct tendency for operators not to ask for help with social problems (50% of the operators said they would not seek help with these problems, compared with 30% for intrapsychic problems). There was no discernible pattern between the three types of problems and in regard to whether operators thought they might seek help "all of the time" versus "some of the time." Rather, certain problems stood out, five in particular. The problem with which operators most frequently sought help was attempted suicide; 84% said they would seek help with all suicide attempts and 14% with some. Only 2% said they would not seek help in such a situation. The next most frequently cited problem for which help was sought was "not paying the rent"; only 16% of the operators said they would not seek help in such a situation. Finally, "refused to take medication," "misbehaved sexually," and "made no sense talking" were problems for which 75% of the operators sought help.

The problems just discussed, which lead to frequent help seeking on the part of the operator, illustrate the practical orientation of facility operators. In general, operators of small family-care facilities are more likely to seek help when residents misbehave sexually or do not pay rent. Because operators and their families live in the facilities, the primary impetus for seeking help in these situations is the threat to the operators' livelihood and the disruption of family life caused by nonreceipt of rent and resident's sexual misbehavior.

The practical orientation of operators toward services was further evidenced by the analysis of resident's "refusal to take medication." Request for service when residents refuse to take medications is more likely if there have been complaints to the authorities by neighborhood people than if complaints are made just to the operator. This is true because, with the former action, a *situation of operator accountability* has been set up. Operators seek help to cope with the *publicly* defined responsibility. Operators' accountability also figures into the frequent requests for services related to suicide attempts.

The high frequency of requests for help when residents "made no sense talking" is associated with operators who (1) have received complaints about their facility, (2) have had problems recruiting residents for their facility, and (3) are dependent upon the facility for their income. The motivation here is to prevent rehospitalization of clients, which might cause significant financial problems.

Operators depend heavily on social-work help. The one exception is that police are called to help with suicidal patients, because police are always available and, as Bittner (1967) observes, will in almost all cases take the suicidal resident immediately to an inpatient facility (see Table 6.2). (The hospital is also frequently used as a help source for suicide attempts. This request usually results, however, in police involvement where the hospital calls the police to deal with a person considered a danger to himself.) The reason for the greater reliance of operators on social workers as a help source is probably their familiarity with them. The social worker is responsible for most placements and is therefore in a position to offer service to the facility operator. Further, general practitioners and psychiatrists are a more expensive, less numerous resource in community mental-health centers.

The importance of the operator's focus on keeping his facility running smoothly—as evidenced by his willingness to use services in situations that practically threaten his financial stability and the social stability of his home or make him publicly accountable—must be taken into account in designing a more effective service system based on priority of residents' needs. Any service delivery designs not taking these factors into consideration are likely to be unsuccessful.

Conclusion

The negotiated character of the placement process has not changed with the passage of the 1969 mental-health reform. What has changed are the roles of the participants. Former mental patients no longer have to be the system's commodities (its object of barter). Their status has been changed to service consumers. They are not, however, prepared, and they do not actively exercise the rights and responsibilities that result from their status change. Failure of residents to exercise their consumer prerogatives has been reflected in the low level of quality of care in many facilities. This situation has been a major reason leading the state to move toward regulations.

Placement and services in sheltered care are currently dependent upon social contingencies that to a large extent are independent of residents' needs. Future planning of a sheltered-care service system must not only take account of the social contingencies that now operate in the system but also become more focused on clients' needs.

REFERENCES

Apte, R. Z. *Halfway Houses: A New Dilemma in Institutional Care.* Occasional Papers on Social Administration No. 27, London: G. Bell and Sons, 1968.

Aviram U. "Mental Health Reform and the Aftercare State Service Agency: A Study of the Process of Change in the Mental Health Field." Unpublished doctoral dissertation. Berkeley: University of California, 1972.

Bardach, E. *The Skill Factor in Politics.* Berkeley: University of California Press, 1972.

Barton, R. *Institutional Neurosis.* Bristol, England: Wright, 1959.

Bittner, E. "Police Discretion in Emergency Apprehension of Mentally Ill Persons." *Social Problems,* 14 (3), 278–292 (1967).

Caffey, E. M., C. R. Galbrecht, and C. J. Klett. "Brief Hospitalization and Aftercare in the Treatment of Schizophrenia." *Arch. Gen. Psychiat.* 24(1), 81–86 (1971).

Caffey, E. M., R. Jones, and K. Diamond. "Brief Hospital Treatment of Schizophrenia: Early Results of a Multi-hospital Study." *Hosp. Community Psychiat.* **19**, 282–287 (1968).

California Administrative Code. (Title 22, Division 6 "Need Assessment Act" #80329).

California Legislature, Legislative Analyst, Budget Analysis 1970–1971, pp. 631–651.

California State Employees Association. *Where Have All the Patients Gone: A Report on the Crisis of Mental Health Care in California,* Sacramento, January 1972.

Craft, M. "Psychiatric Day Hospitals." *Am. J. Psychiat.* **116**, 251–254 (1959).

Crockett, H. M. "Boarding Homes as a Tool in Social Casework with Mental Patients." *Ment. Hyg.* **18**, 189–204 (1934).

Crutcher, H. B. *Foster Home Care for Mental Patients.* New York: The Commonwealth Fund, 1944.

Cumming J. and E. Cumming. *Ego and Milieu: Theory and Practice of Environmental Therapy.* New York: Atherton, 1967.

Ellenberger, H. "Zoological Garden and Mental Hospital." *Canad. Psychiat. Assoc. J.* **5**, 136–147 (1960).

Fairweather, G. W., D. Sanders, H. Maynard, D. Cressler, and D. Blech. *Community Life for the Mentally Ill: An Alternative to Institutional Care.* Chicago: Aldine, 1969.

Farber, L. "Casework Treatment of Ambulatory Schizophrenics." *Social Casework,* **39**(1), 9–17 (1958).

General Licensing Information for California Community Care Facilities Handbook, Sacramento: California State Department of Health, 1976.

Glick, I., W. Hargreaves, and M. Goldfield. "Short Versus Long Hospitalization. *Arch. Gen. Psychiat.* **30**, 363–369 (1974).

Goffman, E. *Asylums: Essays on the Social Situation of Mental Patients and Other Inmates.* Garden City, New York: Doubleday, 1961.

Gruenberg, E. M. *Evaluating the Effectiveness of Community Mental Health Services.* New York: Milbank, 1966.

Herz, M. I., J. Endicott, R. L. Spitzer, and A. Mesnikoff. "Day Versus Inpatient Hospitalization: A Controlled Study." *Am. J. Psychiat.* **127**, 1371–1382 (1971).

Hollis, F. *Casework, A Psychosocial Therapy.* New York: Random House, 1964.

Kaplan, A. "Psychiatric Syndromes and the Practice of Social Work." *Social Casework,* **37**(3), 107–112 (1956).

Kramer, M. "Statistics of Mental Disorders in the United States: Current Status, Some Urgent Needs and Suggested Solutions." *J. Royal Stat. Soc.* **132**, 353–407 (1969).

Lamb, H. R., D. Heath, and J. Downing. *Handbook of Community Mental Health Practice.* San Francisco: Jossey-Bass, Inc., 1969.

Lamb, H. R. and V. Goertzel. "Discharged Patients—Are They Really in the Community?" *Arch. Gen. Psychiat.* **24**, 29–34 (1971).

Langsley, D. G., P. Machotka, and K. Flomenhaft. "Avoiding Mental Hospital Admission: A Follow-Up Study." *Am. J. Psychiat.* **127**, 10, (1971).

Lee, D. T. "Family Care: Selection and Prediction." *Am. J. Psychiat.* **120**, 561–566 (1963).

Miller, D. *Worlds That Fail: Retrospective Analysis of Mental Patient Careers.* Sacramento: Department of Mental Hygiene Research Monograph No. 6, 1965.

Morrissey, J. R. *The Case for Family Care of the Mentally Ill.* Community Mental Health Journal Monograph No. 2, New York: Behavioral Publications, 1967.

Olshansky, S. "The Vocational Rehabilitation of Ex-Psychiatric Patients," in A. J. Bindman and A. D. Spiegal (Eds.). *Perspectives in Community Mental Health.* Chicago: Aldine, 1969.

Pasamanick, B., F. R. Scarpitti, and S. Dinitz. *Schizophrenics in the Community: An Experimental Study in the Prevention of Hospitalization.* New York: Appleton-Century-Crofts, 1967.

Smith, S. and E. Cross. "Review of 1000 Patients Treated at a Psychiatric Day Hospital." *Internat. J. Soc. Psychiat.* 2, 292–298 (1957).

Wilder, H., J. Kissell, and S. Caulfield. "Follow-Up of a 'High Expectations' Halfway House." *Am. J. Psychiat.* 124, 103–109 (1968).

Wing, J. "Institutionalism in Mental Hospitals." *Brit. J. Soc. and Clin. Psychol.* 1, 38–51 (1962).

Zusman, J. "Some Explanations of the Changing Appearance of Psychotic Patients," in E. M. Gruenberg (Ed.). *Evaluating the Effectiveness of Community Mental Health Services.* New York: Milbank, 1966.

SEVEN

The Community-Based
Sheltered-Care Facility

The community-based sheltered-care facility is a residential setting that purports to provide a supervised living arrangement to a handicapped group. Three types of facilities were included in our study—family-care homes, halfway houses, and board-and-care homes. The oldest form of facility is the family-care home (Morrissey, 1967), this form of placement traditionally being aimed at the chronic mentally ill in an attempt to maintain them in the community. Later the halfway-house movement entered the scene (Apte, 1968), and with its development the goals of rehabilitation and transition back into the community became a more important part of the program than in the older family-care program. Most recently the family-care home and the halfway house have been supplemented by the development of the board-and-care facility, which has taken on all three functions of community-based sheltered-care facilities—that is, long-term care, transitional care, and placement of first resort. The increment in the number of facilities available as a result of this entrance is impressive.

In California there are approximately 1155 facilities in the state serving nonretarded individuals between 18 and 65 years old who have had some experience in a psychiatric inpatient facility. Family-care homes account for 26% of the facilities in California and serve 14% of residents in sheltered care. Halfway houses, which have by far received the greatest attention from mental-health professionals, constitute only 2% of facilities and serve only 3% of the population in sheltered care. Board-and-care homes, which have developed in an unplanned, *ad hoc* manner, service 82% of the California sheltered-care population and comprise 72% of the state's facilities. The extent of service now provided by board-and-care facilities leaves little doubt that an entirely new residential-care system for the mentally ill is emerging. The more familiar and well-defined facilities—halfway houses and family-care homes—have only a minor role in this new system.

In this chapter we describe the sheltered-care facility environment, focusing on the range of life experiences it provides, its major functions as a residence, and the characteristics of its facilities.

LIFE IN SHELTERED CARE

Life in community-based sheltered care is not a uniform experience but varies considerably along several dimensions. If by chance you found yourself in the position of a recently released mental patient and were fortunate enough to have a social worker who would take you to three facilities to choose from (residents are supposed to be given a choice of the next three facilities on a rotating list), you might be faced with three totally different potential life experiences. As a prospective resident you could find facilities varying in size from 1 person to 280 persons. You could observe a facility functioning like a boarding house or one run like a mini-hospital. You could come across a place looking very much like a flophouse or one looking like a fancy resort. You could find a home, a commune, or a therapeutic community.

After the interviewers in our study completed their interviews in a facility, they were asked the following question:

What would be your reaction to moving into this facility tomorrow as a resident if you had to make such a move?

A comparison of the desirable and undesirable facilities from the interviewers' point of view demonstrates the diversity of sheltered-care environments. At the positive extreme one interviewer notes:

The house is the most beautiful I have yet seen. Residents live in cottages, each having a living room. The interiors of all the cottages are incredibly beautifully decorated with beautiful carpets and wall paper. All are neatly kept. I should only live in a place like that!

There is an orchard and garden which the residents care for. Gardening and occasional games appear to be the only activity within the house. Although one resident goes to a sheltered work shop, one resident goes to the mental health center, and one goes to real estate school, many residents, especially the elderly ones, apparently lead a sedentary existence. [There are fourteen residents in this facility.]

The operator has several residents who pay large sums of money which compensates for SSI residents. The operator feels he loses money on the place—that it's a tax write-off.

Although initially there were problems with one neighbor, most neighbors supported the operator when he applied for a conditional use permit—a significant fact, since the facility is located in a wealthy area (F.N.).*

This type of facility is unique in its physical characteristics but shares with other good facilities an operator dedicated to serving the residents in the best possible manner. Describing a facility with less physical attractiveness, another interviewer wrote:

It is a large old single-family home broken into several independent living units with 13 residents. The operator positively impressed me. Her residents were on relatively low medication—as a policy. Residents are involved in activities in the house (cleaning, playing with the operator's children) and outside. The operator's relationships with residents seemed excellent, not put on for my benefit. This operator says she "punishes" by taking away chores, which residents like to do.

Mentally retarded and mentally ill live here together, but the operator says she insists on only taking mentally ill who can fit with the retarded. The ambiance of this facility is "one big family": lots of noise, visitors, children, little resident sitting and staring (F.N.).

In another facility in which an interviewer was willing to live, we again find a committed operator in a very different social environment:

This facility has 22 men and women. The youngest resident is 48 years old. The operator expects residents to come dressed neatly to meals and put on makeup. She addresses them by surnames to teach them manners. There are few activities at the house. The operator feels that this is due to a lack of resident interest.

The operator feels compassion for residents—most of whom she feels are very sick. She feels as able to handle their problems as a psychiatrist.

The facility atmosphere is calm. The house is very neat and has a very good location. There are lots of places to go on a nearby boulevard and residents tend to use them quite frequently during the day (F.N.).

*F.N. refers to field notes taken at the time of a structured or open-ended interview.

In examining the facilities about which the interviewers had reservations, their judgments appeared to be influenced by three factors: (1) a high general degree of psychological disturbance manifested by the facility residents, (2) poverty in the physical environment of the facility, and (3) lack of personal concern for the residents on the part of the facility operator.

Describing a facility into which he would not want to move, one interviewer wrote:

The residents . . . were very disturbed. The operator must have gotten most of the very sick ones when the hospital closed.

I was *very* impressed with the facility. It had some of the sickest residents I had seen, yet it was very clean, neat and pleasant. The men seemed happy there. The place was full of chickens, geese, ducks and cats. It was a large house with added living units surrounded by trees and plants.

A church group supported the facility. The residents' money was supplemented by church money. The residents could choose what they wanted for meals and were taken around in a bus that the manager owned. I found this to be a very excellent facility—particularly in consideration of the type of resident they were looking after (F.N.).

The observation that the more severly psychologically disturbed residents are concentrated in one facility is common in several areas of the state. Certain facilities will accept the more disturbed resident while many will not. This results in a selective system that concentrates the more severely disturbed in particular facilities.

In describing an old hotel that had been converted into a sheltered-care facility to house 23 men, one interviewer had the impression that the residents had never left the hospital's back ward:

The house had a depressing atmosphere—residents sitting around near the entryway looking bored. It's a large facility—very gloomy and "dusky"—cold and damp. Although there is an outside area for sunbathing (chai$e lounge and some greenery); it is not used. The operator, while concerned with the residents' nutritional needs (she feeds them well), has little contact with them. She says residents pay for room and board (F.N.).

Finally the following describes one of the poorest facilities visited:

The facility is located in an industrial area of an urban ghetto. The streets are dirty in the area. There is no public transportation in reasonable walking distance. All the buildings on the block are quite old and very run-down.

This facility has a bed capacity of nine, yet currently has only two residents—both of whom had on disheveled looking clothing and were heavily medicated. The facility has large rooms with high ceilings. The largest room has been partitioned into three bedrooms with three beds to a room. The beds were old hospital beds. The furniture in the TV room was very old (the stuffing was coming out of the couch).

After completing the interview, the patient thanked me profusely for coming out to talk with him. He said he was so lonely! All his friends had been at the hospital and now he had no one and nothing to do (F.N.).

THE CHARACTERISTICS OF SHELTERED-CARE FACILITIES

In considering the characteristics of sheltered-care facilities, one must take account of the functions fulfilled by the system as well as the character of the population served. Given the stable character of the population and the tendency for the use of sheltered care to lead to a new residual population similar to chronic mental-hospital patients (discussed in Chapter 8), we describe the facilities in terms of their habilitative and rehabilitative potential as long-term "homelike" settings. Thus, for our purposes, a "better" facility is defined in terms of characteristics that promote social functioning on a long-term basis.

In addition the facility is often conceived of as a necessary compensation for the family (Apte, 1968). In Chapter 8, however, we point out that family support to the population is minimal if not totally absent. It seems, therefore, that the environment should be seen, not so much as a means of compensating for the failure of the family at a particular time in the life of these individuals, but as a substitute for many for a family-like situation. This is true even for those facilities whose operators conceive of care as transitional.

We describe sheltered-care facilities from four perspectives: (1) their neighborhood environment, (2) general characteristics of facilities such as size and service targets, (3) characteristics of the people who operate the facilities, and (4) the internal operating procedures employed by facilities.

Neighborhood Characteristics

The neighborhoods in which we find sheltered-care facilities provide the context of habilitation. We must consider how neighborhood characteristics, such as type of area (e.g., suburban, domestic), social-class composition, type of housing available, and racial composition, are related to factors such as distance of a neighborhood from community services, the availability of services and other important influences on the everyday lives of facility residents.

The types of neighborhoods in which most facilities are located clearly show the placement bias toward the middle-class, suburban, single-family home ideal (see Table 7.1). In fact the family ideal is an often-stated goal of placement in this type of environment. Whether this environment is conducive to achieving the goal must be weighted against other factors, such as the availability of community resources and community receptivity.

Community Resources.   The relationship between neighborhood characteristics and the availability of community resources to a facility reveals some interesting consequences of family-oriented placement policy. Generally 36% of the facilities in the state (serving 31% of the sheltered-care population) are located at least a long walking distance from community resources. Given the level of psychological disability of the population being dealt with, this is certainly unfortunate. For some individuals, a trip to a supermarket is a sufficiently threatening experience in itself, without the added burden of a long walk or bus ride through an unfamiliar environment.

Distance to community resources was assessed on an 11-item scale measuring distance to a local shopping area, park, library, community center, public school, theater, restaurant or coffee shop, bar, place of worship, an organization offering opportunities for volunteer work, and a barber or beauty shop. With respect to each item, operators of a facility were asked whether residents "definitely needed transportation" to get there, "usually use transportation," "it was a good long walk," "was within easy walking distance," or "was only one or two blocks away."

Table. 7.1   Neighborhood Characteristics of Sheltered-Care Facilities

Neighborhood Type	% of Facilities (N = 1155)
Social character	
Suburban	44
Downtown	28
Rural	18
Urban ghettos	3
Other	7
Housing characteristics	
Single family	37
Single family, duplexes, and apartments	32
Stores, businesses, and residences	18
Other	13
Social class	
Upper	4
Middle	47
Working	46
Lower	3
Racial composition	
Primarily Caucasian	31
Primarily Black	9
Primarily Chicano	3
Mixed	56

The total score on the distance-to-community-resources scale is a summary score of the 11 items just noted. In suburban areas at least 42% of the facilities are situated a long walk from community resources. This was true in 59% of facilities in rural nonfarm areas and 93% of facilities in rural farm areas. In contrast only 6% of facilities in the urban ghetto or 5% of facilities in downtown areas are a long walk from community resources. But 58% of facilities in suburban areas are within easy walking distance of community resources. Thus the suburbs offer an environment that can, if selected appropriately, provide good accessibility.

Of the facilities in single-family areas 50% are situated a long distance from community resources and 50% within easy walking distance. As might be expected, no facilities in areas composed primarily of farmhouses are within easy walking distance of community resources. In contrast, however, to the single-family and farm-housing areas are those with a combination of single-family homes and apartment houses, those with a small number of businesses, and those with a large proportion of stores or businesses. In these areas 5% or less of the facilities have residents who require transportation to community resources. It would seem that the likelihood of fostering independent outreach by the sheltered resident is greater in the latter types of environments.

Medical and Social Services. Only 21% of the facilities in our study reported that formal medical and social services were inaccessible or unavailable. Approximately half report that they were available, and 30% that they were easily available. It is possible that such formal medical and social services are of higher priority than general community resources in considering the community placement of the mentally ill.

Our measure of medical- and social-service availability is a summary score of 11 specific services, including day-hospital and day-care treatment, psychiatric inpatient care, general medical care from a private physician, general medical care from a public facility (e.g., a county hospital), community volunteers who visit and take the resident out of the facility, paid helpers who give residents advice and do things on their behalf (such as help in filling out forms), public-health nurses who visit the facility, social-work visits, socialization programming, vocational rehabilitation programming, and workshop-type programs.

Geographic location of facilities plays a significant role in the availability of medical and social services. At least a third of those facilities in suburban areas and a third in areas with only single-family housing report that services are difficult to obtain, if not unavailable. The relationship between neighborhood class structure and service availability substantiates the importance of area characteristics. For example, facilities in upper class areas are most likely to report that services are unavailable to them. This type of placement, then, while quite attractive in terms of physical surroundings, may have significant drawbacks.

Looking at the relationship between service availability and the racial composition of a neighborhood, we found that facilities in areas with a predominantly black population were most likely to report that they had difficulty obtaining services; 41% of the facilities in this type of area reported difficulty, compared with 15% in white neighborhoods, 12% in Chicano neighborhoods, and 18% in mixed neighborhoods.

Neighborhood Receptivity. Another important neighborhood characteristic is receptivity, one indication of which is the frequency of complaints about facilities; 19% of our sample of facility operators have received complaints from their neighbors, 14% have had complaints about their facilities made to the local authorities, and 4% of the interviewed operators indicated that they had been threatened or harassed by neighbors.

Contrary to the popular conception that complaints occur only at the time the facility opens and that afterward the neighborhood adapts to the presence of the mentally ill, our findings indicate that 80% of complaints to the operator and 68% of complaints to local authorities occurred after the facility had been opened awhile; this may indicate that those facilities that have complaints before being opened are prevented from opening. Subsequent complaints do not rule out the ultimate adaptation of the community to the mentally ill, but they do show that this adaptation may be a long and arduous process.

The majority (66%) of complaints received by facilities are made against those in suburban areas, while they constitute only 44% of the total facility population.

Complaints to or about facilities are made differently in different types of neighborhoods. Whereas 23% of the facilities in the ghetto have had complaints made to authorities about them, only 5% of the facilities in suburbia have had these complaints. These figures are further highlighted by the observation that ghetto facilities report that no complaints were made directly to them by neighbors. Thus the formal social-control system has proportionately greater involvement with facilities in ghetto areas than in the suburbs. This social pattern of response may erroneously lead to a conclusion that the problems related to community reaction to sheltered-care facilities are greater in ghettos as opposed to suburban areas.

In summing up our findings on the relationship between area characteristics and the location of sheltered-care facilities, we note that the suburban area, which is often held as an ideal resource for the sheltered-care facility, may in fact be quite problematic if not carefully selected in terms of availability of medical and social services and in terms of its relationship to general community resources. Greater consideration should be given to these facts in location decisions to ensure the proper social context for a long-term habilitation program.

Facility Types

Many characteristics can be used to distinguish different sheltered-care environments. Here we present only the beginnings of our research group's efforts to consider different facility types and their implications for sheltered care. Typing allows us to consider some of the diverse dimensions of the facility.

Previously we discussed the familiar types, that is, the halfway house, the family-care home, and the board-and-care home. In this section we continue our focus on these familiar types and then consider other characteristics of sheltered care that might be used for classifying facilities.

Board-and-Care, Family-Care, and Halfway-House Facilities. Looking first at the relationship of these facilities with their respective community environments, we note that a large percentage of the halfway houses in this state tended to be a long walk from community resources, as opposed to family-care homes and board-and-care homes, which show a greater variance in their distance from such resources. This is contrary to what had been expected, because it was assumed that the outward-reaching orientation of the halfway house would lead them to emphasize their relationship to community resources more than our data indicate. A finding more in line with our expectations is that the halfway houses, the professionally sponsored facilities, all found medical and social services easily available. We observed that 17% of the board-and-care facilities found services either difficult to obtain or unavailable. A full third of the family-care facilities have this problem. This latter statistic represents a very interesting finding, because traditionally family-care facilities are sponsored by social-service organizations and have all their service needs brokered by a social worker from the organization, and thus have a direct line of access to professional services. Perhaps the dependence of the family-care operator on his social worker as a broker for medical and social services makes obtaining these services more difficult than they would be if the operator in fact contracted for his own services. In such a situation the operator would not have the added factor of limitation on the social worker's time—due to other job demands on the worker—to influence the delivery of services. Depending upon the social worker as one's only broker for medical and social services may be unrealistic given worker caseloads.

Family-care homes, in contrast to board-and-care and halfway houses, tend to be situated in suburban and single-family areas as opposed to downtown and multiple-dwelling areas; 49% of the family-care homes in our sample were in single-family areas, compared with 34% of the board-and-care facilities and none of the halfway houses. We note that, complementing this finding, 57% of the family-care facilities are situated in suburban areas, compared with 41% of board-and-care homes and 20% of halfway houses.

A relatively large percentage of the halfway houses are situated in ghetto areas where there is a combination of businesses and residential dwellings; 30% of the halfway houses in the sample were in the area they described as a ghetto, compared with 3% of the board-and-care homes and none of the family-care homes. Moreover, 70% of the halfway houses indicated they were in commercial areas. The location of a large proportion of halfway houses in ghetto and commercial areas may account for the finding that these facilities tend to be far from general community resources.

The halfway house shows itself to be quite different from the board-and-care and family-care homes. Why should we emphasize these differences when halfway houses constitute only 2% of the sheltered-care facilities? The halfway house is singularly important because it represents, more often than not, the professionally initiated and community-sponsored facility. Such facilities are held up as models of care and are more likely than other types of facilities to have direct access to community funding sources. Unlike the board-and-care and family-care homes, they are less likely to operate solely on a fee-for-service basis. Given these characteristics of the halfway house, it should be noted that, as community-sponsored facilities—thus more public in their inception—they may be less able to open in nonghetto or noncommercial areas. The technique of "sneaking" a facility into a given area to avoid community confrontation is one that is less available to them compared with the family-care and privately owned board-and-care facilities (which often open as an extension of one's residence).

One important facility characteristic based on the aggregated characteristics of individual residents* is the degree of psychopathology present in the facilities' populations. Two measures of individual resident psychopathology have been aggregated to provide facility indices.

The Langner Scale involves interviewee response to 22 statements regarding specific symptoms—for example: I feel weak all over much of the time; I have had periods of days, weeks, or months when I couldn't take care of things because I couldn't "get going"; Are you the worrying type? (Langner, 1962). Positive responses to these 22 symptom statements by interviewees were found, in the Mid-Town Manhattan Study, to be most predictive of psychiatrists' ratings of the interviewee's degree of psychological impairment

---

*Classification of sheltered-care facility by aggregated individual characteristics is not the best use of our data, because a facility may be characterized on the basis of a single interview or an average of two interviews. This analytic procedure does, however, point to some important findings.

(Srole et al., 1962). Several studies have since shown the ability of this instrument to discriminate between hospitalized inpatients, outpatients, and the general public but have also generated some anomalies—such as college students scoring higher on this scale than patients about to be discharged from a mental hospital (Langner, 1962; Manis et al., 1963). In our study the California sheltered-care population had an average score on the Langner Scale of 5.13. This was found to be significantly lower than that reported from a mental-hospital receiving-ward group (a difference of means test being used) and significantly higher than that reported for a predischarge-ward group (Langner, 1962).

The Overall and Gorham Brief Psychiatric Rating Scale (BPRS) is a direct assessment of the serverity of 16 discrete psychiatric symptoms—somatic concern, anxiety, emotional withdrawal, conceptual disorganization, guilt feelings, tension, mannerisms and posturing, grandiosity, depressive mood, hostility, suspiciousness, hallucinatory behavior, motor retardation, uncooperativeness, unusual thought content, and blunted affect (Overall & Gorham, 1962). Symptom severity assessments on the BPRS are derived from clinicians' ratings (in our study they were made by clinically trained interviewers) of interview interaction and interviewees' descriptions of their behavior during the week before the interview. The overall assessment of an interviewee's severity of symptom manifestations on this scale is considered an indication of the individual's degree of psychopathology.

Whereas Langner Scale ratings are positively related to BPRS ratings ($r = .22$, $p < .01$), they do not mean the same thing. The Langner Scale is based solely on interviewee response to a specific set of symptom statements. The BPRS is a clinical assessment of psychopathology. It is our observation that the Langner Scale is more a measure of the interviewee's level of psychological distress than of the severity of his psychopathology. In addition the Langner Scale requires an ability to verbalize such distress since it is a self-report questionnaire. Such ability requirements, incidentally, might explain the high scores college students obtain on the Langner Scale (Manis et al., 1963).

Table 7.2 shows the relationship between the facility scores on the Langner Scale and the facility type. Table 7.3 presents the relationship between the facility ratings of resident psychopathology on the BPRS and the facility type. The findings summarized in these tables with respect to halfway houses are very interesting. Given the Langner items, we see that more than three-quarters of the halfway houses would be classified as accommodating a seriously disturbed population (that is, having scores of 5 + on this scale).

On the BPRS, on the other hand, we see that almost none of the halfway houses are classified as serving the mild to severe range of psychological disturbance. It is our observation that this is a true finding, reflecting a segregation of clients into different facilities. Often prospective halfway-house

Table 7.2 Aggregate Langner Score as a Measure of Level of Psychological
Disturbance in Board-and-Care, Family-Care, and Halfway-House Facilities

Langner Score	Facility Type		
	Family Care (N = 297)	Board and Care (N = 831)	Halfway House (N = 26)
Low (< 5)	70%	53%	21%
High (≥ 5)	30%	47%	79%
	100%	100%	100%

Table 7.3 Aggregate Brief Psychiatric Rating Scale Scores as a Measure of Level of
Psychological Disturbance in Board-and-Care, Family-Care and Halfway-House
Facilities

BPRS Disturbance	Facility Type		
	Family Care (N = 297)	Board & Care (N = 831)	Halfway House (N = 26)
Not present	42%	25%	69%
Very mild	18%	40%	30%
Mild to moderate	27%	33%	0%
Severe	13%	2%	1%
	100%	100%	100%

clients will have to be interviewed by other residents as part of their entry
into the house. Halfway houses are more prone to accept clients who have the
insight and the ability to verbalize their problems; consequently the clients'
scores are high, and the halfway houses are classified as serving very disturbed clients according to the Langner items. The characteristics observed
in an interview on the BPRS, which are more visual and interactive indications of disturbance, are not present in halfway-house populations. Halfway
houses cannot be characterized by the BPRS criterion as serving very disturbed clients.

On the BPRS family-care homes and board-and-care homes serve a similar clientele. Family-care homes, given the Langner criterion, are less likely—perhaps because they have traditionally served a more chronic population—to serve the more verbal psychologically distressed group than
board-and-care homes are. These latter facilities serve a broader population.

An aggregate rating of consumer-response scores as they relate to facility
types indicates that board-and-care and family-care facilities generally do
better than halfway houses. While 60% of the former two facility types are
rated very good, only 20% of the halfway houses are rated this high. In
addition 30% of the halfway houses are rated as poor, compared with only 5%

of the family-care and board-and-care facilities. Consumer-response ratings must, however, take into account the resident's feelings of obligation to the facility operator. Whereas no halfway houses could be characterized as having clientele with strongly felt obligations, 25% of the board-and-care homes and 36% of the family-care facilities had clientele who felt a strong obligation to operators. The more severe ratings on the consumer-response scale toward halfway houses could be interpreted as a result of fewer feelings of obligation to facility operators. It is difficult to interpret this finding, however, because the obligation-to-operator rating might be genuine or clouded by fear or simply indicate gratefulness to operators of board-and-care and family-care facilities for a job well done. It is the consensus of our research group that a combination of these interpretations is closer to the fact. The positive internal environment of halfway houses leads to a high valuation of these facilities. Their transitional nature may, however, detract from a high valuation for residents who wish to use these facilities as long-term placements. Halfway houses also tend to serve bright and articulate psychotics who are more critical of their care, often promote the "politicization of madness" approach, and thereby encourage skepticism and critical response.

Facility Size. Another classification for sheltered-care environments is facility size. Small facilities (one to six beds) under state zoning laws qualify as single-family units and operate as family-oriented facilities. Facilities with 7 to 50 residents (mid-sized facility) may be viewed as those emphasizing a group-living situation, commonly focusing on a single "resident group." Finally, large facilities, with more than 50 beds, are more likely to have multiple groups or to focus on the individual as a boarder or patient. Whereas family-care homes have usually been identified with the small facilities, halfway houses with the mid-sized, and hotels and boarding and nursing homes with large facilities, board-and-care homes come in all sizes.

Half of the facilities in the state have between one and six beds. These facilities serve 22% of the sheltered-care population; 43% have from 7 to 50 beds and serve 51% of the population; and 6% of the facilities have more than 50 beds (and as many as 280 beds) and serve a quarter of the population. Thus mid-sized facilities, often family homes, boarding houses, or to a lesser extent halfway-house environments, have become the primary providers of sheltered care.

As might be expected, facility size is significantly related to the area in which a facility is situated. More than half of the small facilities are found in single-family areas. In contrast 46% of mid-sized facilities are located in areas with a combination of apartments and single-family dwellings. Those facilities with 51 beds or more are primarily located in commercial areas or those areas with small businesses and larger residences.

The BPRS being used as a measure of psychopathology, approximately 75% of the larger facilities serve a less severely disturbed population, compared with 65% of the mid-sized and 64% of small facilities. No differences were observed with respect to facility size when the Langner scale was used as an index of pathology.

In terms of consumer response smaller facilities tend to be characterized by greater degrees of satisfaction. Whereas 69% of the small facilities are characterized as very good, this is true of only 53% of the mid-sized and 36% of the large facilities. Again, however, this finding is somewhat clouded by the extent of residents' feelings of obligation. Whereas 40% of small facilities promote such an obligation, only 15% of the mid-sized and 8% of the very large facilities are so characterized.

Target Population.   Another means of typing facilities is by whom they serve. Before this study we thought we would be investigating facilities that serve the mentally ill in a sheltered living environment. We found, however, that this broad typing did not accurately describe the new system of community care. Of the 1910 facilities that claim to offer service to the mentally ill between 18 and 65 years of age with a past history of hospitalization, 40% had no residents with these characteristics. In addition, while the primary service population of 72% of the 1155 facilities studied actually was the mentally ill between 18 and 65 years of age, the primary service population of the remaining 28% was some other disadvantaged group, including the mentally retarded, drug abusers, alcoholics, physically disabled, and the aged.

Most sheltered-care facilities tend to service multiple groups: 75% of the 1155 facilities studied actually serve more than one category of clientele. This policy may indicate a step back to noncategorical care, perhaps to the old poorhouse concept where individuals are served indiscriminately. The selection criterion is simply the inability to "make it" in society—that is, social dependency.

Sheltered Care as a Large Business Enterprise.   Another new and important aspect of the sheltered-care system is the entry of business enterprises into the service of the socially dependent; 9% of the facilities we interviewed in, serving about one-fifth of the population, were, in fact, part of a larger business enterprise (a corporation dealing either primarily in sheltered care or in multiple enterprises). Whereas there is no relationship between whether a facility is operated as a business and its distance from community resources, it does seem that medical and social services are more easily available, or at least reported to be more easily available, to the facility operated as a business. Only 2% of these facilities reported that services were difficult to obtain or unavailable to them, contrasted with 23% of the facilities not run as business enterprises.

Facilities that are part of a business enterprise are more likely to be located in commercial areas than nonbusiness-related facilities are. To some extent this is due to their size; they tend to be larger than nonbusiness-oriented facilities and therefore do not qualify for operation in residential neighborhoods, owing to zoning regulations. Facilities run as businesses tend to evoke a more negative response from their clientele than other facilities do. Whereas only 37% of facilities run as businesses were favorably viewed by their clientele, 62% of facilities not run as businesses were so rated. Thus negative consumer response to facilities run as businesses is an important statement on the type of sheltered care we can expect if more business enterprises become involved in the field.

Male/Female.   Of the facilities studied, 55% indicated that they admit both men and women; 20% responded that they would take women only, and 24% serve only men. Although several facilities are inclined to serve both sexes, once they have a preponderance of one sex in the facility, it is difficult for them to reestablish a balance because facilities with a larger percentage of residents of one sex find it difficult to attract the opposite sex.

Operator Characteristics

Recent exposés of the ill treatment of sheltered-care residents have given a negative connotation to the term *facility operator*. Yet, while exploitation does exist in the system, the majority of operators are well-meaning people who, in the process of earning a living, are attempting to offer a service to the individuals in their facilities.

Approximately 80% of sheltered-care facilities are run by female operators. Three-quarters of the facilities are owned by the person who runs the facility. Unlike their residents, 68% of the operators are married, while only 5% have never been married. Their age distribution approximates that of the people for whom they care: 65% of the operators are over 50 years of age, and only 7% are under 33 years of age.

From a socioeconomic perspective the operation of sheltered-care facilities represents a step upward for most operators. A large proportion of this group have had related backgrounds in roles such as hospital attendants and vocational nurses. Three quarters of them would score lower in their previous occupations than they would as sheltered-care operator by use of Reiss' (1961) Socioeconomic Index (SEI) as a measure of status mobility.

Racial composition of the operator group is another indicator of status mobility. A full third of the operators of sheltered-care facilities are black, compared with only 9% of the residents they serve; 7%—the same percentage as the population they serve—are Spanish speaking; and 2% come from other minority backgrounds, compared with 3% of the sheltered-care population. These figures are in marked contrast with the proportion of white operators to white residents in the sheltered-care business: Only 58% of the operators are white, compared with 81% of the residents they serve.

Sheltered-care operators are somewhat more educated than the residents they serve: 50% have completed high school and some college; 14% have completed college and some graduate work.

Regarding the motivation for becoming a sheltered-care operator, almost half say that they did so primarily to help people; another fifth responded that they joined this profession because of their experience in the service professions before entering the sheltered-care field; 6 percent claim that they became operators for companionship, 10% for income, and another 12% for other or a combination of reasons.

True motivation is difficult to assess. In interviewing operators, we asked them a series of questions from the Marlow Crown Social Desirability Scale and found that many of their answers were directed toward providing what they thought were socially desirable responses. Our observation was that many operators tried to conform all of their behavior to "socially acceptable" norms—not just their responses in this context to make a good impression on us about their facilities.

Although there is no doubt that one can make money in sheltered care (and many do, even to the extent of diminishing the well-being of their residents), it seems that there is also great commitment on the part of many operators, often a deep and sincere religious commitment. Nan Elizabeth Adrian, in her book *House Full of Hope* (1970), summarizes this commitment very well in her description of taking one of her residents—a woman who had been in a mental hospital for 25 years—to a supermarket. "We walked around . . . I watched her face come alive. Somehow between the soup and the canned fruit, I had one of those sudden, rare moments of true self-knowledge and self-determination. *With God's help, I will go on doing all that I can for people like Evelyn*" (p. 46).*

In viewing the facility operator as a business person, we find that 28% claimed that their income was totally derived from the facility, 19% said it was primarily derived, and 58% said it was partially derived from their facility. (Many in this last group run a facility in their retirement for "something to do" and do not depend upon it for income.)

Sources of facility-operating funds, aside from the income of the facility, are primarily obtained on an individual basis unrelated to facility opera-

---

*The emphasis is Adrian's.

tions—for example, a husband's income, since some facilities may operate at a loss. Only 3% of the facility operators responded that they were receiving grants or subsidies to enable them to continue their facility operation work. A third of the operators said that they are members of a local board-and-care operators' association. From the point of view of professionalization, this is only a small representation.

Facility-Operating Procedures

To describe the operation of a sheltered-care facility, we must consider the statement of purpose outlined by the facility owners and operators. As a goal or stated purpose 75% of the facilities answered that they hope to provide a family-life environment, 18% wish simply to provide a nice place to live, 5% want to provide a treatment environment, and 2% have multiple purposes involved in their environmental conception. In line with these statements of purpose a third of the operators see themselves as "parents" to their charges; more than half see themselves as friends and advisors; other roles seen to a lesser degree are caretaker, landlord, and therapist. In this family-oriented system 60% of the operators have their families with them at the facility, and two-thirds eat with their residents regularly; 60% of the operators report that no places in the facility are off limits to their clientele. Given the family orientation, it is no surprise that only 1% of the facilities report that they have a stated time limit on a person's residence in their home.

Given this family-oriented atmosphere, it is interesting to note the extent of disagreement between operators and residents on positive assessments of the social-psychological characteristics of the facilities. The Community Oriented Programs Environment Scale (COPES) provides a means by which to assess the social-psychological environment of the sheltered-care facility (Moos, 1974). This 100-item scale breaks down into ten 10-item subscales (nine of which were used in our study) involving three different aspects of the facility: the quality of relationship between staff and facility residents, the treatment effort in the facility, and the efforts at system maintenance made by the facility. We had the residents and the operators of each facility we studied complete the COPES to evaluate the extent of agreement between them on the nature of their facility's environment. Taking the average rating of a facility by the residents in that facility, we compared this to that of the facility operator on each of the subscales in the COPES. In Table 7.4 we compare the percentage of average resident ratings and facility operator ratings that were high (i.e., above half the total score possible) on each of the subscales of the COPES. The greatest amount of agreement between operators and residents occurs on the relationship scales. Residents and operators are in closest agreement on the extent of program involvement in a facility (e.g., the extent to which the members put energy into the program, think the

Table 7.4 Extent of Disagreement Between Average Resident Ratings and Facility Operator Ratings in Positive Assessments on the Subscales of the Community Oriented Psychiatric Environment Scale (COPES)

| Involvement (Relationship) | Support (Relationship) | Spontaneity (Relationship) | Autonomy (Treatment) | Practicality (Treatment) | Personal Problems (Treatment) | Anger and Aggression (Treatment) | Program Clarity (System Maintenance) | Order and Organization (System Maintenance) |

Rating values shown: 4.5%, 47.3%, 34.3%, 19.6%, 52.9%, 58.8%, 68.3%, 77.1%, 47.9%

R[b] and O[b] endpoints marked.

% Rating high[c]

[a]Scale Group

1. Relationship: Average Disagreement (Residents more favorable) 28.7%
2. Treatment: Average Disagreement (Operators generally more favorable except for autonomy) 50%
3. System Maintenance: Average Disagreement (Residents more favorable) 62.7%

[b]R: Resident responses
O: Operator responses

[c]A facility is rated above one half the total score possible on a given COPES subscale.

facility a lively place, volunteer for facility activity, or are interested in discussions with the other residents). Other relationship scales show more disagreement (though less extreme than the nonrelationship scales). Spontaniety (e.g., the degree to which members are encouraged to express themselves) in the facility shows a 34% disagreement between operators and residents. The extent of support available (e.g., staff encouragement, concern, empathy) shows a 47% level of disagreement. Residents are much more positive in their responses on the relationship scales than the operators are. On the other hand, residents are much more negative in their responses (and tend to disagree much more with operators) on the treatment scales: "Autonomy" (e.g., expectations for members to take leadership in the program), "Practical Orientation" (e.g., facility expectations that members will make detailed plans for the future), "Personal Problems" (e.g., members talk about personal problems openly and talk about their past and are encouraged to do this by staff), "Anger and Aggression" (e.g., staff think it's healthy to argue and encourage residents to express anger openly). Operators tend to rate their facilities very high in meeting treatment demands; residents tend to see them as quite low in this area. A reversal of this trend occurs on the "Autonomy" subscale, perhaps because the content of this subscale is close to the relationship dimension as well as being an aspect of the treatment dimension. On two system maintenance subscales, "Program Clarity" (e.g., members know consequences of breaking a rule, or rules are clearly understood) and "Order and Organization: (e.g., activities are carefully planned, the place is neat), residents tend to rate the facilities high, whereas operators tend to rate them rather low.

The positive orientation toward the facility expressed by residents on the relationship scales appears to depend on the amount of support that residents in such facilities tend to offer each other—a supportive system to a large extent independent of the operator in many facilities. At the other end of the spectrum residents tend to report a much less treatment-oriented environment than that perceived by the operators. To some extent the high disagreement reported on treatment-oriented activity may be representative more of what operators hope to achieve than what they actually have achieved; however, such a large difference of opinion should be explored further in terms of the types of treatment programs being implemented in facilities.

Finally the disagreement on system-maintenance factors is best described as one of stated versus unstated perceptions. Residents in sheltered-care facilities seem to develop very quickly an understanding of the expectations and limitations of their facility operator. These expectations are quickly but informally conveyed within the resident peer group and very often remain verbally unstated by the operator. Their unstated nature may account for the low ratings of the sheltered-care operators and the high ratings of the residents who, as we have indicated, seem to respond clearly to the informal demands of the system.

A number of facility rules have a significant impact on residents' functioning. Approximately half of the facilities do not exercise any curfew. Of those that do, 40% do so on an indiscriminate basis, while only 10% make clear distinctions between residents. Most facilities use a set of rules to supervise dispersal of medication: 82% of the facilities set up a supervisory system for all their residents, 10% for some of their residents, and only 8% for none. There can be no doubt of the perceived importance of medication as part of the aftercare environment. Certainly, even though facilities claim to emphasize a family style of life, there is a significant trend toward more institutional demands. This institutional overlay is supported by the fact that only half the residents actually control their own spending money; the remainder either request money from the operator on a daily, weekly, or monthly basis or, in a few cases, receive no money at all. This type of supervision, while in many cases necessary and part of sheltered care as a quasi-familial institution emphasizing the parental role of the operator, must be closely managed to avoid carry-over of the institutional rules from the hospital.

TYPICAL SHELTERED-CARE FACILITIES AND THEIR ENVIRONMENTS

Two typical sheltered-care facilities help delineate the targets for service development: (1) the single type of facility serving the greatest proportion of residents in sheltered care and (2) the single-type facility that is most available or of most frequent occurrence.

The typical facility serving the greatest proportion of residents in the sheltered-care population is a board-and-care home with a bed capacity of approximately 18. It often operates with the conflict of attempting to provide a family environment to a group that is too large to accommodate such an effort. The facility is run on residents' payments and therefore has limited staff. It is located in an area with a combination of apartments and single-family dwellings, close to general community resources. This board-and-care facility does not report that it is difficult to obtain social and medical services. The operators of this facility have a procedure for medication supervision and perceive their program as being significantly more treatment oriented than the residents do. Clients in this facility are generally unable to verbalize their psychological problems but are moderately satisfied with the facilities.

The typical facility that occurs most often is a small home with one to six beds. Its operating budget is obtained almost entirely from residents' payments. This facility is either a family-care home or a board-and-care home, run by a family, as a family, and located in a single-family housing area. This type of facility services a full range of behavior disturbance. Yet, if it is a family-care home, it may find obtaining medical and social services difficult. It may or may not be near community resources. Consumers feel most positive about this type of environment but are likely to develop strong feelings of obligation to the facility operator. Such obligation is engendered both by dependence and genuine gratitude.

Given these composites, the detailed characteristics of sheltered care, and the range of possible life experiences open to a resident, we now consider how residents currently relate to their social environment.

REFERENCES

Adrian, N. E. *House Full of Hope*. Valley Forge, Pennsylvania: Judson Press, 1970.

Apte, R. Z. *Halfway Houses: A New Dilemma in Institutional Care*. Occasional Papers on Social Administration, No. 27. London: G. Bell & Sons, 1968.

Langner, T. S. "A Twenty-two Item Screening Score of Psychiatric Symptoms Indicating Impairment." *J. Health and Human Behavior*, 3, 269–276 (1962).

Manis, J. G., M. G. Bruner, C. L. Hunter, and L. C. Kercher. "Validating a Mental Health Scale." *Am. Sociological Rev.* 28, 108–116 (1963).

Moos, R. H. *Evaluating Treatment Environments: A Social Ecological Approach*. New York: Wiley, 1974.

Morrissey, J. R. *The Case for Family Care of the Mentally Ill*. Community Mental Health Journal Monograph, No. 2. New York: Behavioral Publications Inc., 1967.

Overall, J. E. and D. R. Gorham. "The Brief Psychiatric Rating Scale." *Psychological Rep.* 10, 799–812 (1962).

Reiss, A. J. *Occupations and Social Status*. New York: The Free Press, MacMillan, 1961.

Srole, L., T. S. Langner, S. T. Michael, M. K. Opler, and T. A. C. Rennie, *Mental Health in the Metropolis*. New York: McGraw-Hill, 1962.

PART FOUR

STARTING WHERE THE RESIDENT IS

Programs demanding greater degrees of involvement or competence than clients are capable of usually fail to reach their target populations—that is, they end up attracting individuals not originally thought of in the conception of the service but capable enough to benefit from the program's content.

A basic principle of social work practice, whether it involves establishing a direct helping relationship or determining the nature of a policy program, is to start where the client is. To approach the goal of integrating the mentally ill in the community, it is necessary to understand how involved individuals have been in the past with their social environment and what for them are the relative levels of difficulty currently associated with different types of social involvement. We therefore turn to an effort to pinpoint where the client is with respect to social integration.

In Chapter 8 we discuss the descriptive characteristics of the sheltered-care population. Lacking longitudinal assessments, we use demographic factors as social indicators of social integration. In doing so, we outline what we believe to be the past level of social integration of the sheltered-care population and the major constraints they have with respect to facilitating their social integration and speculate on their current potential for becoming socially integrated.

In Chapter 9 we discuss how residents currently use their environment, indicating the relative difficulty of different types of social involvements for individuals in sheltered care.

EIGHT

Who Are the Mentally Ill in Sheltered Care?

In asking who are the mentally ill in sheltered care, we are concerned with what their experience has been with respect to social integration, what their current potential is for becoming socially integrated, and what seem to be the most formidable obstacles to integrating them into the community.

The data we present in this chapter indicate that the mentally ill population in sheltered care are a residual group, never integrated into society's mainstream, with few prospects for complete economic and residential independence—that is, complete social integration into the mainstream of society. Our data show that the social-integration goal for this population should involve efforts to develop independent outreach and social involvements both within the facility or in the external community, on the assumption that the facility will be a base of operations.

We do not wish this rather strong statement to invoke the pessimistic attitude that assumes these residents cannot be helped. We believe their social integration can be greatly enhanced. We wish, however, to help define realistic expectations and prevent the disillusionment with helping efforts that has so often in the past led to the neglect of the population's needs.

We have defined social integration in terms of five levels of involvement—that is, presence, access, participation, production, and consumption. The social characteristics of the sheltered-care population offer some significant insights into their past involvements and future opportunities for developing these types of involvements.

DEMOGRAPHIC CHARACTERISTICS: A UNIQUE POPULATION

Comparison by age, sex, and marital status with the general population of California demonstrates that the mentally ill in community-based sheltered care are a unique group with unique needs. Their social characteristics place them at a disadvantage with respect to integrating themselves into society's mainstream.

Age and Sex

Almost half (46%) of the sheltered-care population between 18 and 65 years of age are 50 years old or older, compared with 25% of the general population in California and approximately 25% of the general population of mental-hospital releases (Heckel et al., 1973; Miller, 1965). This is extremely important in considering the feasibility of transition back into the community: These individuals are in need of support at a time society expects them to be most self-sufficient and is least willing to tolerate a lack of self-sufficiency.

The sex distribution of the sheltered-care population is equally balanced between male and female; yet our analysis reveals that females in the sheltered-care population are significantly older than males: 54% of them (compared with 39% of the males) are now between 50 and 65. In contrast the youth of this population are predominantly male: Almost 33% of the men are 18 to 33, compared with 19% of the women. We thus have two subgroups—older women and young men—who socially and economically have the most difficulty in finding a place in society's mainstream.

Despite the concentration of younger males in sheltered care (33%) their numbers are smaller than would be expected, given the concentration of younger males in the general population (42%). Also, mental-hospital releases, while slightly older than the general population (regardless of sex), are not as old as the sheltered-care population (Heckel et al., 1973; Miller, 1965). Thus there can be little doubt that problems will arise for this population in relation to their seniority—for example, they will need more transportation aid to make use of community resources.

Marital Status

Marital status is an index of social participation. The marital-status characteristics of the sheltered-care population indicate a lack of resources available to facilitate community transition. Table 8.1 vividly illustrates this by comparing this population with California's general population and with releases from state mental hospitals serving the Bay Area. While the general population figures in California show that 70% of the individuals between 18 and 65 years of age are married, this is the status of only 5% of those individuals in sheltered care. Conversely 18% of the general population compared with 60% of the sheltered-care population have never been married; and 12% of the general population as opposed to 35% of those in sheltered care have had marital relationships that have since been dissolved. Without speculating on the etiologic relationship between marriage and mental disorder, one thing seems sure: Individuals who lack the support of a spouse are more likely to seek social support in a sheltered living environment.

Two trends relating to marital status in addition to the very high proportion of "never marrieds" within their ranks seem to indicate that individuals in sheltered care have never been integrated into the mainstream of social life. First, follow-up studies of released mental patients show a tendency for groups of individuals returning to the hospital to be increasingly composed of "never marrieds" and people with dissolved marital relationships (Davis et al., 1974; Heckel et al., 1973; Miller, 1965; Pasamanick et al., 1967). Thus, as a group, individuals in sheltered care are a residual population of many cohorts of mental-hospital admissions. The second trend is illustrated in Table 8.2, which presents a breakdown of marital status in this population by

Table 8.1   Comparison of Marital Status in California's General Population, a General Population of Mental-Hospital Releases, and Individuals in Sheltered Care.

	18-to-65-Year-Old Population Group		
Marital status	1970 Census of California Population (N = 11,652,082)	General Population [a] of California mental-Hospital Releases (N = 1039)	California Sheltered-Care Population (N = 12,430)
Married	70%	39%	5%
Never married	18%	21%	60%
Dissolved relationship (separated, widowed, divorced)	12%	34%	35%

[a] Miller (1965) pp. 116-117 (marital status was unknown for 5%).

age and sex. This table points to the high percentage of never-married males (73%) and the high percentage of females from dissolved marital relationships (50%). Specifically these two figures are indicative of how males and females fail socially to integrate into today's society.

These marital-status figures are not unique to California sheltered-care facilities but seem in fact, to have much greater generality. Apte (1968), for example, in a study of transitional hostels in Great Britain, finds that 71% of his study population (both male and female) were single, but only 17% came from dissolved marital relationships. The difference between our population and that studied by Apte seems to lie in the fact that he chose to consider only the "transitional hostel," the hostel that had at least a 50% turnover in a given year. Apte notes that this choice of a study group made a significant difference in the age of his target population. Those individuals living in the transitional facilities were significantly younger than those living in hostels he eliminated from his study. We would therefore expect him to find a smaller concentration of dissolved marital relationships than we found because at least a third of our female population who had experienced a dissolved marital relationship were over 50.

The major indication, in terms of future potential for enhanced social integration, of the marital-status characteristics of the mentally ill in sheltered care is that as a population they lack support even from the most immediate of family members—a spouse. In addition they are limited in access to two major sources of social involvement—that is, interaction with a spouse and couple-based interaction.

SOCIOECONOMIC CHARACTERISTICS OF THE POPULATION

In looking at the socioeconomic characteristics of the sheltered-care population, one is again struck by the extent to which individuals in this group have withdrawn from, or have never been involved in, the mainstream of social life.

Work

Work or "production" as a type of social involvement is one of the most important aspects of everyday social life in the United States. It is important, therefore, to look into this aspect of the lives of sheltered-care residents.

Study data demonstrate that 15% of the individuals in sheltered care are in fact in the labor force. This compares with 67% of the general population in California (as found by 1970 U.S. Census figures, U.S. Bureau of the Census, 1973). Moreover, 11% of the sheltered-care population is actually employed and 4% of the population is looking for work. Whereas 4% of the general population in this age group in California were looking for work in 1970, 63%

Table 8.2 Distribution of the Sheltered-Care Population by Sex, Age, and Marital Status

	Sex					
	Males			Females		
Age	Single (n_1 = 4870)	Married (n_2 = 300)	Dissolved (n_3 = 1540)	Single (n_4 = 2520)	Married (n_5 = 290)	Dissolved (n_6 = 2910)
18-33	29%	1%	2%	16%	0%	3%
34-49	20%	1%	7%	13%	1%	13%
50-65	24%	2%	13%	15%	4%	34%
All ages	73%	4%	22%	44%	5%	50%
	n = 6710			n = 5720		
	Males (100%)			Females (100%)		

133

were employed. Thus the percentage of sheltered-care residents looking for work is equivalent to the general population, while the number who have found work is much lower than in the general population.

Working residents and job-seeking residents appear to be different groups in a number of aspects. Workers are equally male and female, single, white, young if female, and middle aged if male. Job seekers, on the other hand, are two-thirds male and more likely to be young, married, or formerly married. Job seekers are also more likely to be minority-group members than workers are. Residents in sheltered care tend to look for work more, and work more, if they have more education. It is also true that the less time elapsed since previous employment, the better the chance that a resident will look for work. These characteristics parallel those of workers and job seekers in the general population, yet the majority of the sheltered-care population (85%) are neither working nor looking for employment.

Workers in the sheltered-care population are different from job seekers in some other important ways. Workers come from more skilled and high-status occupational backgrounds than those people do who are looking for work and those not working. None of the sheltered-care residents who actually have a job report that this is their first working experience. These job holders are more likely to report that they have previously worked in skilled occupations such as carpentry or skilled sheet-metal work or are members of some professional group (e.g., teachers or social workers). In most cases these individuals are no longer employed in their previous vocation; often they are employed at their residence in a more menial job such as cleaning, cooking, washing, or general repair work. They have obtained their work by virtue of previously acquired and generalized work skills (such as the ability to complete an assigned task). Job seekers are more likely to report that they have had no work experience at all.

The significance of these work-related statistics for understanding the potential of the sheltered-care population to become involved in "production"-type activities as a means of enhancing their social integration lies in the observations that those with the most potential for such involvement have shown a significant drift from stable to marginal employment; those with interest in obtaining employment—the job seekers—given their backgrounds, have little chance of obtaining employment; and the majority of the population have not expressed serious interest in this type of social involvement.

Work-Related Characteristics of the Sheltered-Care Population.   The lack of involvement of the sheltered-care population in production-type activities is to a large extent a function of atrophied work skills and past failures in the area in addition to their psychiatric disability. More than half of this population have been out of the labor market or away from full-time employment for 6 years or more; only a tenth were employed during the past year. In a population of which three-fourths of the individuals are over 34 years of age, only one-third have had full-time employment for 6 years or more. The employment prospects of this population are further hampered by the fact that only 66% have ever had steady employment for a year or more.

A Comparison with the General Population of Released Mental Hospital Patients. If we look at previous studies of released hospital patients, we again see that individuals in sheltered care comprise a unique population in relation to employment. Both Freeman and Simmons (1963) and Miller (1965), reporting on studies of released state-hospital patients, indicate that significantly smaller numbers of people who return to the state hospitals are employed before their return than those who manage to stay out of the hospital during the studies' follow-up period. Freeman and Simmons note that, as a total group, 33% of their study population were employed at the time of the community follow-up interview. However, 41% of those released individuals who managed to remain out of the hospital during the follow-up period were employed in some manner, compared with 20% of their hospital returnees. Miller's findings are similar. Her study found a total employment rate of 32%; she also found that 40% of those individuals who managed to stay out of the hospital during the follow-up period were employed, compared with 29% of those who returned to the hospital. Since a large portion of our study group have had several readmissions to state hospitals—a point discussed in greater detail later in this chapter—we might speculate that sheltered-care residents are, in fact, a group with a greatly diminished employment potential, at least as indicated by their employment histories. This potential is, however, indicated solely by employment history; other indicators of work potential must be considered before any final conclusions are drawn about ultimate employability.

A Perspective on Work Potential. Despite these bleak employment statistics, there is some evidence on sheltered care pointing to the possibility of improvement in California: Apte's (1968) findings show that, with a concentrated effort, as much as an additional 31% of California's sheltered-care population might be employed.

Apte (1968) reports that only 46% of the residents in the transitional hostels he studied were, in fact, totally unemployed. It is not clear what Apte means by "totally unemployed"—for example, does this mean that any type of money-making activity, even running errands, would be considered employment? If so, and this criterion is used for the California population, it could be said that 23% of the population are making some money, though the amount of work involved with 12% of the population is minimal and would not normally be considered as even part-time employment. At any rate, given Apte's criteria, we would conclude that 77% of the California sheltered-care population are totally unemployed.

Apte's population differed from the California population in two respects important in assessing employment potential: (1) Apte's subjects lived in Great Britain at a time when there was full employment (i.e., anyone who wanted a job could get one—if one could stand, one could work); (2) they lived in a subset of "transitional" sheltered-care facilities that had a turnover rate of 50% per year and emphasized employment as a program requirement for residents. Brenner (1973) has pointed out the significance of economic factors in relation to mental hospital admission, noting that in hard times there are greater numbers of admissions to mental hospitals. We thus would expect that differences in the economy and the transitional nature of the facilities that Apte studied might well account for a portion of the 31% difference in total employment between his group and the one reported on in California. In any event, even with full employment and with facilities that emphasize employment as a requirement, some residents remain unemployed in Apte's sample. In Great Britain, as in California, the types of jobs obtained by residents are menial; they tend to have little possibility for advancement and seem most vulnerable to hard times.

Education

Education speaks to potential for involvement in productive-type activities. Educationally the mentally ill in sheltered care are not very different from the general population. Though there is a tendency for them to be slightly less educated, they are also much older within the same age limits, and people get more education now than they used to; 7% of the sheltered-care population have finished college, compared with 13% in the general population. Of those completing college, slightly more are male. Both males and females in this educational group are middle aged. While this population is educated similarly to their own age group, their lack of competitive experience in the labor market would force them to compete with younger, more educated individuals for employment. Thus they in fact may be educationally handicapped in the labor market.

Socioeconomic Status

A comparison of the socioeconomic status of the resident population with that of their fathers, as demonstrated by scores on Reiss' (1961) Socioeconomic Index (SEI), reveals that this particular population is downwardly mobile. That is, of five possible index categories (professional, business/managerial, skilled worker, semiskilled worker, and unskilled worker) we find proportionately more fathers of sheltered-care residents in the professional category and proportionately more residents in the unskilled-worker category of the SEI. In general a clear downward drift is apparent from fathers of residents to the residents themselves.

Income

Income is primarily an index of ability to participate as a consumer. Only 6% of the sheltered-care population are supported solely by private funds (family, savings); the rest are supported totally or in part by welfare grants. Currently three-quarters of the residents are receiving financial support from the Supplemental Security Income (SSI); 19.5% have multiple financial sources other than SSI. To a large extent consumptive patterns in this population are determined by factors external to their control—the policies of their benefactors.

Future Prospects

Although the future prospects for social integration seem bleak, they are bleak only from the perspective of the goals of achieving totally independent living and full participation in the competitive labor market for those individuals in sheltered care. Goals emphasizing more modest achievement, such as maintaining adequate levels of social functioning and maximizing the strengths of this population for all types of social involvement, seem much more attainable and realistic. The achievement of these latter goals will, however, be most affected by current constraints on social involvements.

CONSTRAINTS ON SOCIAL INTEGRATION

The major constraints on social involvement for the former mental patient include geographic mobility, chronicity, psychopathology, and violence. Each of these four factors has been viewed as a characteristic of the former mental patient that detracts from his level of social integration. How do these constraints relate to the social integration of the mentally ill in sheltered care?

Geographic and Mobility Characteristics

Two geographic-mobility characteristics have been considered as important in affecting the social integration of the former mental patient. First the loss of social roles due to treatment outside of one's local area was one of the primary reasons for the initiation of the community mental-health movement (Joint Commission on Mental Illness and Health, 1961). Second, mobility itself has been viewed as in indicator of mental disorder that inhibited people from forming close relationships (Ödegaard, 1932).

Providing Care Close to Home. Fully 53% report that they are currently living in a place that they consider to be their home town. In fact 80% live within 50 miles of what they consider to be their home town. This finding must be tempered by the observation that "psychiatric immigration" may occur whereby long-term hospitalized patients come to view the area around the hospital as "home" (Satin & Gruenberg, 1975). However, since the description of the current area of residence as one's home town was in our sample, a response no more characteristic of the long-term than of the short-term hospitalized group, we would conclude that "psychiatric immigration" is not a factor in the resident's report of residing in his home town. Thus our findings indicate strongly that the community mental-health movement is meeting its goal of providing care for the mentally ill close to their actual home environments and that this constraint to social integration may be minimized.

A Relatively Stable Population. The population currently living in sheltered care is relatively stable; 60% have lived in their current facilities more than a year. Discounting rehospitalization as a move to a different living situation, only one-third of the group had moved within the last year. Yet a small portion of the population changes its residence frequently. For example, 16% of the group made several moves in the past year, and 23% lived in more than one facility in addition to their current placement.

Comparing the total sheltered-care population with 1970 U.S. Census figures for the general population in California, we note little difference between these two groups in view of their stability, though there is a slight trend for individuals in sheltered care to be more mobile. This mobility differential, however, may be a slight artifact of the overall newness of the sheltered-care system.

Young males are definitely the most mobile in the sheltered-care population; 63% of the young males have been in facilities for less than a year. In comparison we find that only 42% of young females have been in facilities for less than a year. Being female (in all age categories), as well as increasing age, is associated with residential stability. These findings regarding the mobility of young male residents are congruent with those of Segal, Baumohl, and Johnson (1977), which report a high rate of mental illness in the young, primarily male, vagrant population.

The findings that people in sheltered care are generally stable and that a small group of them tend to be more mobile are consistent with the expressed desire of residents for a stable life-style; 55% say that they wish to stay on at their facility for a long period of time.

Ambivalence about moving and its meaning is reflected in the following example:

Judy, age 34, is one of the few board-and-care residents who is working. If she scrimps and saves, the money she makes is enough to live on. She thinks that eventually she might like to be a psychiatric nurse; her experience in the hospital prompted her interest in that field.

Judy thinks that it would be wise for her to wait another year before going out to look for an apartment of her own. She has been living here since she left the hospital three years ago and is quite satisfied with her present living situation. "Like I say, it's something like taking the place of a family, although you know deep down it never could be. It's just someone to talk to, someone that knows and understands and yet keeps their nose to themselves. So that means a lot" (F.N.).*

Some mobility within the sheltered care system results from a very small number of disruptive residents who have been bounced from facility to facility within a given geographic area, usually ending up in a particular facility informally reputed to accept more difficult individuals. In addition to movement of difficult and hard-to-handle residents within this primarily stable system, there is apparently also movement of a small group of individuals out of the system. (This latter conclusion is, however, based primarily on open-ended data and is not accounted for in geographic-mobility statistics provided by the survey data.)

Those individuals moving out of the system do not necessarily move into stable life situations. They gain a modicum of independence often connected with their efforts and those of their former sheltered-living environment. For example:

Two months before the interview, Kenneth, 32, had made his move from sheltered care into an apartment. He shares his new home with a long-time school friend, a fellow with similar interests. Moving out was not an easy task for Kenneth; the longer he stayed, the more difficult it was to leave. This difficulty was attributed to the feeling of security that he derived from his former living situation, a feeling that prevailed despite the constant turnover of residents.

It was Kenneth's intention to move out with other residents as apartment mates, but these plans fell through. Fortunately for Kenneth, he grew up in this area and has a father living near the sheltered-care facility. When he first moved out of the facility he arranged to live with his father until he could move into his new apartment. Kenneth has maintained a long-term relationship with a woman who often visited him while he was living in sheltered care. Although he had little contact with the people from the facility during the first couple of weeks after he left, some new problems in his relationship with this woman have prompted him to turn to them for emotional support. The facility has hired him to work on their staff on a part-time basis; he attends staff meetings and seminars (F.N.).

*F.N. refers to field notes taken at the time of a structured or open-ended interview.

Given the data on geographic mobility in the sheltered-care population, we currently think that this is not a major constraint for the social integration of this group.

Chronicity: History of Mental Hospitalization

Chronicity, that is, long-term hospitalization leading to the termination of social contacts, is another constraint on social integration. In considering the history of the sheltered-care population's involvement with the state mental hospital, we should note that a quarter of the population currently in these facilities did not have their first admission to a mental hospital until after the enactment of the Lanterman-Petris-Short (LPS) legislation in 1969. Thus whereas a significant portion of the sheltered-care population is new to the state hospital system, it seems that the policy of community care for the mentally ill has the potential for producing its own residual or chronic population: The recent admissions may now represent the same residual population that in the past filled the back wards of the state mental hospitals. The possible substitution of long-term community-based sheltered care for long-term hospitalization is reinforced by the fact that a full 35% of the individuals currently living in sheltered care have cumulatively spent a year or less in a mental hospital. In fact 57% have *never* spent 2 or more continuous years in a mental hospital. Such a history is not characteristic of the former long-term mental patients who were admitted under indefinite commitment to a state hospital.

In general we found that women residents were more involved with both the sheltered-care and the hospital-care systems: Women had slightly more admissions to the mental hospitals in each age category than their male counterparts; they were more likely to be in the chronic-hospital category than men—that is, they were more likely to have spent 2 or more continuous years in a state hospital (35% of young females versus 27% of all women also spent more years in sheltered care and had been in more sheltered-care homes).   In all of these figures age is an important factor. The older one is, the longer one tends to have been involved with the mental-health system. This is a traditional and expected trend. An opposite trend emerges, however, from the initiation of a revolving-door policy (i.e., a policy of easy admission and quick release, often applying to the same individual over many experiences with the mental hospital) precipitated in California by the 1969 LPS Act. For the younger and middle-aged residents we see an increase in admissions over the older group. For example, 46% of the young residents, but only 39% of the old residents, have between 3 and 25 admissions.

The effects of the 1969 LPS changes in admission and retention policies of state hospitals were studied by cross-tabulating the "years since a resident's first admission" (the assumed date of onset of his illness) with "whether or not he had spent 2 or more continuous years in a state hospital." In this analysis we are particularly interested in comparing the group of individuals whose illness began after LPS as compared with the group whose first hospitalization was before 1969. Controlling for age, we find that only 11% of the people within each age category whose first admission was since 1969 report having been hospitalized 2 or more continuous years, but within the group hospitalized before 1969 a minimum of 41% in each age category are likely to report having 2 years of continuous hospitalization. Furthermore, the earlier the first hospitalization, the higher the percentage of each age category reporting continuous hospitalization of 2 years or more. In general we find an increased number of admissions for those who have spent less than 2 years continuously in a state mental hospital in the group of more recent onsets. This is true for both sexes and all ages. We conclude that LPS has prevented the negative effects of long-term hospitalization on social integration but that, in doing so, it may be helping in the creation of a new separate system of social integration—the sheltered-care facility. Individuals may now give up their community contacts to become chronic sheltered-care residents. We consider this question in looking at those factors that facilitate and hinder the social integration of the resident.

Psychopathology

Psychopathology can be considered a major constraint on social integration in the sheltered-care population. Psychopathology has a negative influence on specific types of social involvements for a large part of the population. Our data lead us, however, to believe it is significantly handicapping—that is, an overriding factor in their daily interactions—for only a small portion of those in sheltered care. Our interviewers eliminated as too emotionally disturbed only 8% of the people we tried to interview. Indications of disturbance included a great amount of nervousness and agitation on the part of the interviewee. (In one situation the prospective interviewee hid in the closet because he was afraid of the interviewer.) In such cases no attempt was made to force the interview. The interviewers also observed that 18% of the interviewees were delusional at some time during the interview period. An additional reflection of psychological disturbance was that 10% of the population admitted that they had actually contemplated suicide during the past month.

In looking at the level of disturbance in the population, our ratings on the 16 symptom categories in the Overall and Gorham Brief Psychiatric Rating Scale (BPRS) reveal that only 16% could be considered severely disturbed, while 56% might be termed as mildly disturbed, and 28% could be regarded as lacking any overt psychological disturbance. It would appear from these data that the majority of the sheltered-care population should not find psychopathology a major constraint to attaining moderate levels of social integration. In our next chapter we discuss more specifically the relative difficulty of different types of involvements for residents and the effects of psychopathology on such involvements.

Sheltered-Care Residents as a Community Threat

We have discussed the public conception of the mentally ill as the "raving maniac"—one whose acts have no rational basis and are, therefore, unpredictable. How much of an actual threat do the mentally ill in sheltered care pose for the community? How does the perception of them as a community threat act as an impediment to their social integration?

Perhaps more directly related to age, though supported by the "revolving-door" hospitalization policy, is the finding that older residents tend to be hospitalized fewer times than younger residents with equal dates of first admission. This seems to be a function of the tendency of younger residents to pose a more active threat to the community and therefore to be more susceptible to hospitalization; 11% of the sheltered-care population reported having been arrested in the past year. The arrests were for minor offenses, primarily disturbing the peace, loitering, drunken and disorderly conduct, petty theft, and destruction of property. This may be a somewhat biased response group, however, because residents involved in the past year in serious crimes would probably no longer be living at the facility. Assuming this bias, we asked facility operators if any of their residents had been picked up by the police in the past year and what the reasons were for these police contacts; 40% responded that at least one of their residents had been picked up by the police in the past year. Only one operator (out of 92) reported that the reason for being picked up by the police was the commission of a violent act (specifically charges of armed robbery). Only 4% of the police contacts involved bizarre behavior.

The most frequent reason given for a resident's being picked up by the police—40% of the affirmative responses—involved a resident "lost and wandering around the neighborhood." It is not known whether this happened because the resident was actually lost or because a neighbor worried about the resident's standing in front of his or her house.

These statistics should lead to an appreciation of the vulnerability of this group rather than of its dangerousness. It would seem that fear of released patients' going to sheltered care is based on unfounded stereotypes rather than on actual threat to the public and that the constraint on the social integration of this population derives from these stereotypes or residents' vulnerability. With respect to the latter observation, 16% of the residents do not feel safe on the streets at any time, and another 34% feel safe only during the daytime hours. This is a significant constraint on their mobility and thus on their social-integration potential.

THE MENTALLY ILL RESIDENT IN SHELTERED CARE

The typical sheltered-care resident is between 50 and 65 years of age, white, Protestant, has less than a high-school education, and has been out of the labor market for several years. The resident is generally not living far from his or her home town and is fairly settled into a stable life situation in the sheltered-care facility. The major source of financial support for the typical resident is SSI. The resident does not provoke much trouble for the community from the perspective of social disorder and manifests a mild level of psychological and emotional disturbance. Prospects for making the transition to full community life in terms of obtaining gainful employment seem small, as are prospects of establishing some sort of conjugal unit on which to base social life.

The impediments to social integration of the sheltered-care resident are those relating primarily to establishing himself more as an independent self-supporting individual. Constraints on social interaction, such as severe psychopathology, community reaction to patient stereotypes, or lack of social contacts due to mobility or long-term hospitalization, must be viewed as factors adding to the difficulties posed by a lack of previous social integration. Our efforts emphasize, therefore, the basics of social integration. The goal of our study, then, is—current constraints being taken into consideration—to assess those factors that can help improve the sheltered-care experience of these individuals and promote their efforts to reach out in a more independent manner to the external community. With this goal in mind, we now turn to a consideration of how residents use their environment.

REFERENCES

Apte, R. Z., *Halfway Houses: A New Dilemma in Institutional Care*. Occasional Papers on Social Administration, No. 27, London: G. Bell and Sons, 1968.

Brenner, M. H. *Mental Illness and the Economy*. Cambridge, Massachusetts: Harvard University Press, 1973.

Davis, A. E., S. Dinitz, and B. Pasamanick. *Schizophrenics in the New Custodial Community: Five Years After the Experiment*. Columbus, Ohio: Ohio State University Press, 1974.

Freeman, H. and O. Simmons. *The Mental Patient Comes Home.* New York: Wiley, 1963.

Heckel, R., C. Perry, and P. G. Reeves. *The Discharged Mental Patient.* Columbia, South Carolina: University of South Carolina Press, 1973.

Joint Commission on Mental Illness and Health. *Action for Mental Health.* New York: Science Editions, 1961.

Miller, D. *Worlds That Fail: Part 1. Retrospective Analysis of Mental Patients' Careers.* California Mental Health Research, Monograph #6. Sacramento, California: California State Department of Mental Hygiene, 1965.

Ödegaard, Ö. *Emigration and Insanity: A Study of Mental Disease Among the Norwegian Born Population of Minnesota.* Copenhagen, Denmark: Evin Munksgaards Publishers, 1932.

Pasamanick, B., F. R. Scarpitti, and S. Dinitz. *Schizophrenics in the Community.* New York: Appleton-Century-Crofts, 1967.

Reiss, A. J. *Occupations and Social Status.* New York: Free Press, MacMillan, 1961.

Satin, M. S. and E. M. Gruenberg. "Immigration and Insanity: The Dutchess County Experience." Paper presented at the Fourth Tromsø Seminar in Medicine, June 5–8, 1975. Tromsø, Norway.

Segal, S., J. Baumohl, and E. Johnson. "Falling Through the Cracks: Mental Disorder and Social Margin in a Young Vagrant Population." *Social Problems,* **24**(3), 387–400 (1977).

U.S. Bureau of the Census. *Census of population: 1970,* Vol. 1, Characteristics of the Population, Part 6, California—Section 2, Part 1. Washington, D.C.: U.S. Government Printing Office, 1973.

NINE

How Do Residents Use Their Environment?

The primary goal of community-care advocates has been to help formerly hospitalized patients involve themselves in the social world as average community participants. The achievement of this goal has been measured by the extent to which there is no longer a need for an advocate or mediator to facilitate the individual's involvement. We have defined five levels of community involvement: presence, access, participation, production, and consumption. These levels characterize an individual's interactions with the community outside the facility and within the community of the facility itself.

In speaking about interactions outside the facility, we have discussed the concept of external integration. In this chapter we discuss not only the extent of involvement with both internal and external communities but also the types of involvements that are absent among the sheltered-care population.

EXTERNAL INTEGRATION

Our analysis of residents' responses to questions relating to the five levels of involvement in the external community showed that in this population these levels were neither independent of each other nor all present. Levels of involvement showed different relationships in different aspects of community life. For example, while it was possible to speak about access to community resources independently of participating in community groups—that is, individuals had such resources available but often did not choose to use them—access to friends and family implied actually interacting with them. We also found that so few people in the sheltered-care population were involved in "production" activities (i.e., the extent of their involvements were so marginal) that we could not view this as a characteristic level of community involvement at all.

Components of External Integration

Seven components of external integration were derived, based on the relation of four levels of involvement (presence, access, participation, and consumption) with various aspects of life in sheltered care. The seven components of social integration are:

1. Attending to oneself (i.e., being *present* and *consuming* in the community).
2. Having *access* to community resources.
3. Having *access* to basic and personal resources.
4. Having *access* to and *participating* in family life.
5. Having *access* to and *participating* in friendship relationships.
6. *Participating* in community groups.
7. Using (i.e., *participating* in) community recreational facilities.

A resident's level of external integration is expressed in terms of his total score on all items in all seven component subscales.* (All the items in the external and internal scales, organized by their respective subscales are listed in Table A.5, Appendix A.)

Table 9.1 summarizes the extent of residents' involvement on each of the component subscales. The subscale means listed at the far right of the table offer an indication of the relative difficulty of the specific types of involve-

---

*In collecting our data on the ease of access or on the extent of any activity, we requested responses on a five-point scale: "very easy" ("very often") (5), "easy" ("often") (4), "not much trouble" ("sometimes") (3), "difficult" ("rarely") (2), or "very difficult" ("never") (1).

In discussing resident's total score on the external-integration scale and the relative contribution of each of the seven component subscales to the overall external-integration assessment, we assume that the degree of external involvement, like the response to a single question, can be discussed within a continuous five-point range where five means "very high involvement" and one means "no involvement." Working with this assumption, we divided the range of the total scores on the external-integration scale into five equal segments. The segments were numbered 1 to 5 from the low to high ends of the scale, respectively. The same procedure was employed with each subscale score so that comparisons could be made across subscales and between the total external-integration score and subscale scores.

ment measured by the scale—the higher the mean score, the easier the type of involvement for the sheltered-care-resident population. Thus access to community resources and to the basic and personal resources is easiest to obtain. Participatory activities involving families, friends, and attending to one's own basic needs are somewhat more difficult for sheltered-care residents. The most difficult types of participation involve interaction in community groups and use of community facilities. It is in these latter types of involvement that there is also the most room for improvement. Participation in community activity might be the focus of social programming, which, as we will see from our discussion of the content of each subscale, will have an impact on further enhancing resident scores on the friendship access and participation scale.

Differing amounts of psychopathology have a significant impact on the degree of difficulty associated with each type of involvement. Those residents with higher levels of psychopathology have increasingly greater difficulty with each type of involvement in the external-integration scale. But higher levels of psychopathology most adversely affect friendship access and participation. These types of involvements are significantly easier than familial access and participation involvements for those without significant amounts of psychopathology, have about the same level of difficulty for those with a moderate degree of disturbance, and are more difficult for the severely disturbed group. The greater ease of friendship access and participation involvements for those without significant psychological disturbance should pinpoint this subgroup as the target population for programs emphasizing community involvements—programs in which there is most room for improving residents' social integration.

Attending to Oneself. This first subscale combines the concept of presence (simply being out in the community rather than staying inside the facility) with consumption (shopping or eating outside the facility); 16% of the population fell into the "never" category in the total subscale score. The average level of participation (on our five-point scale) is between "rarely" and "sometimes" (see Table 9.1).

The most frequent activity in this subscale is going to a local shopping area on a typical day. The most infrequent activity is spending time outside the facility between 5 p.m. and 11 p.m.

The attending-to-oneself subscale as a description of interaction adds depth to the initial notion of "presence" as simply being in the community—that is, outside the facility. A person interacting this way is "present" in the community, and though he may also be isolated from other forms of interaction, he at least obtains meals and goes shopping. For example, an elderly woman in one facility spent most of her time at home sleeping. Rather than eat with

Table 9.1 Distribution of Resident Involvement on the External-Integration Subscales

Subscales	Distribution of Resident Involvement					
	1	2	3	4	5	
	Never/Very Difficult	Rarely/ Difficult	Sometimes/ Not Much Trouble	Often/ Easy	Very Often/ Very Easy	Subscale Mean
1. Attending to oneself	16%	35%	40%	8%	0.3%	2.4
2. Access to community resouces	4%	17%	24%	41%	14%	3.4
3. Access to basic and personal resouces	6%	13%	32%	38%	12%	3.4
4. Familial access and participation	26%	25%	29%	16%	4%	2.5
5. Friendship access and participation	30%	22%	29%	14%	4%	2.4
6. Social interaction through community groups	65%	22%	10%	2%	1%	1.5
7. Use of community facilities	50%	35%	12%	2%	1%	1.7

other house residents, she preferred to walk to a local luncheonette where she could eat alone. She also purchased her toilet articles herself at a local store. This resident thus satisfied her immediate needs independently of the support of the facility.

Access to Community Resources. The second subscale, "access to community resources," determined how easily residents could obtain access (without any help from the facility) to a shopping area, park, library, movie, community center, restaurant, bar, public transportation, place of worship, volunteer organization, barber shop or beauty parlor, and a pleasant walking area; 4% of the population fall into the "very difficult" category on the total subscale score. The average level of access is between "not much trouble" and "easy" (see Table 9.1). Taking a walk in a pleasant area was the most available resource; the local bar was the least accessible.

Access to Basic or Personal Resources. The subscale "access to basic resources" reveals how easy it is to get basic goods and services without the operator's help. Such services include laundry facilities, clothing store, telephone, meals outside the facility (or inside without the operator's help), and getting medication outside the facility; 6% of the sheltered-care population fall into the "very difficult" range. On the average these goods and services are available "easily" or "without much trouble" (see Table 9.1). A telephone and toilet supplies are most accessible to the average resident, although medical care and laundry services are easiest to get for residents who have access to only one or two of the items in this scale. If one has minimal access, it is not to social elements such as a telephone or toiletries but to illness-related necessities—medical care and laundry. Clothing and meals outside the house are the least accessible items in this subscale.

Family Access and Participation. The data did not indicate that access to community or personal resources implied their actual use by residents. There was, however, a link between access to and participation in family and friendship activities. The subscale "family access and participation" refers to both the ease of contact with one's family by phone call and visit and the frequency of such contacts; 26% of the population are in the "very difficult" access or "never" contact category on this subscale. The average accessibility is between "difficult" and "not much trouble" (see Table 9.1). Only 29% have at least minimal access to or contact with family on *all* items in this subscale (see Table A.5, Appendix A). In general, phoning is easier than visiting. Half the residents either have no contact with family or their contact is limited to phone calls. The other half of the population visits at least "rarely" with family.

"Family access and participation" is related to access to "basic and personal resources" and to a lesser extent to "access to community resources" and to "attending to oneself." Relationships with the immediate family are largely confined to providing basic needs and "duty" calls. Relationships with more distant relatives begin to shade into the more active involvement characteristics of friendship relationships. Visiting with immediate family is related to stereotype "Sunday activities"—that is, going to church, going to a movie, to a restaurant, to a sports event. Visits with more distant relatives are associated with activities more characteristic of friendship—such as working at a volunteer agency, interacting in community groups, participating in sports, and using a bank account. These latter activities require more initiative. Thus contact with relatives may signify a more active person rather than a more concerned family.

Friendship Access and Participation. The subscale "friendship access and participation" refers to how often and with what ease residents interact with acquaintances and close friends. Like the subscale "family access and participation," access to friends implies interaction. This subscale describes access by phone or visit and actual visiting patterns with friends and acquaintances; 30% of the population find access "very difficult" and "never" have contacts with friends. The average level of access is between "not much trouble" and "difficult" (see Table 9.1).

Only 34% of the population have at least minimal access and participation on *all* items in this subscale (see Table A.5, Appendix A). As is true of "family access and participation," phoning is easier and more frequent than visiting. Generally, close friends are more accessible than acquaintances; however, for those who find all friendship access and participation difficult, it is more difficult to have contact with close friends than with acquaintances. Indeed for these individuals it is easier to visit with an acquaintance than to phone or visit a friend.

Although individual items in the family-access-and-participation subscale are related primarily to basic resources, the individual variables in this subscale are related to access to community resources and to a good range of community-participation variables. It seems that interaction with the immediate family centers around a minimal set of duties, while relationships with friends both imply and provide greater access in the community.

Social Interaction Through Community Groups. An important source of friendship is participation in community groups—interaction as a volunteer worker or in a social organization or a community club. This kind of activity is important in the sheltered-care environment, because it represents the reaching out of the resident for friendship, independently of the facility.

This subscale includes two variables from the friendship-access-and-participation subscale—visiting with friends and visiting with acquaintances—as well as doing volunteer work and participating in activities of social and political groups outside the house.

As might be expected, almost two-thirds of the population fall in the "never" participate category on the subscale. The average level of participation is between "never" and "rarely" (see Table 9.1).

Use of Community Recreational Facilities.   The seventh external-integration subscale is "use of community recreational facilities" and describes actual participation in the activities available in the community. Although a wide variety of community recreational facilities is accessible, only a few are used often enough to be included in the participation scales. The activities included in this scale are going to a park, to a library, or to a sports or entertainment event and participating in sports activities. Half the population are in the "never" participate category on this subscale. The average level of participation is between "rarely" and "never" (see Table 9.1).

In addition to a strong relationship with the friendship-access-and-participation and interaction-with-community-groups subscales, "use of community recreational facilities" is also related to "attending to oneself." This may indicate that these activities are semisolitary, requiring access to community resources but not reflecting as much social interaction as the interaction-with-community-group subscale.

Variables Excluded from the External-Integration Subscales.   All variables excluded from the external-integration scales to some extent share the common dimensions of greater social involvement, greater participation in the community, and some disassociation from the residents' group (see Table 9.2). They are underrepresented or not related to the scales that describe the sheltered-care population, because of the relatively small number of individuals in sheltered care who have achieved the kind of social integration these activities indicate. Emphasis on these types of activities must follow the development of the more

Table 9.2   Poorly Represented External-Integration Activities

Activities	% Never	Item Mean
Educational activities	89	1.289
Going to a bar	75	1.416
Using credit	93	1.128
Going on a date	70	1.504
Using a bank account	64	1.744
Working	75	1.677

basic types of involvement represented in the seven components of the external-integration scale.

External Integration: An Overview

The external-integration scale as the summation of seven component scales
represents four dimensions of social integration into the life of the community: *access* to community and basic resources independent of operator or the
facility, *presence* in the community, *participation* in various activities and use of
community resources, and to a lesser degree *consumption*. This scale delineates
the ease and frequency of contact with friends and family. (Only 0.5% of the
population have no access or never participate in any of these activities, while
19% show some activity or access to all.) We can now describe the sheltered-
care population on a five-point continuum from least integrated (Level 1) to
most integrated (Level 5) based on the total external-integration score.

Level 1.   Of the sheltered-care population, 1460 members (12%) fall into the
group that is least integrated. They rarely or never participate or find access
difficult or very difficult on all the external-integration subscales. Residents
in this least externally integrated group find it difficult to get community
resources or basic resources on their own and very difficult to contact family
or friends. They never or rarely go out of the facility to shop or eat, never see
family or friends, never interact in community groups, and never use community recreational facilities.

Mitchell is a 50-year-old sheltered-care resident who *on his own* does not go
out of his facility or have access to or get to use community resources. He does
not obtain his own food, clothing, or toilet supplies and finds it difficult to
contact family and friends.

Mitchell attributes his choice of board-and-care facility to his mother's fussiness; his
present home was the first to meet his mother's strict standards. This maternal concern, however, does not appear to carry over into other aspects of their relationship.
Mitchell has seen his mother once during the past two years because she has been
hospitalized. She writes to her son that she is getting better. Mitchell has a married
sister whom he last saw "quite a few months ago." When asked if he had plans to visit
her Mitchell replied, "I can't very well invite myself. I have to be invited . . . you just
can't do something like that."
Mitchell's days are spent reading *TV Guide* and watching television. Because he dis-
likes buying things without his mother's approval, he doesn't go shopping. Mitchell
talks to his friends who live in the house. Recently, he went to the circus with a group
of residents, an uncommon event (F.N.).*

*F.N. refers to field notes taken at the time of a structured or open-ended interview.

Level 2. Moving up on the external-integration scale, the Level 2 group—that is, those who find external integration difficult and who rarely participate—are the largest group in the population; 5000 individuals (40%) in sheltered care are members of this group. The responses in this group are varied, including the full range (1 to 5) in the access-to-community-resources subscale; a range of 1 to 4 (excluding very often-very easy) on "attending to oneself," "family," "friends," and the "use of community recreational facilities," and a range of 1 to 3 on "socializing through community groups."

Residents in this group do not have much trouble getting to community resources or obtaining basic and personal resources; they find it more difficult to contact family and friends, rarely go out of the facility to shop or eat, and never interact in community groups or use community facilities.

The last eleven of John's sixty-one years have been spent in the same board-and-care home. After leaving the state hospital he lived with his sister for two years, an acceptable arrangement until she moved out of state to be near her children. On her last visit five years ago, his sister and a friend took John on a trip that included an airplane ride and a tour of the tourist spots in southern California. John has some relatives living up north, but he hasn't seen them for a long time. He has no friends in the area.

Some of John's time is passed in conversations with the other people in the house. When he goes shopping, he goes alone. He takes public transportation to a downtown area and checks out the windows of the big department stores. There was a social worker who used to come to the house to take the residents on outings, but she doesn't come anymore. A community center that provides recreation and arranges outings for board-and-care residents is within walking distance, but John finds it difficult to get there and hasn't used the center for a year. "They have asked me to come back. Every time I do want to go, something comes up . . . just deciding whether you want to go today or deciding whether you want to wait until tomorrow and stay. 'Course I think if somebody came by in their State automobile and they took me, I'd be going"(F.N.).

Level 3. At the third level of external integration, we find 4680 individuals (38% of the population) who indicate little trouble in terms of access and who "sometimes" interact with the outside world. This second largest group in the external-integration scale covers all response ranges on six of the seven subscales—excluding only "very often" responses on the use of community facilities subscale. The majority of responses were in the sometimes (not much trouble) and often (easy) categories.

This large group of residents find it easy to get to community or basic resources and do not have much trouble contacting family and friends. Sometimes they go out of the facility to shop or eat but "rarely" use any community facilities and "never" socially interact in the community.

Marian, age 35, is working in a sheltered workshop. She obtained this position through her social worker shortly after being released from the hospital and travels to work on the city bus. In the workshop her day is spent tying strings on price tags; she admits having been rather bored with this task at first, but has somehow come to accept it. She is also learning how to use a typewriter at a rehabilitation center.

Marian last saw her family at her mother's house four months previous to the interview, on her birthday. Last June her mother had promised Marian that she would be able to attend her brother's graduation, but at the last moment her mother telephoned to say that she could not arrange a ride. Marian was extremely disappointed.

Marian describes her co-workers at the workshop as being "independent." "They get done what they have to do." She doesn't talk to people at a local rehabilitation center because she believes that they are prejudiced. "They talk to you if you talk to them but they don't say nothing if you don't." The other residents in the house were also described as "independent." She does talk to them about television shows, but the only place she goes with them is "to the store and back."

When asked where she could meet people she replied that one could go to the park and get involved in activities there, or sometimes one could meet people in church. Marian thought that it would be difficult to meet people alone and had no friends to accompany her in this pursuit. She said that she had gone to the park and back once or twice.

Marian has limited contact with her family members, and apparently no close friends outside the house. Although she has access to community resources, the park and the rehabilitation center, she does not use them to increase her social contacts (F.N.).

Level 4. Moving to the fourth level of external integration, where individuals find access easy and participate often, we find 1160 people (9% of the sheltered-care population). Responses are concentrated in the higher ranges here. This smaller group of residents find it very easy to get to community or basic resources, easy to contact family or friends, and sometimes go out of the facility to shop or eat, interact in community groups, and use community recreational facilities.

Michael, 24, has been living in California for a year and a half. Although his family lives on the East Coast, communications have been maintained without much trouble. His brothers and sisters write regularly, and an older brother visited a few weeks before the interview. Michael recently spoke (on the telephone) to an old friend who proposed taking up a collection among Michael's family and friends to buy him a plane ticket home, hopefully in time for a Christmas visit. His parents have told him that he can live with them if he returns to his home town, but this offer is not very appealing to Michael.

Michael estimated that "most of the time" he was happy with his living situation. "I'm starting to like it more because I'm starting to get out and do things more." Two weeks before the interview he had gone dancing with a woman he met outside of the house. A summer job provided opportunities for Michael to meet people. He does part-time work landscaping and cleaning apartments, jobs arranged through a friend of a former resident. Michael has a couple of friends who live outside the house, one of whom is an old friend of his sister. He has enrolled in a local college and is hoping to make new friends in his classes. He believes that he would feel a lot more settled in this area if he could meet more people. His living situation makes it harder for him to meet people, particularly women. He hopes to buy a car, and sees this as a solution to his problem (F.N.).

It is easy for Michael to get to many community and basic resources because they are within walking distance. He uses community facilities and goes outside of the facility to shop and eat.

Because many of his social activities and therapy are arranged through the facility rather than community groups or services, Michael would be classified as Level 4, rather than Level 5 of external integration.

Level 5.   In the highest range of interaction, where people interact very often with others and find it very easy to obtain access, we find only 120 individuals, 1% of the population. This tiny percentage scored in the "easy-very easy" range on all the scales except "family," "social interaction through community groups," and "use of community facilities," where they dipped into the "sometimes" category.

The very small percentage of residents who are highly integrated in the external community find it very easy to get community and basic resources and to contact families and friends. They very often use community facilities, go out of the facility to shop or eat, and socially interact in community groups.

Linda, 53, exemplifies a person at Level 5 of external integration. Tuesday through Friday she may be found at one of several community centers. She spends one day at each center learning to make ceramics, jewelry, and candles, and participating in a singing group. Saturdays are for shopping at the local shopping center and Sundays are for going to church. Linda uses public transportation. Some of the other members of the house participate in the same program as Linda, and she has made friends at the community centers also with people who live in other board-and-care homes.

At the time of the interview she was eagerly anticipating her birthday and planning a party which the other members of the house, Linda's stepmother, and a neighbor would be attending. Linda's stepmother visits her about every five or six weeks. She also has an aunt that visits. Linda and her aunt sometimes go out for dinner; the last time they did that was two weeks previous to the interview. Linda has a boyfriend whom she met when they were at the state hospital; they see each other every two or three weeks.

It is very easy for Linda to get to community resources and facilities, and she uses them almost every day. She frequently goes out of the facility to shop and eat and has no difficulty contacting family and friends (F.N.).

INTERNAL INTEGRATION: A LIFE CENTERED AROUND AND MEDIATED BY THE SHELTERED-CARE FACILITY

The basic social arrangement in modern society is that the individual tends to sleep, play and work in different places, with different coparticipants, under different authorities, and without an overall rational plan. The central feature of total institutions can be described as a breakdown of the barriers ordinarily separating these three spheres of life. (Goffman, 1961, pp. 5–6).

To the extent that all aspects of a resident's life are centered in a sheltered-care facility or that a resident's use of the outside environment is mediated by the facility, the facility is itself a self-contained community. A group of residents who board a bus with a sign reading "Happy Mountain Sheltered Care Facility" to go to church on Sunday have not, in fact, participated in the broader external aspect of church interaction. They have attended church as a group of outsiders, perhaps viewed benevolently by other church members, but nevertheless not viewed as part of the general community. A sheltered-care operator observed that the church group near his facility treats residents like:

one or two pets that they sort of bring into the church, but when you want to bring a large amount they discourage you. . . . One particular church . . . invited our people down for a luncheon, which is fine and they went down and they gave them a nice luncheon and everything was just great. However, on Sunday when a large group of our people wanted to go, they discouraged this, they said, why don't you break it up, between the other two same sect churches in our community, just bring a few of them here and a few of them there. . . . In other words, don't make our congregation all mental or look like it's all mental (F.N.).

It thus appears that, even when a few individuals attend a social event, if their attendance is mediated by the facility, they are perceived as outsiders, and the focus of their interaction can be directed only inward toward the facility. Internal integration, the extent to which a resident's life is centered around and mediated by the facility, is not necessarily a pejorative concept. The community of the facility can be extremely benevolent and, depending upon one's values, provide a very satisfying and fulfilling life. At issue here is the policy of the facility on encouraging integration into the broader outside community and the dependence it may create and reinforce.

Components of Internal Integration

We have empirically identified five components of "internal integration" by which we can measure levels of involvement in facility life:

1. Operator will transport resident to community resources.
2. Operator facilitates activity.
3. Operator provides basic necessities.
4. Socializing with other residents and the operator.
5. Supplies purchased at the House.

These components define three levels of internal integration: access, participation, and consumption.

While external integration involves access and participation in the life of the community independent of the support of the operator of the facility, internal integration covers access to community life with the active support of the operator, as well as social interaction and consumption within the facility.

Presence in the facility is assumed, and this is not reflected as an independent factor in internal as it was in external integration. Access relates to the availability of goods and services, similarly to external integration, but through the operator, who provides transportation to the resources or supplies the goods and services directly through the facility. Access is described in three subscales: (1) operator will transport resident to community resources, (2) operator facilitates activity, and (3) operator provides basic necessities.

Participation in the internal-integration scale refers to social interaction or friendship activities within the facility and is measured in the subscale "socializing with other residents and the operator."

Consumption indicates making essential purchases from the facility and is described in the subscale "supplies purchased at the house." Table 9.3 summarizes the extent of residents' internal involvements, and the mean scores on the five subscales are an indication of the relative difficulty of each type of involvement. The lower the mean score, the more difficult a given type of internal involvement. Thus it is easiest to get access to basic necessities through the facility and most difficult to purchase supplies at the house. Whereas increased psychopathology makes all these types of involvements more difficult, the relative difficulty of each remains the same within each level of disturbance. This latter finding is important because it indicates that support within the facility is not selective—that is, those who are more disturbed require increased access to basic necessities through the facility and perhaps more opportunity to purchase supplies through the facility. The data show, however, a general decrease in internal integration with increased psychopathology. Thus, developing more selective use of facility social supports should be a goal in the development of future facilities and in the modification of current efforts.

Table 9.3 Distribution of Resident Involvement on Internal-Integration Subscales

| | Distribution of Resident Involvement | | | | | |
| | 1 | 2 | 3 | 4 | 5 | |
Subscales	Never/Very Difficult	Rarely/ Difficult	Sometimes/ Not Much Trouble	Often/ Easy	Very Often/ Very Easy	Subscale Mean
1. Operator will transport residents to community resources	8%	21%	43%	23%	5%	2.92
2. Operator facilitates activity through the facility	10%	27%	41%	19%	3%	2.78
3. Operator provides basic necessities	1%	6%	17%	48%	28%	3.94
4. Socializing with other residents and the operator	7%	16%	28%	36%	14%	3.34
5. Supplies purchased at the house	40%	30%	17%	11%	2%	2.05

Operator Will Transport Residents to Community Resources.   This subscale describes how easy it is for residents to get transportation from the facility (the operator, the operator's family, or a staff member) to various places in the community (a park, shopping center, restaurant, etc.) (see Table 9.3); 8% of the residents find access to community resources very difficult to obtain through the facility. The average level of access is "not much trouble."

Places that are most easily available (in order of accessibility) are: a barber shop or beauty parlor, a supermarket or large shopping center, public transportation, a preferred place of worship, a park, and a restaurant or coffee shop. Less accessible places are a library, a community center, volunteer work, a movie, and adult education. These items are divided between more and less accessible items as in the external-integration scale, although ease of access is somewhat less through the facility operator than independent of a facility.

Operator Facilitates Activity Through the Facility.   The second access subscale of internal integration is "operator facilitates activity through the facility." This subscale describes how easy it is for residents to get rides from the facility to sports events, social activities, vocational training, religious service, or therapy (see Table 9.3); 10% found it "very difficult" to arrange such activity. The average level of access is "not much trouble."

The most easily arranged item is in-house activity, which on the average, residents feel is "easy" or "not too much trouble" to arrange. Individual therapy at the house, trips to sports events, vocational training at the house, and religious services at the house follow (in order of decreasing ease of arranging).

Operator Provides Basic Necessities.   The third subscale in the internal-integration scale is "operator provides basic necessities." This subscale describes how easy it is for the resident to get laundry service at the house; help from the operator in getting clothing, toilet supplies, and incidentals at the house; and use of facility's telephone; 1% of the population find that obtaining basic necessities at the facility is very difficult. The average level of access is "easy." The most accessible service is laundry at the house: 42% find it very easy. For the items "use of the telephone," "toilet supplies at the house," "help from the operator in getting clothing," 60 to 75% of the population find it "easy" or "very easy" to get these at the house.

There is a strong relationship between the provision of basic resources in the house and socializing with the facility operator. This relationship is much stronger than it is with respect to any of the other access subscales in internal integration. It seems that interaction with the operator is initiated over these daily basic needs when the facility takes responsibility for their provision.

Socializing with other residents and the operator. This subscale describes the frequency of social interaction within the facility: playing card games or other activities with fellow residents; making friends, sitting, and talking with other residents; talking with the operator, house visitors, or staff; 7% fall into the category of "never" socializing at the house. The average frequency of participation is between "sometimes" and "often" (see Table 9.3).

Residents talk with each other slightly more than they try to make friends and interact with each other, and slightly more than they talk with the operator or facility staff. The least frequent activity is engaging other residents in activities. While on the average residents talk with each other and the operator or try to make friends "sometimes" or "often," they engage in activity "rarely" or "sometimes." More than 50% "never" or "rarely" play cards or games with other residents.

Supplies Purchased by the House. This scale is both the least frequent and most independent of the internal-integration subscales. It describes how often residents purchase laundry services, clothing, toilet items and incidentals, or grooming services at the house or from the operator of the house; 40% of the residents fall in the "never" range on this subscale. On the average, residents "never" or "rarely" purchase these items through the facility (see Table 9.3).

The median level of purchase is one item: Half the residents purchase laundry or no services from the facility, while the other half purchase at least laundry services and perhaps other items. It is important to view these subscale results against the reported ease of obtaining basic resources outside the facility (see Table 9.1). Whereas we would not want residents to go without such resources, the apparent focus of the population on obtaining such items without the aid of the facility is itself a step away from dependence on the service of the total institution.

Items Excluded from the Internal-Integration Scale. Two groups of items were excluded from the internal-integration scale by the statistical analysis: variables describing typically solitary activities—that is, reading, watching TV, sleeping during the day, keeping to oneself; and variables describing activities largely absent in this population, and at the opposite end of the spectrum from solitary activities—that is, dating other residents, activities with other former patients, and working at the house. It might be argued that these latter activities are not well represented in the sheltered-care population, because participating in them would represent acknowledgement by a resident of "out-group" membership; that is, by dating another mentally ill resident one would risk social identification with the group.

Internal Integration: An Overview

Internal integration describes the amount of access to community resources, basic necessities, and social activities that residents have with the help of the operator and through the facility. It also describes social activity within the facility and consumption of basic goods and services through the facility. Virtually all the residents have at least minimal access to participation in one of the subscales; 48% have access to or participate in all the subscales.

We can now describe the internally integrated on a five-level continuum from least (Level 1) to most integrated (Level 5).

Level 1. The residents who are the least integrated into the life of the facility—the 2% of the sheltered-care population scoring at Level 1 on the internal-integration scale—have almost no access to community resources or activities through the operator and have minimal access to basic necessities through the facility. These residents also rarely socialize with anyone in the facility. In addition most find it very difficult to get the operator to transport them to community resources or to arrange social activities or therapy at the house. It is also difficult for the resident to get laundry services or use the telephone at the house and very difficult to get toilet supplies or clothing through the operator. Social activity is also very infrequent; whereas residents may rarely talk to the operator or staff, they never talk to other residents, try to make friends, or join in activities with other residents in the house.

Interestingly the lack of ability to obtain necessities through the house or little socializing within the house are less the marks of a very *poorly* internally integrated resident than are the lack of access through the operator to social activity through community resources and not purchasing supplies through the facility. It may be that the ability to establish a relationship with the operator is most important in enhancing internal integration.

Joe is a veteran and lives in a house in an urban ghetto area. While the house has the capacity to handle 9 people, only Joe and another man live in this facility. Joe spent over 12 years in a VA hospital, where he participated in many activities and had many friends. He indicates that there is nothing for him to do at the house; he sits around all day looking at the four walls. His relationship with the other man in the house is minimal. The operator of the facility has no transportation; therefore when anything is required, Joe and the other man in the facility must walk with her to do the shopping or to complete any other house activity.

Joe was poorly dressed for the interview. He indicated that it would be very difficult for him to go on any trips because of the lack of transportation, and that he really had never considered asking the operator about any activities. He simply wished to return to the hospital where all his friends were and where he had in the past found things to do (F.N.).

Level 2.   The second level of internal integration describes a group of people who find access difficult and participate only rarely in activities in the house. This group constitutes 16% of the sheltered-care population. The resident who is somewhat internally integrated has the most difficulty getting the operator to take him to community resources or to arrange social activity at the house and rarely socializes at the house. These residents do not, however, have much trouble getting basic necessities through the operator; they "never" or "rarely" purchase these supplies at the facility. Mitchell, exemplifying Level 1 on external integration, would be considered a Level 2 on the internal-integration scale (see p. 152).

Level 3.   The third level of internal integration constitutes the largest group of this population (50%), who find it not much trouble to gain access to things through the facility and sometimes become involved in the activities of the facility. Residents in this category scored in the full range of all subscale items but three (all had at least some access to necessities through the house, and none had very easy access to social activity through the house or purchased supplies through the house).

Martha, age 59, suffers from arthritis in her legs. Because the disease limits her mobility, she is dependent upon the operator of the board-and-care home to take her to visit her only relative, a stepmother. The last time Martha saw her stepmother was about a month before the interview.

No member of the house was described as being a special friend; "we just all sit in the sitting room." She says that everybody in the house is pretty busy; most of the residents, including Martha, work in sheltered workshops during the day. Martha describes her co-workers in the workshop as "just everyday folks." About all they do together in the house is play cards. She has no friends in the neighborhood or from her life before entering the home.

On Sundays, Martha and the other residents are taken to church by the operator of the house. The operator has also taken them to the zoo and to a fair, trips which Martha enjoyed (F.N.).

Level 4.   Residents in this category (29% of the population) are more internally integrated than average. They find it "easy" or "not much trouble" to get the operator to transport them to community resources or to organize activities and "very easy" to obtain necessities from the operator. They often socialize in the house, and 46% sometimes purchase supplies through the house.

Bob, age 18, last had a visit from his family "a long time ago, to take me to a clinic or something." He did go to visit them last Christmas, but most of the time he "just doesn't relate to them."

He speaks of his present living situation with great satisfaction. It is here that he feels he is loved. "People here don't yell at you when you make a mistake." John, Thomas, and Peter, other residents of the house, are his special friends. Sometimes they play football together out in the street. Last week Bob and John went to a concert together.

Although Bob says that he would like to meet people living outside of the house, he has no clear way of accomplishing this. His neighborhood is a "rough place," and "not a proper neighborhood in which to make friends."

Camping trips and other activities such as weekend marathons are arranged for Bob through the house, as is his schooling. Group therapy at a nearby community counseling center is arranged by the house for all residents (F.N.).

Level 5. The highest level of internal integration is achieved by 3.5% of the sheltered-care population. This level corresponds to having very easy access or very often participating in social activities in the facility. Residents in this category find it easy or very easy to get access through the operator to community resources, social activity, or basic resources; all socialize in the house often or very often, and 50% purchase supplies through the house often.

Hannah is highly involved in the life of her facility. She, in her early 50s, is the oldest person in the facility, the other women in her house being in their early 30s. Hannah has been living in the house for 10 years, and has a very close friendship with the operator. She has achieved the status of an informal house supervisor, helping orient new residents, making sure that all the tasks around the house are completed, and to some extent becoming an informal member of the facility operator's family. She has accompanied the facility operator on vacations along with some other residents, and in return for her cooperation and help she is able to obtain the things that she needs—whether they are necessities or involve transportation to community resources.

Hannah is quite settled in her current placement; she is very happy there and feels a responsibility for new residents. In line with this responsibility, she often attempts to build friendships with these individuals, socialize with them, and help them adjust to the community (F.N.).

The Relationship Between External and Internal Integration

Table 9.4 outlines the relationship between the internal- and external-integration scales. As can be seen, a low score on external integration is much more frequent than a low score on internal integration. Only a quarter of those with low external-integration scores also had low internal-integration scores, while 70% of those with low internal-integration scores also had low external-integration scores. In looking for the really isolated individuals then, low internal integration seems to be the key factor. In looking for well-integrated individuals, the reverse is true: three-quarters of those high on external integration were also high on internal integration.

Table 9.4   Relationship of External and Internal Integration

Internal-Integration Level	External-Integration Level			
	Low	Medium	High	Total
Low (1-2)	12.9	5.4	.2	18.5
Medium (3)	30.1	18.5	2.5	51.1
High (4-5)	9.0	13.7	7.7	30.4
Total	52.0	37.6	10.4	N = 12,430

The relationship between internal and external integration can be of three types. In the first situation the social skills inherent in interacting within a facility will also be manifested outside that facility, and therefore both internal and external integration will be positively enhanced by these skills. In the second situation internal and external integration may be somewhat independent of each other; the resident may simply enjoy being involved in one area, with no cross-over or contribution to another area of one's life. Finally, a third type of relationship is one of conflict, where either external or internal involvements must be sacrificed to enhance the other. This is traditional social dependency as it relates to the conflict between living in a sheltered environment and attempting to leave that environment. It is hypothesized in this situation that the involvement within the facility will be counterproductive to one's reaching out to the external community. In Part V, which considers factors that facilitate and hinder an individual's level of social integration, we consider how these factors function and what their roles are in the sheltered-care environment.

REFERENCE

Goffman, E. *Asylums: Essays on the Social Situation of Mental Patients and Other Inmates.* Garden City, New York: Doubleday, 1961.

PART FIVE

FACTORS THAT FACILITATE AND HINDER SOCIAL INTEGRATION

Part V focuses on those factors that facilitate or hinder the integration of the mentally ill in the community. We enumerate the factors that are significantly related to external and internal integration and then indicate the variables most related to the facilitating or hindering factor. For example, it is not sufficient to say that an "accepting community environment" is a factor that enhances social integration. We must also discuss the variables that define an "accepting community environment."

Chapter 10 enumerates factors that facilitate or hinder external integration of sheltered-care residents. Chapter 11 considers factors that facilitate or hinder internal integration. In Chapter 12 we discuss the relationship between internal and external integration as a function of their facilitating or hindering factors.

TEN

Involvement in the Outside World

The most difficult problem for community-care advocates in striving toward their goal of integrating formerly hospitalized patients has been to know what to emphasize programmatically in the absence of clear specifications of those factors most important in enhancing external integration. In this chapter we attempt to specify the factors that facilitate or hinder an individual's external integration, discuss how the influence of such factors can be increased or decreased in the lives of sheltered-care residents, and indicate which factors are most influential for different types of people.

FACTORS-THAT FACILITATE OR HINDER EXTERNAL INTEGRATION

This study deals with three types of facilitating or hindering factors in relation to external integration. In order of importance for the total sheltered-care population, they are (1) community characteristics, (2) resident characteristics, and (3) sheltered-care facility characteristics (see Figure 10.1). The simultaneous or joint influence of all characteristics was evaluated after controlling for the degree of individual ability and psychological disturbance of residents. Our goal was to find factors modifiable through social-policy action.

In looking first at the figures for the total sheltered-care population, community characteristics were found to have the most important influence on external integration. It has long been established that the characteristics of the larger social group influence the internal dynamics and membership patterns of its subgroups (Cartwright & Zander, 1953). It therefore seems obvious that the characteristics of the external community would be very important in determining the level of social integration of sheltered-care residents. Yet the emphasis in mental-health programming to date has been on the design of the facility's internal environment, such as its social structure (Caudill, 1958; Stanton & Schwartz, 1954) and pattern of interrelationships (Fairweather et al., 1969). Although these internal factors are statistically significant predictors of external integration, we find them least important

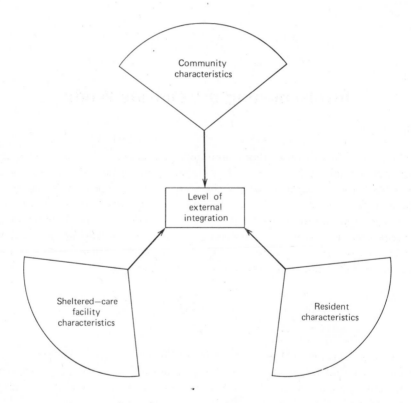

Figure 10.1   Types of factors that facilitate and hinder external integration for the total population in sheltered care.

among significant predictors in achieving the goal of external integration. In large part this focus on the internal environment is most immediate, easier, and fits well within the clinical orientation, exemplified by attempts to build a therapeutic community within the facility to ameliorate the significant psychological problems of this group. This orientation is centered on the individual's changing to cope with the community and makes no demands on the community to respond to the individual. The results of this study point to the need to broaden our focus beyond the internal facility environment if community integration is to be achieved.

The predominant role of community factors in influencing external integration was evident even in looking within subgroups in the resident population. The two characteristics, used to divide the population into subgroups that have the greatest effect on the relative priority that could be accorded to factors predicting external integration, are degree of psychological disturbance (measured by the Overall and Gorham Brief Psychiatric Rating Scale (BPRS) (Overall & Gorham, 1962) and resident age.* Yet only for the subgroup evidencing no overt symptomatology was there any question of the major import of community factors. For this subgroup individual characteristics were almost as important as community characteristics.

The nine community, individual, and facility characteristics considered as significant predictors of external integration are described in Figure 10.2. They are, in order of their overall importance: neighborhood response to residents, resident perception of having sufficient spending money, frequency of community complaints about the facility, involuntary placement in the facility, rural location of the facility, ideal psychiatric environment, distance of the facility from community resources, resident control of spending money, and isolated resident group. These factors were chosen because they were significantly related to external integration and because they were considered modifiable by policy action. The joint effects of these characteristics and their individual importance in promoting or detracting from an individual's external integration need to be discussed, for while each variable is related significantly to external integration, their simultaneous effects upon external integration reveal that their relative importance as predictors of external integration varies a great deal (this was true both in considering the entire sheltered-care resident population and its major subgroups).

*In dividing the population into subgroups reflecting different levels of psychological disturbance, we divided the sum of the ratings on all 16 symptoms of the BPRS into three categories, category three characterizing the most disturbed, and category one, the least disturbed. (In controlling for psychopathology in our regression models, we residualized predictors by a composite of both the BPRS and the Langner scales.)

Residents were divided into three age subgroups—young (18 to 33), middle aged (34 to 50), and old (51 to 65).

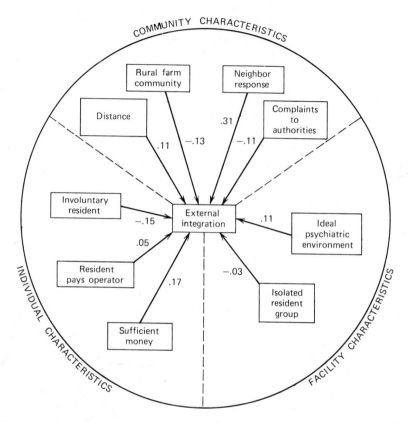

Figure 10.2   Factors facilitating or hindering involvement in the outside world for the total sheltered-care population (after controlling for individual ability and psychological disturbance). All variables are significant (p < .05). The numbers attached to each arrow are the significant standardized partial regression weights. Since all predictors were residualized by individual ability and psychological disturbance and were evaluated in our equation, their absolute size indicates the relative importance of each factor controlling for the impact of the others as a predictor of external integration. The external-integration model accounted for 27 % of the total variance.

Community Characteristics

The community characteristics found to facilitate or hinder the external integration of an individual were, in order of their importance for all sheltered-care residents: (1) response of neighbors, (2) rural-urban location of the facility, (3) complaints from neighbors made to authorities about the facility, and (4) distance of the facility from community resources.

Response of Neighbors.   All variables being taken into account, positive response from neighbors—that is, inviting residents into their homes and having more than casual conversation with them—was most important in promoting the external integration of the individual. This finding holds even when the ability of residents to elicit such a response is taken into account. Residents who reported these positive responses from their neighbors were more likely to live in neighborhoods where facilities had not elicited any serious complaints and were also least likely to be located in totally Caucasian neighborhoods. These findings lead us to the simple hypothesis that neighborhoods that interact with residents have a greater tolerance of deviance than neighborhoods in which there is no response. Our results do not, however, support this.

Using a newly developed technique to study cross-level inference, we studied the response of communities (measured in terms of the neighbor-outreach variable) to individuals in the facility *as individuals,* and to them *as members of a group* (Boyd & Iverson, in press). Our findings indicate that the efforts of neighbors to interact with residents as individuals tend to increase residents' social integration; however, when neighbors' response is directed at the whole group of residents in a facility, we found that the impact of this response is negative and leads to a reduction in level of social integration of house residents as a group. It thus appears that the effect of neighbors' interaction with the residents as a group is opposite from such interaction when directed toward the individual. Encouragement of increased neighbors' response to residents as a group may have a negative impact on residents' social integration.

One operator exemplifies the significance of these findings as they relate to neighbors' response to the individual. When asked what reintegration into the community meant, this operator replied:

it means interaction with a community. . . . the first half is you go out and you go shopping and you get involved, you go to the movies, you walk on the street. . . . On top of this, people . . . come in just the same as if you, as an individual, move into a neighborhood, as long as you don't have a visitor, at least one neighbor coming in or what-not, you don't feel that you really belong to the community. . . .

I would say that the amount of participation by our patients with the neighbors is in the minority. . . . I have a home where the neighbors get along very well with our people. . . . one of them even made a buddy—one of the women in the home. She is a lonely widow that lives nearby. She often has her come over, she may pay two or three dollars for help with her home and takes this resident wherever she goes. It's a very pleasant arrangement (F.N.).*

Although this is a pleasant arrangement for one member of this facility, interaction by other residents with other neighbors is limited. The crucial question posed by our data is the extent to which the community can reach out to the residents of the facility as a group without depressing their social

*F.N. refers to field notes taken at the time of a structured or open-ended interview.

integration. Outreach to residents as a group is usually a response to them as former mental patients. This approach may cause residents to withdraw and thus reduce their overall social integration.

Positive community response remained the most important factor predicting external integration across all age categories and all categories of psychopathology, except for those individuals showing no overt symptomatology. In this subgroup of residents, it ranked second to the involuntary resident—that is, a situation wherein the residents did not choose their facility. Being placed without having a chance to participate in the choice of one's placement tended to depress an individual's social integration. This finding simply emphasizes the importance of self-determination for the asymptomatic group. This group, unable to rationalize a lack of self-determination due to illness, may thus be more affected by such deprivations than the groups with mild or severe symptomatology.

Rural Location of the Facility. The negative influence of the rural farm facility—leading to a reduction in external integration—was primarily related to the location of the facility, which makes it difficult for residents to move out independently and interact in the community. They are dependent—especially for transportation—upon the services of the facility.

Although individual ability is controlled for, the effect of group characteristics of residents in rural facilities must be considered as they relate to the social integration of any individual. Residents of rural facilities are generally more chronic and older. Operators of these facilities tend to be less educated, and the neighborhoods in which these facilities are located tend to be less open, socially, for residents (i.e., community members not living in sheltered-care homes are part of established social networks offering little access to sheltered-care residents as independent people seeking to enter) (cf. Cumming & Cumming, *Closed Ranks,* 1957). Even with these limitations, however, the asymptomatic individual may find such an environment conducive to community outreach.

Complaints. Complaints to local authorities after a facility has been open awhile have a negative effect on an individual's social integration.

Neighbors who complain about a facility to local authorities are likely to do it frequently. Communities where complaints are made to the police are most likely to be areas with both businesses and residences—areas classified as lower class and ghettos (see Chapter 7).* Facilities in such areas are more

---

*People with lower social status are more likely to report assaults to the police (Banton, 1964; Block, 1974), and lower class community members have been found to have positive attitudes toward the police (Gilbert & Eaton, 1970).

likely to be halfway houses or large treatment-oriented board-and-care homes, which receive more complaints than smaller, family-oriented facilities with earlier curfews.

Facilities having complaints made about them to authorities were also more likely to have had residents picked up by the police in the last year, especially for alcohol-associated arrests. In addition, residents in these facilities were more likely to have been hospitalized in the past year. Although these findings appear to indicate that facilities having more complaints have a more difficult resident population, it is also possible that complaints themselves initiate the arrests, hospitalizations, and a greater reliance on alcohol. A community that reinforces social isolation may contribute to a person's use of alcohol and a reduction in his level of social integration.

Whereas the impact of complaints is generally negative, the predictor was not significant for the old population. Perhaps this is due to the general low level of external involvements of this subgroup.

Distance from Resources and Services. As might be expected, the closer a facility is to community resources and medical and social services, the higher the level of social integration manifested by its residents. Contrary to current belief (cf. Chapter 7) middle-class neighborhoods composed of single-family homes may have a negative impact on the external integration of residents because of their distance from shopping areas, parks, libraries, theaters, and community centers. Facilities in downtown areas are more likely to be closer to community resources and therefore tend to enhance their residents' social integration. This phenomenon is well illustrated in the Charles Schulz strip reproduced on page 174.

The drawbacks of single-family housing areas led us to reconsider the residential zoning controversy (cf. Chapter 5). Certainly it is necessary to protect the rights of individuals in sheltered care and ensure that they are not excluded peremptorily from the life of the community. The location of facilities in single-family housing areas should, however, be carefully considered; the goal of external integration is less likely to be fulfilled in many areas zoned for single-family units. In addition to the distance factor middle-class areas tend to be characterized by more stable family networks. Social integration into such networks for the disaffiliated individual is difficult (Bott, 1971).

Facilities situated closer to community resources (park, library, etc.) and medical and social services (community mental-health center, vocational-rehabilitation center, etc.) are also more likely to rely on programs already existing outside the facility than to develop their own, internally oriented programs. For example, if a resident of a facility close to medical and social

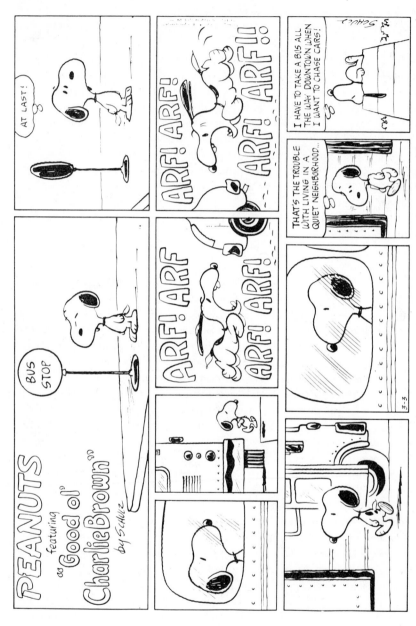

services required treatment after leaving the mental hospital, he would be more likely to receive it as an out-patient than at his place of residence. The closer facilities are to community medical and social services, the more often residents in these facilities tend to make use of these services. Thus we see that focus on the external community (as facility policy), as well as supports for reaching out (available services), are provided in this type of setting.

Facilities close to community resources and medical and social services are more likely to be in a downtown commercial zone, in a non-middle-class, working-class area (as opposed to a lower class ghetto), in a neighborhood with a combination of businesses and residences, often comprising small commercial pockets within residential areas. This type of neighborhood represents a desirable setting for encouraging external outreach of residents.

Proximity of community resources and medical and social services is an independent contributor to external integration, though as we have seen, many community factors associated with the distance of a facility from community services tend to contribute to the impact of this factor. Long Beach, New York, is a good example of the interaction of exclusionary trends in a middle-class suburban area where sheltered-care residents have been placed in hotels a "good long walk" from community resources. In addition community policy confines psychiatric services to the hotels in which residents live—the hotel owners set aside space for hospital personnel to continue medication supervision and a very limited counseling service. Efforts to move these services into the community have been blocked by local government. The result of these actions has been an overall reduction of reaching out on the part of residents in these homes, representing the creation of an informal mini-hospital in the community, where residents are isolated and confined to their facilities (Segal, 1973).

The only subgroup for whom distance is not significant as a predictor of social integration is the most severely disturbed. Their very low level of external integration may imply that they have not reached a point where they are able to take advantage of the opportunities afforded by minimizing distance to resources.

The four community characteristics—neighbor responsiveness, rural location, complaints, and distance—all contribute to the amount of external integration of sheltered-care residents. As already noted, past emphasis on these characteristics has been minimal compared with that placed on the internal environment of a facility; therefore, we again emphasize the need to consider the impact of the community in developing a true community mental-health program.

Resident Characteristics

In looking at resident characteristics—controlling for ability and psychological disturbance—we again selected those that seem to be most modifiable by policy action.

Sufficient Spending Money. The most important resident characteristic is called "sufficient spending money." Residents were asked how often they had enough money to do the things they wanted to do. Regarding sources of funds, residents on general assistance were less likely to have a sufficient amount of money available to do what they wanted. This is to be expected, because the levels of general assistance provided by counties are much lower than those of Supplemental Security Income (SSI) programs. An unfortunate aspect of this differential is that it often takes individuals a good deal of time to be established on SSI, and therefore they must spend the first few months in their placement with minimal financial support for social activity.

The typical resident who reports that he has enough money to do what he wishes to do is single, has been away from his home town for a long period of time, and has chosen to live in the facility that he wants to live in. This resident is engaged in some sort of educational activity program, often a full-time educational experience. Such an individual seems to be quite independent to begin with and is probably facile at obtaining and using his funds. However, since we have controlled for psychopathology and ability already in looking at the impact of the adequacy of the spending-money variable on external integration, we must look further at this predictor and beyond the impact of these two control variables to explain its influence.

We are talking about two phenomena here: an absolute level of financing and whether or not individuals perceive the amount of money they have to be sufficient. For example, how might full-time educational activities of residents contribute to their perception that they have enough money to do what they wish? In California there is an unusually well-developed adult and community-college system with a wide variety of course offerings—many of which are recreational or social (e.g., brush painting, astrology, and ceramics). Such educational activity may provide access to free or inexpensive entertainment. Certainly it provides a good deal of informal, low-cost social contact. Although there is no doubt that $33 per month for spending money (the spending allowance under SSI) is very little in terms of paying for social events, the money can be "stretched" by taking advantage of the low-cost opportunities associated with the student status. In addition the education itself may further enable people to make more efficient use of their social environment.

[Where are good places to meet people?]

[pause] I guess some of the beaches and some of the parks. I thought the bars too . . . but I think it will be better when I get back in school. I think it will be easier for me to meet people in school . . . that's why I'm going back to school. I think going back to school, I'll be able to meet a lot of people—other people around the same age (F.N.).

This resident made significant social contacts and obtained part-time work but was limited by insufficient means in establishing social relationships. Going back to school provided a context for such relationships, though the resident's rationale for attending school had nothing to do with lack of means. Given this example, it appears that other low-cost social opportunities should be considered for individuals who cannot or do not wish to take advantage of a more middle-class educational pathway.

The significance of having money to do what one wants is a strong and positive predictor across categories of psychopathology. However, though strong for all three categories, it is much stronger relative to the other elements of the predictive model for the severe symptomatology subgroup than for the asymptomatic residents. Thus it is sixth in strength for the asymptomatic and second in strength for the mildly and severely symptomatic groups. Apparently, the more symptomatology is present, the less other forms of support in the environment are able to compensate for a lack, perceived or real, of money. This point is reinforced by the observation that making creative use of social resources, as illustrated earlier, is more difficult when one is absorbed in his or her own disturbance.

The Involuntary Resident. This predictor of integration refers to the extent to which people did not choose the facility they were currently living in. Even after individual ability and level of psychological disturbance were controlled for, not choosing the place in which one will live is associated with lowered levels of external integration in the community. The following example is typical of the situation faced by many residents during their placement process.

I: The first house you lived in after you left the hospital, did anybody tell you you were going to go there?

R: The social worker—well, when I was in the hospital, one of the technicians said I was going to be released, and they told me what date the county people would pick me up and take me to the home. That the place was quiet.

I: And did you want to go there?

R: I wanted to get out of the hospital, so I had no choice.

I: Did you have a chance to live anywhere else? If you told them when you got out of the hospital that you wanted to live somewhere else, could you have done that?

R: *I don't know, it never occurred to me.*
I: Was there another place that you wanted to live?
R: No. I just wanted to get out of the hospital, that's all (F.N.).

Residents who did not choose their facility were likely not to have seen the house before they came and to have trusted the person who recommended it to them. They were least likely to have had a social worker from the Community Care Services Section (CCSS) of the State Department of Health involved in their placement. Individuals who did not choose their placement were generally dissatisfied with their living arrangements. They were more likely to be placed in old YMCAs, fraternity houses, boarding homes, and hotels.

Even after controlling for ability and level of psychopathology, we found that involuntarily placed residents are less likely to plan their own daily activities. Perhaps the system's denial of the right of these individuals to choose their own residence encourages a dependence upon the operator to make other important decisions.

The "involuntary resident" was the third most important influence on external integration of the nine factors relating to the total sheltered-care population and open to policy action. One qualification must, however, be added in relation to the impact of failing to choose one's residence on important population subgroups. We have already pointed out that not choosing one's residential facility is the most important factor negatively influencing (i.e., reducing) the external integration of the asymptomatic group. On the contrary the severely symptomatic resident who does *not* choose his/her placement is *more* likely to be externally integrated. Thus it appears that, for the small severely symptomatic subgroup, expert placement is indicated to ensure them maximum opportunities for external integration. Perhaps attempts to accommodate the perceived needs of the severely symptomatic have led to overcompensation—that is, too great a willingness to make important client decisions for all prospective residents—and the concomitant debilitating consequences for the asymptomatic. Certainly, if the negative influence of involuntary placement on external integration is to be avoided, the placement process itself will need careful and planned revision.

Controlling Spending Money.   A factor related to availability of money is exercising control over one's finances. This predictor relates to whether a resident paid his own rent at the sheltered-care facility—that is, a conservator or the operator did not pay the rent, and the operator did not actually appropriate the resident's check when it arrived and take out the rent money. The latter procedure, even when controlled for resident psychopathology and ability, had a negative effect on residents' external integration. When we look within categories of symptomatology, we find a differing impact of this variable on the asymptomatic and mildly symptomatic, compared with the severely symptomatic. For the first two resident groups, having control of their money strongly enhances their external integration. For the third group the influence is not significant.

The most important factor determining the character of this predictor is the presence of some outside influence over the facility operator. Residents who control their own money are more likely to be in facilities where the operators are active in local associations or are affiliated with CCSS of the Department of Health—the aftercare follow-up arm of most state mental-health programs. Such facilities are more likely to be family-care homes than board-and-care facilities. Their operators tend to use the CCSS in emergencies, report that they find the assistance helpful, are likely to have chosen their profession because of companionship and religious commitment, and are in a somewhat better financial position than other operators (their facilities are likely to be subsidized by some outside support such as a working spouse).

Although local operator associations and the CCSS have only limited control over the facility operator, their presence is related to reduced abuse of residents' financial prerogatives. To some extent this may be a result of the more concerned and responsible operators' initiating contact with the organizations. But contact with these organizations renders the operation of one's facility more public and in this respect should be encouraged as a means of preventing abuse of residents' prerogatives.

Internal Facility Characteristics

The internal characteristics of the facility were least important as predictors of external integration when compared with community and resident characteristics. Internal facility characteristics considered (1) the extent to which a facility could be termed an ideal psychiatric environment and (2) the extent to which the residents as a group in the facility were isolated from the external community.

Ideal Psychiatric Environment.   This predictor of external integration refers to the social-psychological environment of the facility, often represented as an ideal in literature on therapy. The ideal psychiatric environment is significantly and positively related to external integration. It emphasizes program involvement, support from staff and other residents, spontaneity (the open expression of feelings), a structured program with clear expectations, a practically oriented program encouraging autonomy, the open expression of anger and aggression, and the open discussion of personal problems. We combined these components, measured by Moos' Community Oriented Programs Environment Scale (COPES) (1974), to create an index called the "ideal psychiatric environment."

There is little consensus about what constitutes an "ideal psychiatric" or "therapeutic environment." In our population of facilities the concept was empirically derived. In sum it emphasized relationship and system-maintenance characteristics of the facility rather than treatment factors (cf. Chapter 7). Since it did, however, include these latter factors, it does seem appropriate to conceive of it as one index of an ideal environment.

In comparing his former family-care placement with the halfway house he lives in, Joe, a halfway-house resident, describes how his former family-care home may by COPES criteria, be considered a more ideal psychiatric environment than the halfway house:

I was living with the S. family since I got here last year. It was a lot more therapeutic than living in the halfway house. Mrs. S. was a therapist and she got training. She runs a group and all that. People come in and live with her and with her natural family. There's a lot less room and a lot more structure than there is here. When I was living with the S. family I knew that the confrontation level was higher than here. The level of involvement of the people with the other people in this halfway house isn't quite as high as it was with the S. family. If you were off by yourself people found out why, told you why you were off by yourself. If you were withdrawn, they told you why you were withdrawing. There's a lot more to it than here—here if you are off by yourself a lot of times, it'll go for a couple of weeks until someone will say something about it (F.N.).

Residents living in facilities with an ideal psychiatric environment are more likely to be satisfied with that environment and less likely to wish to move out of the facility than residents not living in such an environment. Ideal facilities are more likely to be situated outside working-class downtown areas, often in remodeled single-family homes in middle-class neighborhoods.

Operators who run these facilities are likely to make use of the county hospitals in some psychiatric emergencies, but they more often use the social worker at the welfare department. The support services offered by the social worker in emergencies are no doubt an important alternative to rehospitalization.

Ideal psychiatric environments are family oriented more often than not, and their staff (if any) tend to eat with the residents. This pattern of interaction tends to promote a closer relationship between staff and residents—one devoid of many of the status differentials experienced in hospital situations.

The ideal psychiatric environment ranked seventh in importance of the nine predictors of external integration for the total sheltered-care population. Whereas this low ranking is not surprising in view of the emphasis of external integration on community-outreach skills, the ideal psychiatric environment can be crucial in encouraging these skills.

For the most symptomatic resident group, the ideal psychiatric environment was not a significant predictor in promoting external integration. For the asymptomatic and the older population, however, it was a significantly stronger predictor, ranking fourth for the former and third for the latter group. One must hypothesize that the presence of internal support systems to encourage and facilitate external integration is more important for these two subgroups in the population.

Social Isolation of the Resident Group. The extent to which facility residents as a group are isolated from neighbors and abandoned by their families is another factor influencing external integration of the individual. Although this may be a selection factor—that is, people who are isolated tend to be grouped with other isolates—it may also point to the need for a different policy on mixing residents in facilities, placing externally oriented individuals in facilities with at least some similarly inclined individuals. This latter point is emphasized by the observation that the asymptomatic group is most likely to be affected by this social situation. This factor is not significant for the more severely ill.

The following interviewer comment illustrates two forms of social isolation—isolation of the facility in a rural setting and isolation of a particular individual in the facility setting.

There's another lady that I remember . . . because I thought she was terribly misplaced. . . . She was a very well-educated lady, verbalized very well . . . on the nervous side but nothing peculiar about her behavior. . . . She was in a small home with about 15 residents out in an agricultural area. . . . She was 52 years old and all the other residents were over 80 years old. Not many of them could speak very coherently or get around by themselves. She told me she was just literally going crazy because there was no one she could talk to, no one to go places with, no one to really associate with (F.N.).

In this example the rural location of the facility exacerbated the lack of external integration of a resident placed with a group of isolates.

In determining what factors might lead to the social isolation of the resident group, we compared the socially isolated resident group with other indicators in the study. Regarding resident characteristics, we found that the socially isolated group was composed primarily of residents who needed help in their basic life functions and who, by and large, tended not to be mentally retarded. This latter finding is quite interesting. Perhaps the community is less threatened by mentally retarded people and more willing to enter a facility and become involved with them as a group than the mentally ill. Tringo (1970) has in fact established that the retarded are a less rejected group than the mentally ill.

The location of a facility in a predominantly Caucasian neighborhood is positively related to social isolation of residents. This might be a reflection of the class character of the neighborhood and its attitude toward the mentally ill within its boundaries. On the other hand halfway houses in ghetto areas were also apt to have more isolated populations than the many family-care homes we observed. This may be a function of the threat of area crime to residents who engage in outreach activity. Sheltered-care residents are often victims and often confine their activity to the facility for their own protection.

A most interesting finding with respect to social isolation is the clear and strong relation in the data between isolation of the facility operator and isolation of the resident group. Operators who entered the business primarily for companionship do not encourage their residents to reach outside the facility. Those who are not themselves active in state or local associations (except in obtaining information and referrals) are most likely to have residents in their facility who are isolated from the community. We also noted that such operators tend to isolate themselves from the professional service community. They are more likely to view services as harmful to their clients and less likely to call CCSS or to find a psychiatrist helpful in a psychiatric emergency. They are also less likely to transport their residents out of the facility for any type of therapy or rehabilitation program. They rely primarily on private physicians to help them in a psychiatric emergency. This service orientation is devoid of a supportive psychological orientation and holds that physicians deal with physical illness and with serious types of psychological illness. Use of community support services could ultimately reduce the social isolation of the total resident group and contribute to an individual's external integration.

REACHING OUT

Our analysis of predictors of external integration has not only provided an indication of the overall importance of predictors for the total sheltered-care resident population but has also pointed to the significance of two individual characteristics—degree of overt psychological disturbance or symptomatology and age—in distinguishing the needs of specific subgroups in this population.

Comparing subgroups on the basis of their degree of psychopathology—or more specifically their degree of symptomatology as measured by the BPRS—the asymptomatic residents display very different priorities, vis-à-vis predictors of their external integration, than the mildly or severely ill residents do. Having chosen their placement and living in a receptive neighborhood within reasonable distance from community resources is of paramount importance for the former group. There are fewer significant predictors of external integration for sicker residents (only five for the severely ill) and less compensation or facilitation attributable to the facility's internal environment. The strongest factors influencing the sicker residents are whether the neighbors reach out to these residents and whether they have sufficient spending money.

Looking within age groups, we see the importance for the older individuals of the supportive system within the facility and a neighborhood without a distance barrier between residents and community resources. Although these factors are not so important for the younger group, those between 18 and 33 share with older individuals the need to experience a receptive neighborhood and to exercise choice of their placement.

The results described in this chapter relate solely to the goal of promoting the external integration of residents, which, as we see in the next two chapters, is not the only legitimate goal in serving sheltered-care residents and which, to some extent, may conflict with involvement of the resident in the internal environment of the facility.

REFERENCES

Banton, M. *Policeman in the Community.* New York: Basic Books, 1964.

Block, R. "Why Notify the Police?" *Criminology,* **11,** 555–569 (1974).

Bott, E. *Family and Social Network.* London: Tavistock, 1971.

Boyd, L. and G. Iverson. *Multi-Level Statistical Analysis: Concept and Techniques.* Unpublished manuscript. Berkeley, California: in press.

Cartwright, D. and A. Zander. *Group Dynamics: Research and Theory.* New York: Harper & Row, 1953.

Caudill, W. *The Psychiatric Hospital as a Small Society.* Cambridge, Massachusetts: Harvard University Press, 1958.

Cumming, J. and E. Cumming. *Closed Ranks: An Experiment in Mental Health Education.* Cambridge, Massachusetts: Harvard University Press, 1957.

Fairweather, G. W., D. Sanders, H. Maynard, D. Cressler, and D. Blech. *Community Life for the Mentally Ill: An Alternative to Institutional Care.* Chicago: Aldine, 1969.

Gilbert, N. and J. W. Eaton. "Research Report: Who Speaks for the Poor?" *J. Am. Inst. Planners,* **36**(6), 411–416, (1970).

Moos, R. H. *Evaluating Treatment Environments: A Social Ecological Approach.* New York: Wiley, 1974.

Overall, J. and D. Gorham. "The Brief Psychiatric Rating Scale." *Psychol. Rep.* **10,** 779–812 (1962).

Segal, S. *Social Exclusion Revisited: Sheltered Care in California and New York.* Unpublished memo, Berkeley, California: University of California School of Social Welfare, 1973.

Stanton, A. H. and M. S. Schwartz. *The Mental Hospital.* New York: Basic Books, 1954.

Tringo, J. L. "The Hierarchy of Preference Toward Disability Groups." *J. Special Ed.* 4(3), 295–305 (1970).

ELEVEN

Involvement Within the Facility

We define internal integration as the extent to which an individual focuses his life within the sheltered-care facility or lives a life mediated by that facility. The extent to which an individual does this is to some extent determined by what the social setting will accommodate. Many social institutions in our society not only foster but also encourage the focus of one's life within their confines. These include traditional institutions such as mental hospitals and service organizations like Synanon, as well as the military and the church (most notably monasteries and convents). All these examples encourage one to adopt an inward focus in terms of our five areas of social integration—presence, access, participation, production, and consumption.

Focusing one's life inward on the living arrangement is not necessarily negative. It offers a high level of social support for many individuals who, without such support, would be unable to function in our society. Unfortunately internal integration, when discussed with respect to the care of the mentally ill, has taken on a pejorative meaning.

In looking at an individual's involvement in a sheltered-care facility and the predictors of that involvement, we emphasize that higher levels of internal integration may be very desirable for some individuals. Internal integration should be considered positive in its own right and not valued merely for preparation of the mentally ill for a transition to the external community environment.

The notion of mentally ill persons' needing a long-term supportive living arrangement has been given only marginal validation as a goal for their care. Hospitals, the traditional source of care for the mentally ill, historically refer to a place for shelter and entertainment of travelers or strangers (*Webster's Dictionary*, 1971). There is to some extent a connotation of transiency or transition in this concept that can be viewed as somewhat inappropriate to meet the needs of patients for whom the hospital became a permanent home. This problem was recognized, for example, in the Wisconsin system, which was founded on a separation of care for the chronic and acutely mentally ill (Scheff, 1966).

Recent observations are that involvement in one's social group has interesting and positive consequences for the individual, as well as negative consequences often pointed to in the mental-health literature. Whereas writers such as Wing (1962) and Barton (1959) speak of institutional neurosis as a pathology caused by institutionalization, epidemiologists around the world have recently noted that the death rate from malignancy in mental institutions is only a third of that reported for the general population (Rassidakis et al., 1973). The fact that a mental institution provides a structure, role, and group membership, as well as meets all survival needs, may explain this rate. Health statistics on other internally focused groups support the beneficial effects of group involvement. For example, the excellent health statistics of the Mormons and Seventh Day Adventists are better than for the general population (Enstrom, 1975), and church attendance tends to be related to lower death rates due to heart attack (Comstock & Partridge, 1971).

The sheltered-care population cannot get family-type support, because they are not involved in the traditional family (only 5% are still married and only 52% have ever been married). Life in the facility, then, may serve as an important substitute for the family in providing support and in promoting a healthy response to one's environment. Fairweather et al. (1969) found that involvement in the ongoing program of a community facility showed significantly better outcome in terms of community adjustment among former hospital patients. His results also indicate that, once the supportive group was dissolved, the benefit accruing to the members of that group quickly disappeared. This finding clearly supports the need to establish programs that sanction internal integration on a long-term or ongoing basis.

While these are admittedly speculations, they point to the importance of looking at internal integration, not only as a means to the end goal of external integration or as a dependency-producing phenomenon, but also from the perspective of optimizing its positive contribution to individual health.

FACTORS THAT FACILITATE OR HINDER INTERNAL INTEGRATION

Eleven factors were found to facilitate or hinder the internal integration of the total sheltered-care population. They are, in order of their overall importance (measured by their partial standardized regression weights):

1. The ideal psychiatric environment.
2. Positive response from neighbors to the individual resident.
3. Low levels of individual psychological stress.
4. Having the facility located outside of a downtown area.
5. Having a facility operator who perceives community services as helpful.
6. Location of facility in a rural farm community.
7. Character of the facility unlike that of a residence club.
8. Whether the resident has what he perceives to be enough spending money to interact in his environment.
9. Having a female operator.
10. Having other residents in the facility who have community contacts.
11. Resident control of medication.

As was the case with external integration, we found three groups of factors that influence internal integration. In their order of importance, these factors are community characteristics, facility characteristics, and resident characteristics. (Note that these are the same groupings of factors influencing external integration but in a different order of importance; see Figure 11.1.) The importance of community characteristics as a group must, however, be modified by the observation that the single facility characteristic—ideal psychiatric environment—was the most crucial factor determining internal integration. Also community characteristics, while the most important group of factors predicting internal integration for the total sheltered-care population, vary in their order of importance for specific subgroups. For individuals with severe psychological disturbance, and the middle aged (33 to 50), resident characteristics are the most important predictors of internal integration. Facility characteristics are the most important predictors of internal integration for the older population.

Community Characteristics

Community characteristics were found to be first in order of importance in predicting internal integration. The three community characteristics predicting internal integration are, in order of importance (determined by the size of the partial β weight in the total model):

1. Neighbors' positive response.
2. Location in a downtown area.
3. Location in a rural community.

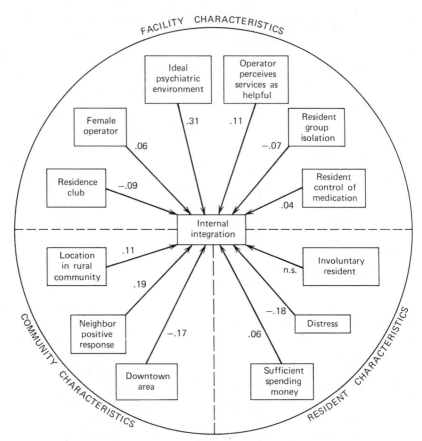

Figure 11.1.   Factors facilitating or hindering involvement in the sheltered-care facility. While all variables are significant when considered individually (p < .10), n.s. indicates that a variable was not significant at at least the .05 level when evaluated jointly with the other variables. All factors with the exception of "distress" have been controlled for "individual ability" and "psychological disturbance." The numerical values are taken from one equation and are the standardized partial regression weights. Their absolute size indicates the relative importance of each factor, controlling for the impact of the others as a predictor of external integration. This internal-integration model accounts for 30 % of the variance.

The first and third factors tend to enhance internal integration for the sheltered-care population as a whole, while the second tends to detract from it.

Positive Response from the Neighbors.   A positive effort on the part of neighbors in a community to reach out to facility residents tends to promote internal integration. This conclusion holds even after level of psychological disturbance and resident ability to reciprocate are taken into account. This finding is crucial in offering an indication of the extent to which community inputs determine interactions within the facility. In Chapter 10 we discussed what leads community residents to reach out to sheltered-care residents. How does this outreach affect interactions within the facility?

Two observations provide insight into the contribution of neighbors' positive response to internal integration. First, the status of individuals within the facilities may increase as a result of neighbors' response. Second, positive social behavior is encouraged by such a neighbor response. The first factor is exemplified by a gentleman who is invited to visit a neighbor down the street. On his return to the facility he has new information and a new experience to convey to facility residents. With reference to the second factor this gentleman's behavior is modeled to meet the demand of normal social interaction. He carries this behavior pattern back to the facility, and it is reflected in his level of internal integration in the facility.

The impact of the community's positive response on internal integration is less on the elderly. Although this factor is still significant for those over 50, they tend to rely less on external contacts for enhancing their internal prestige. Community's positive response has no impact on the internal integration of the severely symptomatic or disturbed. Segal, Baumohl, and Johnson (1977) report that the impact of severe mental disturbance on social relations between young vagrants is pervasive in the sense of limiting opportunities for social contact. It thus seems that more direct influence is needed to promote the internal integration of the severely disturbed than is provided by the positive response of outsiders.

Downtown Location. The second most influential community characteristic, negatively related to the individual's level of internal integration, is the location of his residence in a downtown area. Downtown areas are likely to be commercially zoned and not likely to have a "neighborhood character." Downtown facilities have a more transient quality; they are usually old hotels or old YMCAs. Residents from these facilities are likely to come from county hospitals, and the facilities themselves are likely to have residents who have been picked up by the police in the past year. The transient character of the facility is illustrated by the fact that such facilities have more residents who are supported financially by general assistance or general relief (the county subsistence grant offered as a last resort when the resident is ineligible for state or federal aid programs and most commonly received by transient groups). This type of transient environment leads to a reduction in internal integration, because it offers little possibility for the development of internal commitments on the part of residents. The severely disturbed individual, who is largely turned inward and focused on himself, is not affected by this or other community characteristics.

Rural Location. In contrast to the negative relationship of the downtown urban setting to internal integration a rural setting is found to promote higher levels of internal integration of facility residents—especially those who are younger and who show no overt symptomatology.

Facilities in these areas are likely to be family oriented. The operator and his family often reside in the facility. The focus of life, then, is centered around the facility itself, and residents report feeling "safe" in this environment. One operator of a facility in a rural area had nine men residing there. She arranged special tasks and jobs for each of them and made sure they got up in the morning and were dressed, clean, and socially presentable. To a certain extent she assumed the role of mother for all these men, and a rather strong relationship developed between her and the men. The environment in which this social interaction took place, by virtue of its physical isolation and the absence of outside threats to the social existence of these individuals, was conducive to a high level of internal integration.

Facility's Environment Factors

Six characteristics of the facility were distinguished as predictors of internal integration, in the following order of importance: (1) ideal psychiatric environment, (2) operators' perception of helpfulness of services, (3) residence club, (4) social isolation of resident group, (5) female operator, and (6) resident control of medications.

Ideal Psychiatric Environment. The single factor most related to the internal integration of the total resident group is the extent to which the psychiatric environment in which they live can be described as ideal. As noted (p. 121), the ideal psychiatric environment is a composite score of nine subscales in Moos' COPES Scale (1974). Of interest in terms of the health statistics just discussed is that the subscale most related to internal integration within the COPES scale is "Involvement." This scale inquires the extent to which respondents report that:

1. Members put a lot of energy into what they do around here.
2. This is a lively place.
3. Members are proud of this program.
4. There is a lot of group spirit in this program.
5. Many members volunteer around here.
6. Few members just seem to be passing time here.
7. This program has many social activities.
8. Members are pretty busy all the time.
9. Discussions are very interesting here.
10. Members often do things together on weekends (Moos, 1974, p. 372).

Agreement between residents and operators on this subscale was greater than on the others. Other COPES subscales strongly related to internal integration are (1) a facility environment supportive of residents and (2) a facility with a practical orientation rather than one that related to concern about feelings.

Thus the characteristics of the ideal psychiatric environment most important in predicting internal integration are those related to the relationship between residents and staff—that is, the extent to which the environment promotes involvement, support, and a practical orientation.

Characteristics of the facility other than those in the COPES scales also indicate that the relationship aspect of the ideal psychiatric environment is quite important. The operators and staff in such ideal facilities tend to be more involved with the facility. Operators and their families are more likely to live in the facility, and the staff is likely to eat with the residents.

Facilities with an ideal psychiatric environment are also characterized by factors that tend to reduce personal strain between residents and the facility's operators. Such facilities are likely to have operators with outside financial support, who are not totally dependent upon the facility for their income. In psychiatric emergencies these facilities are also likely to make use of social workers from the local welfare department rather than hospitals. This does not, however, imply that psychiatric treatment is absent. In fact residents in these facilities are more likely to be in some form of psychiatric treatment than other residents.

The tendency of the staff to rely less on psychiatric hospitalization is important in terms of relationship with the residents. Although the psychiatric hospital and the involuntary hospitalization of residents have an important role in the care of the chronic mentally ill, the use of these prosthetic devices by operators creates a significant power differential between them and their clientele.

Residents perceiving their operator as willing to use psychiatric hospitalization are more likely to maintain social distance between themselves and the operators and staff, because of this power differential. Involvement in facilities where there is a major power differential between residents and operators is very difficult; the resident must continually be alert to his status in the facility and his relationship with the operator if he is to "stay out of trouble."

The ideal psychiatric environment is the most powerful predictor of internal integration for all individuals excepting the young (18–33) and the asymptomatic subgroup. For these subgroups the ideal psychiatric environment becomes second in importance to the rural environment. The greater degree of isolation experienced by these individuals in the rural environment encourages their more intensive involvement within the facility.

Only 4 of the 12 predictors of internal integration are significant for the severely ill subgroup. Whereas three of these predictors are individual characteristics, the fourth and strongest factor is the ideal psychiatric environment.

Perceived Helpfulness of Services.   The second most important facility characteristic predicting internal integration is the composite of the operators' opinions about the importance of seven community services in helping residents. The services included in this composite are (1) services under local contract from the State-sponsored follow-up agency (CCSS of the Department of Health), (2) community-mental-health-center service, (3) private psychiatric service, (4) private physician service, (5) welfare services, (6) private social agency service, and (7) services obtained from other operators.

Three factors appeared independently to influence the operators' opinions of whether a service is helpful. The first influence is the operator's familiarity with services. The more operators have services available and use them, the more likely they are to report them helpful to residents. In addition facilities offering in-house therapy and recreation programs, and operators who view themselves as more than caretakers and whose family becomes involved with the residents, are more likely to report that services are helpful.

The second influence on the operators' perception involves the ability of the service to help operators meet immediate demands on their time. Operators are more likely to report that services are helpful if their residents report some psychological upset in the past 6 months requiring the operators' attention. However, facilities having their own work-training programs, exercising less control over medication, and having only selective curfew requirements are likely to report that formal services are not helpful to them. One might conclude that these facilities have a less disturbed population and therefore may find the clinically oriented services in this composite less helpful. Familiarity with and utility of services for the operator produce a service orientation in the facility that requires residents' involvements in facility-mediated service activity and therefore enhances internal integration.

The third influence on operators' service perceptions is social control. Services may be a significant mechanism of social control, as supported by the fact that facilities exercising less control over residents are less likely to report that services are helpful to them. Operators are more likely to report services helpful to them if they received complaints from the neighborhood. It is the attempt of the operator to insulate his residents and his facility through service involvements that enhances residents' internal integration and fulfills the needs of social control.

We have explored the relationship between social control and psychopathology with respect to the benefits offered by services in more detail in Chapter 6. Note, however, that, whether or not a social-control component exists with respect to the offering of services, the operator's perception of services as helpful enhances the residents' internal integration in the facility—an important finding regardless of the social-control implications.

The perceived helpfulness of services was not significant in promoting internal integration for the young and the severely symptomatic. In the latter subgroup, individual characteristics, particularly level of distress, overshadowed almost everything else, excepting the ideal psychiatric environment. For the former group the direction of service efforts is often focused on activity external to the facility. Thus the impact on internal integration of services that are perceived as helpful to the young may be minimized.

Residence Club.   The third most important facility predictor of internal integration is whether or not a facility can be characterized as a residence club. Residence-club facilities have a negative influence on the residents' internal integration. The residence club has a transient quality, or at least an atmosphere in which staff are less involved in the ongoing life of their residents. The lack of staff involvement creates a situation where the responsibility for promoting internal integration falls on the shoulders of other residents who may be either unwilling or unable to carry it. This is why the internal integration of older residents and the asymptomatic is not affected by this predictor—these groups are more likely to desire and to have the ability to accept this responsibility.

Residence-club facilities attempt to provide a nice living environment as opposed to a treatment setting. They definitely are not family oriented in their operation. Residence clubs report several areas in the facility off limits to residents, despite the fact that the operator usually does not live in the facility, and so the areas off limits are not the personal living quarters of the operator.

Operators of residence clubs are in business for income. They tend to view themselves as caretakers rather than therapists. Operators of these facilities are more likely to report religious commitment as a reason for entering the business, rather than seeking companionship or helping people. These operators tend to be somewhat more educated than other operators, and their income comes exclusively from the facility.

Residence clubs rely on the private physician for psychiatric emergencies and general care. These facilities have difficulty getting psychological care for their residents. They do not provide recreation therapy programs at the house, though they are likely to provide some form of work-training program.

A large proportion of residence-club populations are viewed by facility operators as unemployable and as having alcoholic problems. Admittance procedures in these facilities emphasize compatibility with others. Thus the residence club is not much more than a hotel, offering shelter primarily in the physical sense of the term.

Social Isolation of the Resident Group.   The fourth facility characteristic that predicts internal integration is the extent to which the residents as a group can be characterized as isolated from their community. Young and asymptomatic individuals experience the greatest impact of this predictor. This predictor is negatively related to internal integration; isolation of an entire group of facility residents from the external community depresses the level of each individual's internal involvement within the facility.

The factors related to social isolation of the resident group have been outlined in Chapter 10. Individuals in facilities where residents as a group are isolated are older, more likely to be abandoned by their families, and more likely to feel the facility is poor. The younger resident misplaced in a facility with only an aged population develops few internal relationships. The age and degree of handicap of the resident population in the facility are not, however, the only significant variables determining the relationship between the socially isolated group and internal integration. (For example, facilities serving the mentally retarded are less likely to have socially isolated groups.) In addition to resident's handicap we must consider characteristics of the facility leading to increased or diminished social interaction among residents, and situations that are frustrating to both operators and residents and lead to the reluctance on the part of facility operators to promote activities for their residents.

We find that residents will be less isolated as a group when the facility's programs are geared to provide a therapeutic as well as practical orientation to the environment. For example, facilities providing work-training programs for both therapeutic and rehabilitative reasons are less likely to be characterized by overall isolation than facilities that transport their residents to individual treatment or simply provide a nondirected living arrangement.

We also found that too much control of social behavior, as well as too little control, tends to increase social isolation. For example, very early curfew or no curfew at all increases isolation. Appropriate structure and limits are important in the facility's environment if isolation is to be avoided. Unfortunately it is difficult for the operator who wants to be perceived as a "nice guy" to provide appropriate environmental structure. Operators entering the business for companionship tend to surround themselves with relatively isolated (both internally and externally) residents. It does not, however, follow that operators should not become involved with residents. In fact, isolation of the resident group is reduced by the willingness of staff to eat with the residents. The operator must, however, control the temptation to "be just one of the gang."

The impact of social isolation on social behavior was vividly illustrated by Stanton and Schwartz (1954) in their observations of incontinence among hospitalized patients. Incontinence hardly ever occurred off the ward and never occurred at social activities such as dancing or outings. It was most likely to occur in situations of isolation, where individuals were unable in any way to display their social capability. Thus the impact of the socially isolated group on an individual's internal integration in a facility is significant, not only for its immediate outcome, but also for its possible destruction of an individual's social capabilities.

Female Operator.   Female operators tend to run facilities that encourage internal integration. As a facility characteristic predicting internal integration, operator's sex ranks fifth in importance. The major factor in the positive relationship between the female operator and internal integration is the distinction between the types of programs run by male and female operators. Males are more likely than females to be more educated, run a larger program, and have a more professional facility. On the other hand female operators are more likely to run a family-oriented facility and to see their role in the facility as that of a parent. In the parental role the female operator creates a family-oriented atmosphere that tends to enhance internal integration of the residents. These operators are most likely to have a positive impact on the internal integration of the older, less disturbed resident.

Resident Control of Medication.   After controlling for current psychopathology, chronicity, and whether or not a resident has a conservator, we found that, in facilities where none of the residents keep their own medication, there is a tendency for older residents to have increased internal integration and for younger residents to have decreased internal integration. Decreased internal integration of younger residents, owing to total control of medication, results from higher dosing of this population (to a point where they are unable to relate to fellow residents) or from their attempt to avoid involvements with such a controlling environment by not taking their medications and staying away from the facility as much as possible.

Two factors seem to explain how medication control relates to internal integration. First, environments that exercise total control over medication tend to be family-oriented homes. We are more likely to find some residents keeping their own medications in facilities that claim to be therapeutic communities and have a treatment focus. Perhaps these therapeutic communities can more easily afford the "risk" (given the fact that they have a staff and are not concerned with protecting their own families) of allowing some residents to keep their own medications. It is also possible that operators of the family-oriented facilities use the medications as a crutch, deriving a certain sense of safety by the presence of medication. In addition the operators of family-style facilities are often women, who may exercise greater control over residents' medication owing to their own sense of vulnerability.

The second factor relating medication control to internal integration is that facilities that have been complained about are most likely to exercise total control over medication. In these cases control of medication as a safety factor for operators is apparent.

The overall benefit of medications for the resident in the facility is discussed in Chapter 14. It should be noted, however, that total control of medications focuses the life of the older individual inward toward the facility, especially when an individual is required to take several doses of drugs daily, and may force the younger resident to flight.

Resident Characteristics

In predicting internal integration, three resident characteristics were considered:

1. Individual psychological distress.
2. Resident's perception of having sufficient spending money.
3. Whether or not the resident individually chose to come to the facility (involuntary resident).

The first has a significant negative effect on internal integration; the second a significant positive effect; and the third is statistically significant in a negative direction for only a portion of the sheltered-care population.

Individual Psychological Distress.   Psychological distress tended to have a severe negative impact upon an individual's internal integration. While it is the strongest resident characteristic, individual psychological distress is third in importance among all the predictors we considered with regard to predicting an individual's internal integration and becomes increasingly important for those with higher levels of overt symptomatology. This is evidenced, not only by its increased strength as a predictor for the more symptomatic subgroup, but also by the fact that there are fewer significant predictors of internal integration in this subgroup.

A resident's distress level is a combination of his score on the Langner Scale and the Overall and Gorham Brief Psychiatric Rating Scale (BPRS). These two measures focus on internally reported symptoms and overtly observed symptomatology, respectively. Residents in distress are likely to feel unsafe on the streets and to be suicidal, overtly delusional, and depressed. They report a high level of general dissatisfaction and recent upsets, which they attribute to intrapersonal as opposed to interpersonal causes.

Consciously these residents tend to be less concerned about their external environment than other residents. They score lower on the Marlow Crown Social Desirability Scale than others do. They also express less obligation to the operators of their facilities and are less likely to be concerned about violation of social norms—that is, they were more frequently involved in loud arguments and had been picked up by the police more frequently during the past year than other residents.

Despite this conscious lack of concern for conformity to social norms and authority, distressed residents are aware of the character of their environment. They are likely to describe their facility as an environment that tolerates the expression of anger and aggression and has a lack of order and organization about it. These residents also report less of a demand on them for program involvement in the environment they live in than residents of other facilities do.

These observations are important in terms of the distressed resident's unconscious reactions to his/her facility environment. Stanton and Schwartz (1954) and Caudill (1958), in independent investigations, showed the impact of disturbances in the social environment upon the expression of psychological disturbance among mental-hospital patients. Our data are consistent with theirs in this respect. We found, however, that psychological distress tends overall to decrease an individual's level of internal integration in the facility in which he lives.

Sufficient Spending Money. The second most important resident characteristic, positively related to internal integration, was whether or not the resident perceived himself to have sufficient spending money to do the things he wished to do in his environment. To a large extent individuals who reported that they had sufficient spending money were, in fact, not being funded under General Relief or General Assistance Budgets and did have more money than other residents.

Interestingly, for the most severely disturbed population, the direction of this predictor becomes negative—those responding that they had enough spending money to do what they wanted to do and who were severely disturbed had lower levels of internal integration. This finding is consistent with discussions on the mentally ill indicating their wish to avoid personal involvements (Roman & Trice, 1967). We pursue this point in greater detail in our discussion of the relationship between internal and external integration.

Aside from the severely disturbed group, residents reporting that they have sufficient spending money and showing increased internal integration are likely to be independent in their activities and to have chosen the facility in which they are living; they tend to rate the facility positively and wish to stay at the facility.

Involuntary Resident. Involuntary residents did not choose the facility in which they are currently living. Although being an involuntary resident is not a statistically significant predictor of internal integration for the total sheltered-care population when considered jointly with other predictors, it is significant for the asymptomatic subgroup, and the direction of its influence is negative.

Residents who did not choose the facility they were living in are less satisfied with it. They are likely to have trusted somebody else's judgment in the choice of facilities, which involves, at minimum, a period of adjustment to someone else's choice. The anticipation of being involved in such an environment does not exist.

SUMMARY

The predictors of internal integration vary most between the severely symptomatic and the asymptomatic, in that neighborhood reception factors become nonsignificant for the former subgroup. In addition more factors—nine as compared with four—are available to promote the internal integration of the asymptomatic.

The importance of internal integration in our society must not be underestimated, not only because of the health implications of a supportive environment mentioned earlier in this chapter, but also because of the need of people in today's society to seek out supportive relationships. The Community Mental Health movement is attempting to encourage people to reintegrate into a society that is yearly becoming more disintegrated even for the "normal." The difficulty of integration and the need for an alternative community are apparent in the increasing number of people joining organizations such as Synanon (even people with no drug involvement) and religious movements such as that sponsored by the Reverend Moon. These people are seeking a life-style conducive to a higher level of internal involvement and support than they have been able to achieve within the traditional social structure.

In summing up his involvement in the facility in which he currently lives, one young man said, "I've got friends here and I feel loved." This man spends time with his friends in the facility, goes places with them, and enjoys things with them. In doing so, he has achieved an involvement within this facility that would have been extremely difficult for him to achieve without the supportive environment provided by the sheltered-care living arrangement. Such involvement is crucial and should be seen as an end in itself.

REFERENCES

Barton, R. *Institutional Neurosis*. Bristol, England: J. Wright and Sons, 1959.

Caudill, W. *The Psychiatric Hospital as a Small Society*. Cambridge, Massachusetts: Harvard University Press, 1958.

Comstock, G. W. and K. B. Partridge. "Church Attendance and Health." *J. Chron. Dis.* **25**, 665–672 (1971).

Enstrom, J. E. "Cancer Mortality Among Mormons." *Cancer*, **36**(3), 825–841 (1975).

Fairweather, G. W., D. Sanders, H. Maynard, D. Cressler, and D. Blech. *Community Life for the Mentally Ill: An Alternative to Institutional Care*. Chicago: Aldine, 1969.

Moos, R. H. *Evaluating Treatment Environments: A Social Ecological Approach*. New York: Wiley, 1974.

Rassidakis, N. C., M. Kelepouris, K. Goulis, and K. Karaiossefidis. "On the Incidence of Malignancy Among Schizophrenic Patients." *Aggressologie*, **14**(4), 269–273 (1973).

Roman, P. M. and H. M. Trice. *Schizophrenia and the Poor*. Ithaca, New York: Cayuga Press, 1967.

Scheff, T. J. *Being Mentally Ill: A Sociological Theory.* Chicago: Aldine, 1966.

Segal, S., J. Baumohl, and E. Johnson. "Falling Through the Cracks: Mental Disorder and Social Margin in a Young Vagrant Population." *Social Problems,* 24(3), 387-400(1977).

Stanton, A. H. and M. S. Schwartz. *The Mental Hospital.* New York: Basic Books, 1954.

Wing. J. "Institutionalism in Mental Hospitals." *Brit. J. Soc. and Clin. Psych.* 1, 38–51 (1962).

TWELVE

Bridging the Gap: The Relation Between Internal and External Integration

Advocates of community care for the mentally ill have attempted summarily to reduce social dependency by moving individuals into the community. They hoped this tactic would stop the development of institutional neuroses, whereby individuals became so dependent upon the hospital they were unable to leave. In view of the community-care goal of involving individuals in the external environment, the importance of internal integration is the extent to which it "bridges the gap" between the facility and the community.

BRIDGING THE GAP: A PERSONAL EXPERIENCE

It was very hard to leave the house. In fact it took me six months to move out. It was just very difficult for me—difficult for me to move in and when I got settled, it got increasingly more difficult to move out because you get the feeling of security there. The meals are there. It's a kind of psychological bind because I was afraid to move out and yet I wanted to move out. I had been there eight months. Before that there was no pressure, but after six months, there seemed to be more pressure put on the residents to move out (F.N.).*

This quote indicates the difficulty experienced by one former resident of a halfway house in attempting to bridge the gap, to move back into the outside world, the external community. This individual had relatives nearby willing and able to take him in and lived in a community where he had many friends outside the halfway house. In addition to the social supports available outside, the facility itself exerted some pressure on him to move out. Ultimately he was able to share an apartment with a friend who was not in any way involved with the facility.

This chapter, as did our chapter on external integration, focuses on residents' efforts to reach out independently to the external community from the facility. Such efforts are a minimum prerequisite to the more difficult move to independent living reported by this individual.

FOUR COMPONENTS OF SOCIAL INTEGRATION

To understand the relationship between the environment and an individual's level of internal and external integration, we must look at four sets of facilitating or hindering factors involved in internal and external functioning, as follows: (1) social support, (2) social insulation, (3) social facilitation, and (4) social-dependency-producing variables (see Table 12.1). The social-support variables enhance an individual's level of both internal integration and external integration. The social-insulation variables enhance an individual's internal integration but have no effect on his external integration. On the other hand social-facilitation variables enhance an individual's external integration but have no effect on his internal integration. Finally the social-dependency-producing variables enhance an individual's internal involvement in the facility at the expense of his involvement in the external community.

In our data on the sheltered-care environment, social-support variables are found to be the strongest factors influencing both internal and external social integration.† Social-dependency-producing variables are second in importance, social-facilitation variables are third, followed by social-insulation factors.

Given the presumption in the past that social-dependency-producing variables predominate in the mental-hospital environment (Goffman, 1961), our findings indicating a predominance of social-support variables in commu-

*F.N. refers to field notes taken at the time of a structured or open-ended interview.
†The relative ranking of the four sets of factors is based on the size of the average partial beta weights for each group of predictors in the external and internal integration models.

Table 12.1   Four Components of Social Integration [a]

Components of Social Integration	Direction of Relationship	
	External	Internal
1. Social-support factors		
Neighbors' positive response	+	+
Ideal psychiatric environment	+	+
Sufficient spending money	+	+
Distress	−	−
Social isolation of resident group	−	−
2. Social-insulation factors		
Downtown area	n.s.	−
Operator perceives services as helpful	n.s.	+
Residence club	n.s.	−
Female operator	n.s.	+
3. Social-facilitation factors		
Involuntary resident	−	n.s.
Complaints to authorities	−	n.s.
Resident's control of money (resident pays bill)	+	n.s.
4. Social-dependency factors		
Rural area	−	+
Distance (closeness to resources produces a higher score)	+	−
Residents do not control medications	−	+

[a] All plus and minus signs refer to the direction of the relationship indicated by the sign of the standardized partial regression weights in the external- and internal-integration models respectively discussed in Chapters 10 and 11. Relationships are significant at least $p < .10$ on the assumption of a simple random sample; n.s. means not significant.

nity-based sheltered care demonstrate a major difference between these environments in the extent to which the social-dependency-producing variables are influential in the individual's social integration. In fact, because social-support variables predominate, community-based sheltered care is a more desirable context than the mental hospital if the goal is moving someone out into the external community. This is true, of course, only to the extent that Goffman's description of the hospital as dependency producing is correct. Others have viewed the patient's role in the context of the hospital community as a more active one (Braginsky et al., 1969).

The 4 sets of factors relating to external and internal integration involve 15 independent predictors that are open to modification by policy action. In

Chapters 10 and 11 we analyzed these predictors and their separate effects on the internal and external integration of individuals in sheltered care. In this chapter we see how each of these predictors relates jointly to internal and external integration, to determine how they affect one's effort to bridge the gap between the facility and the outside world.

Social-Support Variables

In order of their relative importance for the total resident population (based on the averaged ranked importance of a factor in predicting external and internal integration) the social-support variables predictive of both external and internal integration are "neighbors' positive response," "the ideal psychiatric environment," "sufficient spending money," "psychological distress," and "social isolation of the resident group."

While "neighbors' positive response" ranked first in importance as a predictor of external integration and second for internal integration, the ideal psychiatric environment predictor ranked seventh for external and first for internal integration. Thus, in the overall perspective, the community response to individuals in the facility was most important when considered as a predictor of both social-integration variables. This result is consistent with research on the outcome of in-hospital programs (focusing on the internal environment) developed to promote external integration. Fairweather (1964), in an earlier study, developed a ward-based program that markedly changed the behavior of the residents in the hospital but had little carry-over to the outside community once the patient left the hospital. This result emphasizes again the importance of directing change efforts toward the environment in which the change is expected to occur.

Whereas positive neighborhood response and the ideal psychiatric environment enhanced the internal and external integration of the sheltered-care population when considered as a total group, they cannot be considered social-support variables for those individuals in the population who are most severely disturbed or symptomatic. For this latter group positive neighbor response is a social facilitator—promoting external and unrelated to internal integration—and the ideal psychiatric environment is a social insulator—promoting internal integration with no effect on external integration. In fact, for the severely ill, there are no social-support variables simultaneously promoting internal and external integration! This seems to be due to the fact that internal and external integration for this population subgroup are unrelated to one another. The Pearson Product Moment correlation between internal and external integration for the most severely disturbed group is .11 as compared to .42 and .31 for the mildly disturbed and asymptomatic groups respectively (both the latter correlations are statistically significant).

There are two hypotheses that offer some explanation for the lack of relationship between internal and external integration for the most severely disturbed subgroup. The first relates to the fact that the severely disturbed group has much lower levels of both internal and external integration than the rest of the population in sheltered care. Using the analogy of a developing country in economics, one can argue that, before the impact of development in one area of the economy can be experienced in another, a minimal amount of development is necessary in both areas. In other words, for internal integration to have an impact on external integration (and vice versa), a minimum amount of both assets must be possessed by the individual.

The second explanatory hypothesis involves the observation that internal and external integration have a different meaning for the severely ill population than for the mildly disturbed and asymptomatic populations. This latter argument derives from the observation made in the mental-health literature that the severely mentally ill are running away from close relationships (Ödegaard, 1932) or do better in avoiding intense emotional involvements (Brown, Birley, & Wing, 1972). Thus, for the asymptomatic and mildly ill, internal relationships may be used as a means of gaining experience and enhancing external relationships (and vice versa); for the severely ill internal relationships are avoided through the use of external involvements. For this latter group, encouraging internal involvements depends largely upon the well-designed and supportive ideal psychiatric environment.

The more externally integrated resident in the severe-pathology subgroup is more willing to move out of the sheltered-care facility than other individuals are, less likely to wish to remain at the facility for long periods of time, and more likely to spend time looking for an independent living arrangement. In considering a move out of the sheltered-care facility, this resident seems indifferent to (1) reasonable fears associated with establishing an independent household and (2) positive characteristics of the facility in which he lives. Consideration of the loneliness of living alone, the opinion that the sheltered-care facility he is currently living in is a physically and socially nicer place to live than the place the resident might find on his own, and the belief that the other residents are more of a family than the resident's natural family have no bearing on his decision to move! Indifference to such factors and a mobile orientation are characteristic of the severely ill. They are not characteristic of those individuals in the asymptomatic or mild-pathology subgroups. In fact, the more externally integrated one becomes in these latter subgroups, the more consideration he gives to characteristics of the facility in which he resides. For those with no and mild symptomatology ratings, characteristics of the facility and personal fears become important factors in considering a move.

It is possible that those residents with severe symptomatology do not consider home life to be a positive experience for them, and so they choose to focus on a life outside of the home. It therefore would not matter if an apartment of their own was not as attractive physically or socially as the sheltered-care home. A history of negative experiences with their own families may have helped to develop an external orientation, and so they may prefer to be out of the house as much as possible. It is possible that people in the "severe" group project their own unhappiness onto their immediate environment, and in their attempt to avoid this unhappiness, adopt a mobile life-style. Although Brown, Birley, and Wing (1972) speak of former hospital patients' doing better in environments with less intensive emotional involvements, we would think that the intensity and quality of such involvements need further study, since severely disturbed individuals with higher levels of internal integration wanted to stay on at the facility for longer time periods and the ideal psychiatric environment tended to promote internal integration. It would appear, however, that the severe subgroup has a more difficult time dealing with their internal environment, is in need of a more selectively designed environment, and will use external integration to avoid internal commitments.

The third most important social-support predictor facilitating both external and internal integration of the total sheltered-care population is the extent to which residents perceive they have sufficient spending money to do what they would like to do. With respect to the quality of life, having the amount of money necessary to do what one wishes to do not only bolsters the ability to reach out to the external world but also makes interaction within the facility easier. This observation is, however, true only for the largest subgroup in the population showing mild pathology. For the asymptomatic group, having sufficient spending money is a social facilitator—it promotes external integration with no impact on internal integration. The severe subgroup again differs from the other two in the impact of this predictor. For severely disturbed individuals, having sufficient spending money promotes their external integration at the expense of their internal involvements. This relationship is consistent with our observations regarding the wishes of the severely ill to avoid internal commitments and introduces a new dimension to what we might previously have conceived of as a variable, the opposite of which would have been in the social-dependency class. Given the unique character of the severely disturbed group, variables promoting their external integration at the expense of their internal involvements might be termed *social-flight*-producing factors.

Social-support predictors that reduce both internal and external integration are "psychological distress" and "social isolation of the resident group." We include these factors, most notably, level of psychological distress, as social-support variables because modifying these variables (e.g., reducing individual distress levels) will have a generalized positive impact on social behavior as measured both by internal and external integration.

The concept of "psychological distress" was initially used in the analysis of external and internal integration as an intervening variable (i.e., one that may alter the causal interpretation of the predictors to the criterion). This was done because of the underlying assumption that the disability of the mentally ill stands in the way of their social functioning. Of the 15 predictors considered as facilitators or hindrances to social integration, psychological distress was the fourth most important factor overall, as well as the fourth most important social-support variable. Its importance may be underestimated, however, because 7.6% of the sample population were not interviewed, since they were too emotionally disturbed. Higher levels of psychological distress, even within categories classified by their level of symptomatology, remained a generally negative influence on both internal and external integration.

The extent to which psychological distress can be demobilizing is vividly illustrated by the following interviewer remarks:

The interviewer went into his bedroom to see him at 2:00 p.m. The resident had been heavily medicated and was sleeping most of the day. He was a college student who had withdrawn from contact with other residents in his facility and the social contacts in his environment after continuous unsuccessful attempts to become involved in an "intellectually challenging college career." Each attempt on his part was accompanied by a setback due to extreme psychological problems, leading to admission to a new facility, and to his progressive withdrawal (F.N.).

The negative impact of "social isolation of the resident group" on a given individual's level of internal and external integration is also quite important from a sociological perspective. This factor describes the extent to which all residents of a given facility are characterized by the operator as isolated from families and neighbors. It is a significant factor only in reducing the internal and external integration of the population subgroup having no overt symptomatology. The negative relationship to external and internal integration implies that an individual living in this context will be more isolated from social contacts outside as well as inside the facility. Whereas this could be the result of selection—that is, isolated individuals tend to be placed together in the same facility—it may also reflect an aspect of the "social-breakdown syndrome," a redefinition of one's self as chronically sick. Gruenberg (1963) has offered a tentative seven-stage formulation of the syndrome's pathogenesis:

1. Precondition or susceptibility: deficiency in self-concept (which may be characterological or precipitated by current mental turmoil).

2. Dependence on current cues.
3. Social labeling as incompetent or dangerous.
4. Induction in the sick role—that is, the suggestion that an individual adopt a passive, helpless, perhaps potentially dangerous, certainly "sick" role, with little prospect of change.
5. Learning the chronic sick role.
6. Atrophy of work and social skill.
7. Identification with the sick.

It seems reasonable for a resident to have a lower level of external integration if other residents are isolated from the community, because community rejection of the total group explains reduced acceptance of any given member. But why is there also a withdrawal from the internal community? This withdrawal indicates the existence of an additional step in the "social breakdown syndrome," following Gruenberg's "social labeling" (step three), which we shall call "normalization." Normalization is best explained as the attempt to maintain a normal self-concept by withdrawing from the immediate community associated with illness.

Gruenberg's scheme of the social-breakdown syndrome posits too easily the change in the individual's self-concept to a negative stereotype—despite his dependency and susceptibility. Karmel (1969) found, in an empirical test of Goffman's hypothesis, that self-mortification did not occur during the first month's stay in a mental hospital. Karmel found instead that, during the first month, patients experienced "a slight gain in self-esteem and social identity" (Karmel, 1969, p. 134).

Researchers have also noted the tendency of individuals to "normalize" or interpret mental-illness behavior in a more "normal" frame of reference (Clausen & Yarrow, 1955; Starr, 1955).

Consistent with these research findings, a frequent observation by our interviewers was the tendency of residents to define everybody else in the facility, but not themselves, as "crazy." In an effort to protect their identity and combat the development of the social-breakdown syndrome, residents disassociate themselves from other residents. In an external community that disallows the participation of facility residents because it defines them as mentally ill, the residents can protect this "normal" self-image only by total withdrawal. In the following excerpt the interviewer describes a vivid example of the struggle for "normalization" of one's self-concept:

I remember this late middle-aged gentlemen. We had a hard time finding him. He was standing in the dark in a hall closet, doing absolutely nothing, when we did locate him. Apparently this is something he always does so nobody cares or takes notice of him getting in and out of the closet.

When I inquired why he was in the closet, he said he had been there all morning; he liked it in there because it was comfortable. He said he's either in the closet, in his room lying down, or eating—that's all he does.

I think he enjoyed the interview because it was hard for me to get him to answer the questions. He wanted to talk to me about all kinds of things which I thought was rather strange because he didn't want to talk to anybody else. He said he was just generally tired of the people he was living with and their same old problems. It was his notion that "everybody else was crazy"; he didn't want to talk to patients; he called everybody a patient.

He amazed me with his verbal ability, and though he was a little bit delusional, his affect wasn't that bland for living the type of life he was leading. . . . As soon as I explained the study to him, he just started talking right away, telling me the types of things he didn't like about the place and the improvements he would like to see (F.N.).

Social-Dependency-Producing Factors

The second most important set of predictors we found for the total resident population is social-dependency-producing factors. They comprise the most significant set of predictors from the perspective of the iatrogenic effects attributed to mental-hospital care.

Sheltered-care environments encourage a "settling-in" behavior—a predilection to become attached to one's surroundings—characteristic of the general human condition. The strongest predictor in this group of variables is the rural versus nonrural environment. The more rural environment enhances internal and reduces external integration. A good (albeit lengthy) illustration of this phenomenon emerges from one interviewer's experiences in a rural setting in contrast to a large urban area.

The area is mostly agricultural, quite a way from the city, but there are several facilities in the area. One of the homes that I went to was very pleasing; the operators were cordial, cooperative, and eager to pass along the type of program they had established so that people in other areas might establish the same types of things. The home had a massive program; the residents were much more at ease. There wasn't much tension and there wasn't much nervousness. I don't think that the degree of mental illness is any less. I just think that the atmosphere they are living in is more relaxed and more homey than the facilities I interviewed in the city.

One facility was run by a middle-aged couple. They had mostly older people there but they had a very personal relationship with their people. They have a scrapbook of all the people they've ever had. They have birthday parties for every resident. The residents, although they are elderly, are kept fairly active except for those who can't get around. They have a large garden. All the people enjoy working in the garden. They have fresh vegetables, fresh fruits, and I think the residents are very happy to do this type of work. I say this because they are all very excited and the thing they were most proud of, I could tell, was their vegetables or onions or whatever. I spent about forty-five minutes in the garden with the operators and with their guests showing me their produce. . . .

Very few facilities in this area have that peculiar or particular odor of many of the urban board and care homes that I interviewed in. I didn't see any places that were the least bit messy or dirty. I don't know why this is, but in many of the places in the city I was just really turned off by the smell of the homes and even the people.

There wasn't quite as much idleness with the residents in this area as in the city. Just upon walking into the house, there weren't as many bodies just sitting on the porch in front of the TV. One thing that helped is that many of these places are on farms or ranches. There is plenty of work to be done and a lot of the places have what could be considered work-therapy programs where they help out in digging ditches or planting vegetables or keeping the chickens or keeping the cows. It keeps them busy. It seems very healthy and it gives them some sense of accomplishment. I think a lot of them were glad that they were learning to do new types of things (F.N.).

This interviewer's impression of the rural area versus the urban area may sound like a nineteenth-century tract extolling the benefits of rural life. It does, however, point to the fact that very attractive and supportive environments may, by their location and their all-encompassing help and support, operate to focus all involvements within the facility at the expense of the independent involvement of residents in the outside community (a community that in rural areas is often closed to the sheltered-care resident).

Whereas this observation holds for the general population, it requires some modification for those individuals who show no overt psychological disturbance. The rural environment enhances the external involvements of this subgroup, and thus for those without psychological disturbance the farm facility takes on the character of a social-support factor enhancing both internal and external integration.

Second in order of its importance as a social-dependency-producing variable is distance. The farther the facility is from community resources, the greater the level of internal integration and the lower the level of external integration (and vice versa). While it seems logical that facilities farther away from community resources would have a lower level of external integration, the fact that they also develop higher levels of internal integration is quite interesting. To some extent our figures point out that the reason for this is that facilities removed from a concentration of community resources are more likely to be family-oriented facilities in which the operator and his family live. It is also true that facilities located away from community resources are more likely to have a therapy or rehabilitation program at the house. As a result of these two factors, plus the independent unavailability of outside community resources for residents (unless they have their own transportation, which is unusual in this population), "distance" from community resources becomes a social-dependency-producing variable.

A third social-dependency-producing factor is "resident lack of control over their medication." Facilities in which none of the residents control their own medication tend to foster an environment that increases internal and reduces external integration. The policy of selective control of medication in sheltered care leads, however, to a certain amount of risk. For example, Janet Chase (1973) writes of a patient who saved enough Miltown® to commit suicide. The point of Chase's example was to expose poor medication practices in some sheltered-care facilities. However, a negative consequence of rigid supervision of medications is that residents are tied to the facility by a medication schedule that interferes with their ability to move into the external environment. We observed several facilities where, like the hospital ward, social life was organized around the dispensation of medication. This has the obvious effect of focusing an individual's life inward on the facility and increasing his internal integration.

The issue of medication in general is discussed in Chapter 14. We stress here, however, that a selective policy regarding control of medication requires responsible judgment on the part of professionals who supervise medication. Flexibility in this procedure should be given more consideration because of the impact it may have in encouraging people to move out into the community. It also appears that the type of internal integration sacrificed in the policy is one that is dysfunctional because of its emphasis on the sick role, that is, because it forces interaction around the dispensing of medication.

Social Facilitation

Social-facilitation variables tend to promote an individual's level of external integration without affecting internal integration. Three social-facilitation variables are considered here: "the involuntary resident," "complaints to authorities," and "resident control of money." Being an involuntary resident or living in a facility that has complaints made about it to the authorities leads to a reduction in residents' external integration. Having control of one's spending money increases a resident's external integration.

The involuntary resident is the strongest social-facilitation predictor even after level of psychological distress, chronicity, conservatorship, and individual ability are controlled for. This resident did not choose the facility he is currently living in. To some extent the involuntary resident has given up attempting to influence his own environment.

One resident was transferred to his current facility by the owner of his previous facility, which had gone out of business. He expressed a sense of hopelessness and wondered if anything were worthwhile anymore. He was always bored, and had withdrawn to the point of spending most of his time in bed. Despite his dissatisfaction with his current living arrangement, he accepts what comes (F.N.).

In this case we see evidence of negative impact on external as well as internal integration: The individual is withdrawing into his bed as a result of being involuntarily moved from one living arrangement to another.

Looking within subgroups of the sheltered-care population who evidence differing levels of psychological disturbance, we found that, for those individuals showing no overt symptomatology, being unable to choose their facility is significantly and negatively related to both internal and external integration; thus, not directing or participating in the placement process takes on the character of a social-support variable for the "normals." For the mildly ill this variable takes on the character of a social-dependency-producing factor; that is, it encourages internal at the expense of external integration, and for the severely ill, it leads to social flight (discouraging internal and encouraging external integration).

Changes observed in the character of the involuntary-resident predictor for those with differing degrees of overt symptomatology appear to be related to the different stages of the social-breakdown syndrome (though we have no independent assessment of the latter other than the open-ended observations in interview reports).

We have previously observed that, after the social-breakdown-syndrome stage of being labeled "socially incompetent or dangerous," the individual may enter a stage in which his behavior can be interpreted as an attempt to retain his normal self-concept—a "normalization" stage. We have also pointed out that in this stage the individual can react by withdrawal from both the external and internal environments that have labeled him deviant. Thus the reaction of the resident in the subgroup with no overt symptomatology to the loss of his prerogative of choosing his residence is found to be withdrawal from involvements with social contacts in both the internal and external environments that have sanctioned (at least in the eyes of the individual) his involuntary placement.

Looking at the subgroup showing a "mild" or "moderate" degree of overt symptomatology, we find individuals more likely to be in the stages of (1) "induction into the sick role—that is, the suggestion that an individual adopt a passive, helpless, perhaps potentially dangerous, certainly 'sick' role, with little prospect for change" or (2) "learning the chronic sick role." At this stage the reaction to the deprivation of one's prerogative to choose one's residence leads to a withdrawal from the external community (the "normal" community)—as evidenced by the individual's reduced level of external integration— and an increase in involvement with "all the other crazy people he lives with," an increment in his internal integration. For those with mild symptomatology, then, "the involuntary resident factor" is social-dependency-producing.

Finally those individuals evidencing a high degree of symptomatology are more likely to have actually come to identify themselves with the sick role. Their identification is often, however, tinged with a learned hostility toward the system that seeks to help them. Segal, Baumohl, and Johnson (1977) report the sentiments of an eloquent "adolescent schizophrenic" regarding his unwillingness to obtain disability benefits to which he is entitled. This young man says:

Like I don't think I'm *that* crazy. . . . But they won't give me any money until I confess my sins, man. I gotta say "yeah, man, I'm a fuckin' lunatic," and sign ten forms and see eight doctors to prove it. And then they might really lock me up! (Segal, Baumohl, & Johnson, 1977, p. 394).

For those individuals with overt symptomatology the deprivation of the right to choose one's residence becomes a social-flight variable—a variable encouraging whatever external involvements they can muster (which we noted earlier is minimal) and discouraging their involvements with helpers and an internal environment they mistrust. These individuals have accepted the definition of themselves as sick but are avoiding the social implication of that definition in which all interactions in one's environment are made contingent upon and follow from such a definition.

In the helper's need to help lurks the temptation to take over—a temptation that may result in debilitating effects for the recipient of the help. Only 57% of the sheltered-care population respond that on a typical day most of the things they do are planned by themselves. We found that choosing one's residence is significantly related to whether or not one plans his daily activities. In the following example we note how hospital patients can be socialized into a role of being unable to plan their own activities. In commenting on her treatment at the hospital, one woman said:

I would be out of those treatments they were giving! I have gotten tired and they was running me plum crazy, you know. Treatments, they drive me crazy. I was always shocked up. I was so nervous that I was unhappy there and I was so nervous and upset that I would just sit in one place, scared to look down the hallway because there was the room, and there were those doctors and those nurses down there. They call me at any time to take treatments (F.N.).

This woman spent almost all her time waiting to be called on. To the extent that a resident's time is organized around the needs or demands of the facility, and to the extent that he is asked to acquiesce in these needs, all his activities become contingent upon his illness. It is such an experience that is avoided by the "well" residents through withdrawal, acquiesced in by the "mildly" symptomatic, and avoided through the flight of the most severely symptomatic.

Social Insulation

Social-insulation variables are significantly related to internal integration, enhancing or detracting from one's involvement in the facility, and have no effect on external involvements. The four variables considered, in order of their overall importance as social-insulation predictors, are "downtown area," "operator perceives services as helpful," "residence club," and "female operator."

"Downtown area" and the "residence club" are negatively related to internal integration. On the other hand "perceived helpfulness of services" and the "female operator" tend to increase the individual's level of internal involvement in the facility. Manipulating these factors to encourage social involvement within the facility is expedient, because they have no negative implications for external integration.

CONCLUSION

The positive relationship between internal and external integration and the finding that the strongest predictors of these criteria are social-support factors either facilitating or hindering both leads us to the conclusion that the appropriate focus of the design of a sheltered-care facility does not depend upon choosing between internal and external integration or using one type of integration, internal, as a means of promoting an assumedly more advanced type, external (the transitional goal); the appropriate focus is to determine how to design an environment that is dependent on factors that facilitate both internal and external integration in a manner that compromises neither—that is, does not rely primarily on social-dependency-producing characteristics.

In the designing of sheltered-care environments the needs of specific subgroups in the population must be taken into account both in terms of how characteristics affect internal and external integration in a given subgroup—that is, whether the characteristic is a social supporter, social insulator, social facilitator, or a social-dependency-producing factor—and in terms of changes in the meaning of the relationship between external and internal integration for a particular subgroup (e.g., the change we noted in distinguishing social-flight predictors in the severely symptomatic subgroup).

The danger that long-term sheltered care encourages internal at the expense of external integration will remain as long as social-dependency-producing characteristics are inadvertently allowed to operate, though a moderate level of internal integration in a long-term living arrangement may be more desirable and more realistic for much of the population.

Our goal for this population is, however, to promote both internal and external involvements to the extent possible from within the sheltered-care setting according to individual need and with a limited emphasis on transition to independent living situations.

REFERENCES

Braginsky, M., D. D. Braginsky, and K. Ring. *Methods of Madness*. New York: Holt, Rinehart, and Winston, 1969.

Brown, G. W., J. L. T. Birley, and J. K. Wing. "Influence of Family Life on the Course of Schizophrenic Disorders: A Replication." *Brit. J. Psychiat.* **121** (March) 241–258 (1972).

Chase, J. "Where Have All the Patients Gone?" *Human Behavior*, **2** (October) 14–21 (1973).

Clausen, J. and M. R. Yarrow (Eds.). "The Impact of Mental Illness on the Family." *Contemporary Social Problems*, **11**(4), entire issue (1955).

Fairweather, G. W. *Social Psychology in Treating Mental Illness: An Experimental Approach*. New York: Wiley, 1964.

Goffman, E. *Asylums: Essays on the Social Situation of Mental Patients and Other Inmates*. Garden City, New York: Doubleday, 1961.

Gruenberg, E. M. "Discussion of Critical Reviews of Pueblo, Western, and Denver Tri-County Divisions," in Bernard Stone (Ed.). *A Critical Review of Treatment Progress in a State Hospital Reorganized Toward the Communities Served*. Pueblo, Colorado: Pueblo Association for Mental Health, May 1963 (mimeographed).

Karmel, M. "Total Institutions and Self-Mortification." *J. Health and Social Behavior*, **10**(2), 134–142 (1969).

Ödegaard, Ö. *Emigration and Insanity: A Study of Mental Disease Among the Norwegian-Born Population of Minnesota*. Copenhagen, Denmark: Evin Munksgaards Publishers, 1932.

Segal, S., J. Baumohl, and E. Johnson. "Falling Through the Cracks: Mental Disorder and Social Margin in a Young Vagrant Population." *Social Problems*, **24**(3), 387–400(1977).

Starr, S. "The Public's Ideas About Mental Illness." Paper presented at the Annual Meeting of the National Association for Mental Health. Indianapolis, Nov. 1955.

PART SIX

THE SHELTERED-CARE RESIDENT:CONSUMER OR COMMODITY?

The focus of Part VI is on the consideration of the supportive aids available and how these aids can be employed in promoting successful community care for the mentally ill. We consider these aids and the factors that influence their availability from the perspective of the sheltered-care resident both as a consumer of such aids and as an object of barter in the service system.

In Chapter 13 we develop a typology of service delivery based upon goals shared by residents and service providers and upon the major foci of service (the individual and his interactions with his community).

In Chapter 14 we consider the role of antipsychotic medications—one of the major supportive aids in the sheltered-care system. We look at the impact of these medications on residents' levels of internal and external integration.

In Chapter 15 we consider the role of the resident in the helping interaction, noting those areas in which he/she is able more effectively to adopt a consumer role and describing how adopting such a role may best be facilitated.

THIRTEEN

Developing a Typology of
Sheltered-Care Service

Individuals who become sheltered-care residents are in an ambiguous role vis-à-vis the people who provide services to them. The crucial element of sheltered care involves the provision of some form of resident supervision. As part of that supervision, services are provided to the residents. Insofar as services are a concomitant of supervision, the residents are not consumers who choose the services they wish. In fact they may often receive services they would not themselves select. Yet it is in the consumer role that residents will find services most helpful. When residents are in the role of consumers, social and psychological helping services are most effective (Segal, 1972).

Given this basic role conflict, we propose a typology of sheltered-care service emphasizing two goals shared by residents and service providers: (1) increasing internal and external integration and (2) reducing psychopathology. We take this opportunity to document the components of each type of proposed service with creative attempts we have observed to build the consumer role into the helping relationship.

217

A TYPOLOGY OF SHELTERED-CARE SERVICE

Sheltered-care service has two primary foci—the individual and the community—or more specifically the individual's interactions with his community. The focus of service to the individual is either social or clinical aid. In considering the social-aid program, we are discussing not only the provision of minimal room and board but also a series of service efforts aimed at helping a person maintain a level of social behavior and dignity as a person. A major problem with delivery of services to the mentally ill has been the confusion over services: Those that serve a social-aid function are often thought of as achieving the clinical-aid function—that is, the goal of ameliorating illness. Whereas the former services may in fact have an impact on the illness, their independent social benefits are often overlooked. The consequence has been that, when individuals failed to recover from their mental illness, social-aid efforts thought to have curative benefits were dropped from the service scene, with severe negative consequences for the resident. The classic example of this situation was the abandonment of the environmental tenets of moral treatment.

By clinical aid we refer to efforts relating to the elimination of some intrapsychic disturbance in the individual. In considering clinical-aid programming, we are concerned with services thought to have their primary impact upon residents' psychological disturbance.

The focus of service on the individual's interactions with his community is the attempt to integrate the individual into its ongoing functions. The assumption is that the individual will benefit from such integration. For the resident there are two communities—the internal community of the facility and the community external to the facility. In considering the external/internal focus of service content, we look into the emphasis of services taking place outside and independent of the facility—external programming—as opposed to services centered within and mediated by facility efforts—internal programming. The distinction in service-program focus is similar to that made with respect to internal and external integration—internal programming provides a basis for involvement within the facility and external programming lays the foundation for independent resident outreach. (We have included under the rubric of external programming categorical programs developed for residents when such programs do not serve the facility group as a whole but serve residents of separate facilities who independently participate.)

We thus divide service efforts into four types—internal social-aid programming, external social-aid programming, internal clinical-aid programming, and external clinical-aid programming (see Table 13.1). We look at each type of service as having differential impacts on residents' life situations.

Internal social-aid programs are facility sponsored and help to maintain social behavior within the facility and lay the foundation for resident outreach
as part of a resident group. Such a foundation relies heavily upon a feeling of
community with other facility residents. External social-aid programs focus
on independence-producing social and work skills. They involve independent
resident outreach, and there is an important sense of transition (independent
of the support of the facility) to these programs. Internal clinical-aid programs occur at the facility or under the sponsorship of the facility and focus
on the resident's psychological efforts at problem solving. Such problem-solving efforts enable the resident to begin to relate to other residents and staff in
the facility. External clinical aid is independently obtained outside the facility and focuses again on problem-solving efforts but begins to emphasize
greater exploration of deeper psychological problems.

Table 13.1   A Typology of Sheltered-Care Services

| | | Individual Focus of Service Content | |
		Social Aid	Clinical Aid
Community Focus of Service Content	Internal Community	I. Internal social- aid programming	II. Internal clinical- aid programming
	External Community	III. External social- aid programming	IV. External clinical- aid programming

Under each type of programming effort we consider the components that
are most central to achieving the overall program goals (see Table 13.2)—
that is, respectively maximizing internal or external integration and reducing
psychopathology.

Internal Social-Aid Programming

Looking first at programs conducted at the facility, we found that 18% of the
population of facilities serving our client population offered a rehabilitation/
socialization program that could be classified as fitting into the internal social-aid category (e.g., recreation, general education, work training, or living-
skills training). The focus of these programs was on promoting participation
and production activities within the resident group. The components of these

Table 13.2   Components of Sheltered-Care Program Effort

  I.   Internal Social-Aid Program Components
        1.   Recreation and socializing
        2.   Activity structuring
        3.   Resident responsibility
        4.   Work-training program
        5.   Satellite housing
 II.   Internal Clinical-Aid Program Components
        1.   Therapy from facility staff
        2.   Visiting therapists
        3.   Therapeutic community
        4.   Crisis facility
III.   External Social-Aid Program Components
        1.   Socialization and recreation programs
        2.   Work programs
        3.   Transitional advocacy programs
        4.   Subsidized housing
 IV.   External Clinical-Aid Program Components
        1.   Outpatient treatment
        2.   Short-term rehospitalization

programs include recreation and socialization, activity structuring, resident responsibility, work training, and satellite housing.

The following examples of internal programming illustrate the range of program effort offered in the area of social aid within the facility. Programs vary from simple recreational activity to complex efforts to encourage and maintain good social behavior and to promote community outreach as a group member. Given the programs we studied,* those programs promoting transition to totally independent living report only 15 to 20% success. In addition a large percentage of individuals who actually make the transition to independent living have to return to sheltered care. Therefore, internal social-aid programs emphasizing a transitional goal allow the individual to remain somewhat dependent on the facility for emotional and social support.

Recreation and Socializing.   Whereas some large facilities attempt to provide recreational activities in the house with specialized staff, the community volunteer is an important component of recreation and socialization. One recreation project that was directed primarily at small homes for the aged (but

*We obtained program information from each of the study's sample areas and visited with several programs we judged to be among the most creative.

that reached several younger mentally ill people, owing to mixing of residents in facilities) used volunteers and undergraduate students to provide regular (usually weekly) 1- to 3-hour programs including crafts, music, discussions, and outings. This program is unique in its effort to reach less mobile residents.

We found three other programs, dependent upon volunteers, that provide internal social-aid-type services. One program provides a friend to one particular person in the home for a limited time (usually 3 months). Another program, entitled "Adopt a Friend," functions in a similar manner but does not have a time limit. The third program emphasizes the use of "specialists" who have a specific skill to offer (such as grooming or gardening skills) and function on an on-call basis for one or more facilities.

Project Anchor, a Washington, D.C., program, has failed to show any success in using volunteers to promote community reintegration (Watson et al., 1975). Similarly Gurel (1964) has found a negative correlation between the number of volunteers on a hospital's rolls and effectiveness in returning patients to the community. In Project Anchor little supervision was offered to volunteers. The failure of this project may therefore indicate that responsibility cannot be given solely to volunteers for jobs difficult even for professionals. Gurel, on the other hand, seems to have set his sights too high—that is, seems to be emphasizing total community transition.

Activity Structuring. Activity structuring helps maintain social behavior. The job of the operator was described by one operator as "building a supportive structure that the clients can depend on as one would build such a structure for family members, while at the same time avoiding dependence on the operator and making the home their whole world" (F.N.).* Activity structuring seems to be an important factor in achieving such an environment.

Harmon House, a facility that successfully provides for activity structuring, serves 19 residents between the ages of 21 and 41. When residents first come to Harmon House, they agree to be in a *structured-activities* program between 4:00 p.m. and 10:00 p.m. Monday through Friday. House meetings, recreation, and group meetings are scheduled for 4:00 p.m. to 10:00 p.m. during the week. House chores are scheduled two evenings a week; Friday night clubs meet until 1:00 a.m. (see Appendix B).

Twelve house rules are explained to prospective clients during the screening process (see Appendix C), with the understanding that breaking these rules is grounds for dismissal from the facility. When a client is accepted, a program is worked out jointly between the client and the staff. This struc-

---

*F.N. refers to field notes taken at the time of a structured or open-ended interview.

tured routine is part of the socialization process. The house asks for a 4- to 10-month commitment that, along with a basic understanding of the house organization, is formalized in a *written contract* (see Appendix D).

Resident Responsibility. Promoting resident responsibility is often achieved by involving residents in the management of the facility. In some facilities a limited form of resident control resembles patient government on a hospital ward, consisting of group meetings where social activities, problems of house maintenance, and planning for special occasions are discussed. In one facility the residents decided to do house maintenance chores (e.g., distributing sheets, washing dishes, cleaning, shopping, and organizing trips to local restaurants) to save money that would normally have been paid to an outside person. The salary allotted for these tasks was distributed to the residents participating in the maintenance chores.

Going beyond the basic patient-government plan, one model of delegation of responsibility we observed was a facility actually run by the residents: Major budgetary and staff-hiring decisions are made by the resident group. In fact *only residents vote* on the admission of new individuals and other major house decisions. If a resident is having problems with other residents, the responsibility of finding a solution is delegated to a resident work group (composed of residents and staff).

Residents form teams of two to prepare one evening meal per week; planning, cooking, and cleanup are included. Residents prepare their own breakfasts and lunches and are expected to clean up after themselves. Household work is divided into 15 jobs performed each week by the residents on a rotating basis.

This facility is a model illustrating the large number of areas open for the delegation of resident responsibility that can be employed in promoting social integration.

Work-Training Programs. Some facilities provide work access in facility-operated business. One such facility operates its own restaurant, serving breakfast and lunch 7 days a week; they currently plan to serve a dinner meal. This operation is financed by daily receipts; employees of the restaurant are paid on a profit-sharing basis.

Another approach to in-house work is one in which residents can get on-the-job training as prospective facility staff. Residents take shifts in staff work, and after leaving the facility, they may return as substitute staff members. Facilities also form work crews as jobs develop—for example, one facility maintains contact with an apartment-cleaning business, and crews are formed when jobs arise.

Three important aspects of internal social-aid work-training programs emerge: (1) work opportunities leading to financial reward and development of skills, (2) career opportunities as potential staff within the system, and (3) development of a community among residents.

Satellite Housing.   Another important internal social-aid approach is the promotion of socially independent functioning, whereby the facility does not necessarily provide programs but does provide a living arrangement in which the resident is required to assume increasing responsibility for his residential arrangement. The supervisory component of the residential arrangement is crucial here. Several facilities have set up "satellite housing."

These satellites vary a good deal in the amount of supervision provided. In one situation the facility locates four-unit buildings and rents out three of the four apartments to sheltered-care residents (usually four residents in each two-bedroom apartment). The fourth apartment is retained for house parents; thus residents do not have immediate supervision, but supervision is available on a 24-hour basis.

Other arrangements include the operation of an entire apartment house solely for sheltered-care residents. Some facilities have attempted to place small groups of residents in buildings open to the general public. In such situations, which are quite common, the facility usually leases the apartment and retains responsibility for the rent. Some agencies are using condominiums for this purpose; in these situations the supervision is minimal and often exists only during the day. Individuals living in these satellite housing arrangements return to the sheltered-care facility to participate in programming efforts.

The creative internal socially centered programming we have described is rare in the overall picture of internal programs. Most programming efforts are minimal attempts to provide recreation. Many facilities provide only the *possibility* of engaging in recreational activities and the residents themselves have little initiative to take advantage of the opportunity. One facility had a volleyball net that sagged almost to the ground. The operator pointed to this "volleyball court" as one of the recreational opportunities available to the residents, if they should choose to use them.

Internal Clinical-Aid Programming

Of the sheltered-care facilities in California, 9% are offering in-house clinically centered programming primarily emphasizing individual or group therapy. Residents of facilities with in-house therapy programs are more likely to be receiving treatment than residents of facilities without this therapy. This finding holds except when the facility provides transportation to individual or group treatment programs outside the house, which leads to results similar to those from in-house therapy. Thus the provision of internal clinical-aid programming is perhaps the most efficient way of ensuring that the resident will in fact receive therapy.

Residents of facilities with in-house treatment more often receive group therapy, and those in facilities providing transportation to treatment outside the facility more often receive individual treatment.

Four types of clinical-aid programs are available within the facility aside from psychoactive drugs: (1) individual or group treatment conducted by members of the facility staff (often graduate students or volunteers); (2) a more formal therapeutic program conducted by mental-health professionals who visit the facilities on a regular basis; (3) treatment efforts where the program is seen as the vehicle for psychotherapeutic intervention either with the individual or through the group (using the program as a vehicle for treatment activity being characteristic of the efforts of social group workers in recreation and rehabilitation settings and of the efforts often employed as a part of a therapeutic-community approach to sheltered care); and (4) the crisis setting where the facility may operate its own house separately from the main facility, set up to deal with residents in crisis.

Therapy from Facility Staff. The following is an example of the therapy program offered at a facility where staff members are responsible for conducting therapy sessions:

A. Group Therapy.
   1. Experiential groups.
   2. Psychodrama.
   3. Parent and family groups.
   4. Encounter therapy.
B. Individual Therapy.
   1. Counseling.
   2. Crisis intervention.
   3. Behavior modification.
   a. Reciprocal inhibition therapy.
   b. Token economy (for selective cases).
   c. Behavior monitoring—therapeutic assistance.
   d. Member review.

Psychotherapy at this facility is conducted by psychologists with masters degrees, in consultation with a psychiatrist. In addition undergraduate students from local colleges are used as paraprofessional trainees in the therapeutic sessions.

This type of therapeutic program is most characteristic of facilities that serve a younger nonchronic population. It is also a less common program than the reliance on visiting therapists to provide internal treatment.

Visiting Therapists. Programs in which mental-health professionals enter the facility for the sole purpose of conducting therapeutic sessions, often on an appointment basis, are most common in sheltered care. In states other than California such programs are often sponsored as part of the aftercare provisions set up for former state-hospital residents. In such cases continuity of care is assured when the hospital unit that referred the patient retains responsibility for treatment. This is a program type that tends to follow the unified *clinical-team approach* first implemented at the Duchess County Unit of Hudson River State Hospital, New York (Gruenberg, 1966). In California, where there are no longer two separate systems of care (a state and a locally operated system), treatment personnel for those aftercare programs are likely to be hired by the county and assigned to a number of facilities.

Another common aftercare approach is one in which the caseload of the mental-health professional (usually a social worker) consists, not of facilities, but of individuals living in facilities.

One aftercare clinic is conducted by a team in two meeting rooms of a large New York hotel catering to former mental patients. There are many more individuals in the hotel than can possibly be treated by the small team of mental-health professionals available. The psychiatrist on the team provides primarily medication review and reassurance. For example:

The neatly dressed woman in her mid-sixties poked her head through the open door. She had been in the waiting room for approximately forty minutes while the psychiatrist was busy trying to handle the problems of other hotel residents. He cordially invited her in. She was quite concerned about her son. He was institutionalized, and she wished to take him out of the institution he was in. The psychiatrist assured her that it was best for him to stay where he had been placed, since after she passed on, it would be difficult to have him rehospitalized again. The psychiatrist attempted to elicit her feelings about loneliness and fear of being in the hotel. She admitted timidly that she had never lived with "mental patients" before and was quite frightened. After some initial reassurance, her level of medication for depression was reduced.

When she had left, the psychiatrist said that she was one of many cases in which psychotherapy might have been quite fruitful, had there been sufficient staff time available (F.N.).

Group therapy in small family-oriented facilities should be questioned in terms of its impact on the continuing relationships of the individuals in the facility.

One operator notes:

In-house group therapy was tried in this home by a social worker; the clients did not respond. The caretaker did not think it was a success. Clients felt badly if they said too much, or a manipulative client might take something that was said and use it against another person in the intensive family situation (F.N.).

Therapeutic Community. The third type of approach employed in the sheltered-care facility is the therapeutic-community orientation, which involves the development of a program as a tool or vehicle of therapeutic intervention.

Trute House is a residential facility for 15 residents and provides day-care services for 2 to 6 additional clients ranging in age from 18 to 33. Staff members live in as part of the community on a 48-hour basis to avoid a hospital-like two-shift schedule.

General therapeutic-community meetings are held, and in addition to a personal counselor, each client has a day-group counselor with whom he performs required housework. There are three day-group counselors, each in charge of one required task: housecleaning, grounds cleanup, and meals (both preparation and cleanup). The group meets three times a day: in the morning to organize, in the midafternoon to see that the chores have been done and assign other tasks, and later for therapy. The group stays together for 1 week. The counselors are chosen each week, but the members remain for 3 weeks, giving each member a chance to work with each counselor. At the end of the 3 weeks the groups are reorganized with a different composition of members. Both residents and day clients are in the groups. In this environment the total facility program becomes the therapeutic vehicle.

Crisis Facility. An efficient and effective use of resources employs the high-powered treatment-type facility to treat crises and difficult situations on a short-term basis and confines social care to more homelike settings. One facility we studied, for example, owns a crisis-house "facility" with plastic windows and with the capability of being locked and may transfer unruly residents to it. This crisis facility has a more structured program with an average expected stay of 21 days. It is our observation that the provision of treatment within this type of facility is a positive device for the most disturbed clients.

External Social-Aid Programming

Programs emphasizing social integration in the external community have been used, developed, and in some cases, supported by 42% of the sheltered-care facilities. In addition services have been developed in the community independently of the facility as a means of meeting the needs of the residents. These services are provided outside the home with a focus on encouraging independent social behavior and consequently are described as external social-aid programs. In general these programs are divided into four components: socialization and recreation, work, transitional advocacy, and subsidized housing programs. There is a great deal of overlap. For example, transitional advocacy programs, a form of socialization programming, work to build the client's individual internal strength as he moves into independent functioning in the community. Although achievement of independent functioning is an often-stated goal in the system, much of the programming in these externally oriented programs primarily helps individuals maintain their level of social behavior in the external community while residing within the facility.

Socialization and Recreation Programs. Socialization and recreation programs consist of trips and picnics conducted by local recreation departments, church groups, voluntary organizations, and drop-in centers in churches. Activities involved include arts and crafts, music, and socializing opportunities. Some programs include a "party-of-the-month club," where different voluntary organizations organize a party for residents each month. One social and recreational activity for residents involves a hospitality club; community members are invited to socialize with residents in various recreational activities sponsored by the local recreation department. Such activities have included the development of two theater groups and a film program sponsored with the local library.

Another recreation program tried to cover some of its expenses by involving as staff those operators whose entire clientele attends the recreational facility. Of 15 operators, however, only 4 were found to have sufficient commitment to take program responsibility.

In a rural area a traveling recreation program for residents has been used. It is located in a given small town for 1 or 2 days each week and has a definite catchment area to cover during the week. Although a program like this has a definite socialization component, it is also geared to provide recreation. Two other types of programs that have a more directed socialization focus are those placing residents as volunteers in voluntary organizations or on the boards of directors of programs that serve the sheltered-care community.

Work Programs. Several work programs have developed to meet the resident's needs for a work-related experience. The types of job programs offered to residents include home repair in poverty areas, general domestic service (usually as part of a group that provides continual services), thrift-shop employment, restaurant employment, recycle-center operation, agricultural-equipment assembly, furniture stripping and refinishing, and staffing of residential facilities. Most of these job opportunities are on a group basis; the group is responsible for the job, rather than the individual. In this respect dependence on individual ability to complete the job is much less.

One county service organization has organized a residents' hiring hall where four to six people are taken out on jobs for which they are paid $3.00 an hour. The head of the program is paid half with county mental-health monies and half with the payment for the completed job. Thus the head of the program has incentive to find additional work opportunities. So far this hiring hall has sent out workers for painting, gardening, hauling, and the beginning of a salvage business. An attempt is made to avoid competition with local business. In addition residents are sent to work only on properties where the owner carries liability insurance.

Most residents who work on these projects are on Supplemental Security Income (SSI). They can, therefore, make only $55 per month without deductions from their SSI payments. Since the amount of work one can do in the program is limited by this financial requirement, the program truly becomes one of maintaining behavior and providing supplementary income to the resident (who without this money would have only $30 per month to spend).

Transitional Advocacy Programs.   Some external social-aid programs encourage the resident to maximize his own opportunities in his environment.

We found three programs in this category, with progressively intense efforts to help residents exercise their prerogatives. The first is entitled SSI Alert. It is a program run by the Red Cross, in which volunteers run a hot-line telephone service to give handicapped persons information on SSI (*Health News*, 1974). In the second program Mental Health Advocates trained individuals to help former patients find appropriate help in coping with the demands of community life. Advocates are assigned on a one-to-one basis to residents to maximize their use of social services. The third program involves a more direct effort on the part of residents themselves to organize politically for changes in the system. Project NOVA (New Opportunities through Voluntary Action) is an example of such a program. Although NOVA has a core staff of professional community organizers, the program emphasizes developing the strengths of the residents themselves. In contrast to the former two programs NOVA provides a significant social-aid activity by focusing on improvement of the sheltered-care situation.

Subsidized Housing.   This program component involves the attempt to provide independent living situations to former hospital patients where a public agency holds ultimate financial responsibility for an apartment and may itself subsidize rents to maximize the potential of the resident to enhance his external-integration opportunities. Such housing—often in a public-housing project—involves minimum supervision of residents and requires them to make use of external resources common to the general community.

External Clinical-Aid Programs

The program components of external clinical-aid programming involve outpatient treatment and short-term rehospitalization.

Outpatient Treatment. Provision of treatment in the community on an outpatient basis is less reliable than in-house treatment in terms of actually serving the client. There is, however, a danger in providing treatment within the facility—the danger that the facility will become merely a miniature mental hospital, which the surrounding community can simply ignore. Thus, in an attempt to maintain an environment conducive to external integration, many facilities have deemphasized in-house psychological treatment as counterproductive. One program in particular, an aftercare program in a New York suburb, moved its treatment program out of the residential-hotel facility to an outpatient clinic within walking distance of the hotel.

Of the California sheltered-care population, 19% is receiving some form of outpatient treatment—individual or group therapy or both, outside of the facility. The content of this treatment varies from simple medication reviews to more intensive discussions of personal feelings and psychological problems. A large amount of treatment is devoted to supportive problem solving, with the help of social workers associated with aftercare services of county mental-health departments.

In some communities, however, the local mental-health services have faced a significant problem with chronic long-term patients, who upset the regular clientele of the outpatient facility. One New York clinic prohibited chronic patients from receiving treatment because of the reaction of their other clientele. The community clinic proposed the solution of serving chronic patients in the facilities in which they live. The compromise solution offered by the mental-hospital aftercare service team was the establishment of separate outpatient services for chronic patients. The sanction of a dual system of care—one for the "normal" and one for the "crazy"—seems, however, as counterproductive in view of social stigma as totally confining care to the facility.

Short-Term Rehospitalization. There is no single organized system of providing treatment to residents in California. Presently it is the responsibility of either the operator or the patient to seek help. The result is that the service most frequently used by residents is rehospitalization; 22% of the California sheltered-care population were rehospitalized within the past year (1973).

Short-term rehospitalization is one form of treatment outside the context of the facility. Gruenberg (1970) offers five reasons for short-term hospital treatment: (1) to employ treatment procedures requiring continuous observation (e.g., dangerous drugs and electroshock), (2) to protect a person when he is dangerous to himself or others, (3) to remove a person temporarily from an environmental stress during a period when he cannot cope with the stress or be helped to cope with it successfully, (4) to provide a temporary relief for the patient's associates who are managing to live with him but at a significant cost to themselves (these costs including the loss of the caretakers' free time and the emotional energy mortgaged from other potential forms of emotional investment), and (5) to establish a form of communication between patient and hospital . (Two ideas are frequently communicated by the hospitalization of the patient: The patient's difficulties result from sickness, and the hospital is available to the patient and to his family for assistance in living with chronic incurable disorder.)(p. 123)

The hospital does have a function as a supportive device in the treatment of the chronically mentally ill outside the context of their living situation. Items 3 and 4 of Gruenberg's list are, however, functions that might well be delegated to intermediate nonhospital facilities. A crisis-house-type facility similar to that developed as an internal clinical aid but serving sheltered-care homes in a given catchment area might be best developed as an external clinical aid to serve residents who need temporary respite from a stressful situation at the house. A crisis facility or a mutual-support arrangement between operators (such as providing a bed for residents so that an operator may have time off in his own home or providing coverage at the facility while the operator is away for a few days) would fulfill the respite needs of facility operators.

AN APPROACH TO SERVICE

The service objective of sheltered care for the mentally ill is spelled out, at least tentatively, in California's licensing regulations for community-care facilities:

Basic services shall be conducted so as to promote independence and self-direction in all persons admitted; such persons shall be encouraged to participate as fully as their conditions permit, in daily living activities both in the facility and in the community (California State Department of Health, 1974, p. 36).

As things stand, the people who make the most noise get most of the service. Although some residents are not getting all the service they might, there has been a great upsurge of creativity in the development of services to promote and maintain the social behavior of the resident, both within the facility and in the environment external to that facility. In addition creative treatment has been offered to residents, both within the facility and on an outpatient basis. Yet we certainly have a long way to go before the goal of basic services will be achieved. We must seek ways of optimizing the use of the less available clinical supports for external and internal integration by reducing the reliance on service delivery by the "squeaky-wheel" criterion. Most immediate solutions lie in maximizing the effectiveness of those most involved in placement and service delivery—the social worker and the general practitioner. Long-range solutions must depend on experimental program evaluations within the system. Such service evaluations should be classified according to our typology of service delivery, each type of service being considered with respect to the nature of the goals it is designed to achieve—that is, internal social aid, internal clinical aid, external social aid, and external clinical aid.

REFERENCES

California State Department of Health. "Proposed Regulations for the Licensing and Certification of Community Care Facilities." *California Administrative Code,* Title 22, Division 5, Chapter 6, Article 5, Section 75403, Sacramento, California, September 11, 1974.

Gruenberg, E. M. *Evaluating the Effectiveness of Community Mental Health Services.* New York: Milbank, 1966.

Gruenberg, E. M. "Hospital Treatment in Schizophrenia: The Indications for and the Value of Hospital Treatment," in R. Cancro (Ed.). *The Schizophrenic Reactions: A Critique of the Concept, Hospital Treatment, and Current Research.* New York: Brunner/Mazel, 1970.

Gurel, L. "Correlates of Psychiatric Hospital Effectiveness." Paper read at an American Psychological Association symposium on Assessment of Psychiatric Hospital Effectiveness, Los Angeles, September 4, 1964.

Health News, California State Department of Health, May 1974.

Segal, S. P. "Research on the Outcome of Social Work Therapeutic Interventions: A Review of the Literature." *J. Health and Social Behavior,* 13(3), 3–17 (1972).

Watson, C. G., J. R. Fulton, and L. Gurel. "Project Anchor: A Study of an Unsuccessful Volunteer Program to Help Former Patients." *Hosp. and Community Psychiat.,* 26(3), 146–151 (1975).

FOURTEEN

Antipsychotic Drugs in Sheltered Care*

In the past two decades antipsychotic-drug treatment has become the therapy of choice for psychotic states. Whereas substantial research has been conducted on the efficacy of various drugs, very little research has been done on the social implications of antipsychotic-drug use among the mentally ill. We will examine the influence of these medications on former mental-hospital patients living in community-based sheltered-care facilities.

While acknowledging the demonstrated value of antipsychotic medication in controlling certain psychological disturbances—for example, schizophrenic ideation or mania—individuals who take drugs uniformly find their effects *difficult to tolerate* and report that their experience with them is unpleasant.

In one facility where residents control budget decisions, they voted 15 to 1 to fund a staff member's attendance at a course in orthomolecular psychiatry. Residents expressed a strong desire to obtain dietary information that they

*This chapter was written with Dr. Susan Chandler, School of Social Work, University of Hawaii at Manoa, Honolulu, Hawaii 96822.

232

believed would help them control psychiatric symptomatology and thus reduce their dependence on antipsychotic medications. Many residents in their
early 30s had been on antipsychotic drugs for almost 10 years.

The house vote represented a clear commitment on the part of residents to
invest $80 in staff education rather than entertainment. These same residents
had previously voted down another staff request for training in group psychotherapy; the motivation to reduce their dependence on drugs was the key
distinction in determining the election results.

In another example we see the responses to medications made by a group
of individuals in a community facility with a more socially controlled resident
population. This facility is serviced weekly by a psychiatrist, and the resident
response pattern is more typical of institutionalized populations.

This sheltered-care facility showed a positive orientation to antipsychotic
medications. At the time of the visit the facility was having a group meeting
of residents to discuss problems of the previous week. The interviewer was
introduced as a person conducting research on the effects of antipsychotic
drugs. The resident leader of the group suggested that each group member
tell the researcher about the type of medication he or she was taking.

The majority of the residents not only commented on the type and dosage
of their medications but also added that they liked their "meds" or that their
"meds did them good."

One resident emphatically stated, "I am taking Haldol and I love my
Haldol." The manager of the facility later pointed out that several residents
were resistant to taking their medications, and he often had to check to be
sure that "meds" were indeed ingested. He noted that the woman who "loved
her Haldol" was one of his biggest problems, and he had resorted to putting
her drugs in her coffee (without her knowledge) to ensure that the prescribed
dosage was taken.

The concern expressed in these examples, either verbally or in the covert
actions of residents regarding the taking of their antipsychotic medications,
emphasizes the need for an evaluation of the impact of psychoactive medication on the daily life of sheltered-care residents. Three major questions may
be raised as a guideline for such an effort:

1. Who is taking what type of medication and how?
2. How do dosage levels compare with those recommended by authoritative
   sources?
3. How do antipsychotic medications affect the level of social integration of
   residents?

The answers provided to these questions by our data analyses are quite disturbing in view of the therapeutic goals of drug treatments and offer substantial validation to hypotheses regarding the social-control functions of these medications.

PSYCHOACTIVE MEDICATIONS

Until the discovery of modern drugs, classification of medications was a simple matter of distinguishing between sedative/hypnotics or stimulants. As more drugs were discovered, classification lines became blurred. Psychotropic or psychoactive drugs have the ability to alter the individual's psychological state. They are capable of producing subjective changes in mood, thinking, and level of awareness and of modifying a person's observable behavior (Claridge, 1970). These drugs are assumed to exert their influence on behavior by acting on the central nervous system. Yet, although an entire field of psychopharmacology has developed to study the effects and actions of drugs, information on the exact working of most modern drugs is still limited. We do know that drugs rarely have a single effect on the brain; rather there is usually a complex action involving several nervous-system elements. Even when a drug's action is fairly well understood, its influence on behavior may depend on several factors, one of which is dosage. Effects produced at a high dose may not occur at a low dose. Individual variations are at times considerable. For these and other reasons the classification of psychoactive drugs is at present somewhat arbitrary. An empirical classification has been devised by several psychopharmacologists that groups together drugs with broadly similar characteristics and properties.

Sedative/hypnotics, recently renamed antianxiety medications (anxiolytic sedatives), have the effect of reducing mental alertness and bodily activity, inducing sleep and, with progressively larger doses, general anesthesia and, potentially, death. The sedatives are anticonvulsant and habituating, cause a withdrawal state, and are a spinal-cord depressant (Claridge, 1970; Meyers et al., 1974). The most commonly used sedative is alcohol. Others frequently prescribed by doctors to sedate and to relieve anxiety are the barbiturates such as pentobarbital (Nembutal®), secobarbital (Seconal®), and phenobarbital.

In contrast the antipsychotics (frequently called the major tranquilizers) do not cause general anesthesia. A patient can be aroused even after the ingestion of huge doses. They are convulsant in their action, not habituating, and their therapeutic usefulness is in the treatment of psychotic, rather than of anxious patients (Meyers et al., 1974). The antipsychotics are not effective in reducing anxiety but can suppress schizophrenic ideation and behavior. These drugs are also distinctive in that they produce easily recognizable extrapyramidal signs, parkinsonism, and dystonias. The antipsychotic medications most widely used today are phenothiazine derivatives, but the phenothiazine part of the tranquilizer molecule is not essential and may be replaced by some other chemical group (for a further discussion of the chemical distinction, see Meyers et al., 1974, Chapter 25, "Antipsychotic Tranquilizers"). Commonly prescribed antipsychotic medications are chlorpromazine (Thorazine®), thioridazine (Mellaril®), trifluoperazine (Stelazine®), and fluphenazine (Prolixin®).

Minor tranquilizers or minor antianxiety agents are extremely similar to the sedative/hypnotic drugs in their pharmacologic properties but are often associated with the major tranquilizers because they were introduced at the same time (Meyers et al., 1974). They have the effect of sedation, disinhibition, and relief of anxiety and tension. Commonly prescribed minor tranquilizers are diazepam (Valium®), chlordiazepoxide (Librium®), and meprobamate (Equanil®, Miltown®).

Antidepressants are central-nervous-system stimulants and claim to raise mood in mild or moderate depression. Recent research has, however, demonstrated that the popular antidepressants are not distinct from the antipsychotic drugs just discussed.

Amitriptyline (Elavil®) and imipramine (Tofranil®), though widely used as antidepressants, are similar in property to the antipsychotic medications. The pharmacologic properties of the antidepressants are identical to those of the antipsychotics (Meyers et al., 1974).

Antiparkinsonian drugs have become common among the mentally ill patients, owing to the drug-induced extrapyramidal side effects of the phenothiazines. The manifestations of the extrapyramidal symptoms are (1) akinesia, a paucity of or difficulty in initiating movement; (2) muscle spasms or dystonias; (3) rigidity and tremors. These drugs work to improve the akinesia and the rigidity, but usually a fine tremor remains. Commonly used antiparkinsonian drugs prescribed for mental patients are trihexphenidyl (Tremin®, Artane®) and benztropine (Cogentin®).

Prescribing psychoactive medications for psychiatric patients has become a widespread practice. Whereas the severity of symptomatology of psychiatric patients varies widely, the pattern of prescribing psychoactive medications is almost routine. The vast majority of mentally ill people under care in the United States are taking psychoactive drugs.

EVALUATING MEDICATIONS

As part of our original data collection, information was gathered about the type and dose level of medications that each resident was taking. The information was asked of the sheltered-care operator and verified by interviewers (by examining drug labels). All medications, including nonprescription drugs, were recorded and tallied, so that a total daily dose for each drug was computed. Each resident's medication was coded by name and total dosage level.

To compare the relative potencies of the major antipsychotic drugs, schedules were used to obtain drug-dosage equivalencies. Each antipsychotic drug was converted into a relative-potency dosage equivalent to 100 milligrams of chlorpromazine, by using Hollister's (1973) relative-potency scale. If two or more antipsychotic drugs were used by one resident, a total score was obtained by adding the equivalencies. For comparison purposes a second coding scheme was established by using Meyers (1974) relative-potency schedule. Data were also considered relating to the total number of drugs taken by each resident; the number of "psychiatric" drugs, prescribed antipsychotics, antidepressants, anxiolytics, and anticonvulsants; and the frequency with which a patient takes medications.

Drug Dosage

A comparison was made of the study population's "average daily dosage" with other published dosage levels. The average daily dosage is a recommended range of drug levels within which various authorities suggest the clinician confine his prescriptions. Hollister's (1973) work was again used as an authoritative reference. Average recommended daily dosage ranges were also taken for comparative purposes from the American Medical Association's (AMA) *Drug Evaluations* (1971), and *The Physician's Desk Reference (PDR)* (1974). Each resident's drug prescription was compared with these recommended dosage ranges.

The range of dosage recommendations from all sources was very broad, frequently including disclaimers such as "adjust dosage to individual and the severity of his condition" (*PDR*, 1974, p. 1386). Milligram dosages are, however, suggested. The AMA *Drug Evaluations* discusses "usual" dosage as follows:

For many drugs the correct dose will depend on the size, age, and condition of the patient; his response to treatment; his sensitivity or tolerance; and the possible synergistic or antagonistic effect of concomitant medication. The epitome of dosage is to weigh expected benefits against risks. Accordingly, the usual doses are often given as ranges. Even the limits of these ranges are seldom inviolable: the upper limits stated for most ranges, however, do suggest that larger amounts either may enhance the risks of toxicity beyond what is ordinarily acceptable or may fail to provide additional therapeutic effect in significant degree; similarly, the lower limits often indicate that smaller doses could not be expected to provide full therapeutic effects for most patients (AMA, p. xv).

Few drugs have as extensive a therapeutic margin and such a wide range of therapeutic dose levels as the antipsychotic drugs. Hollister (1973) contends that the requirements of most patients fall within a range of 200–800 milligrams daily based on a chlorpromazine equivalent.

The dosage issue is complicated for several reasons. A drug can be effective only if delivered to the appropriate cells in the body at the appropriate time and with the appropriate strength. Individuals vary in their absorption rate and probably in the function of dose actually observed and thus have varying responses to the same dose. Measurement of drug concentration in the blood plasma (most drugs must enter through the bloodstream) is extremely difficult, and so doctors must rely on clinical signs and adjust dosages accordingly. Oakley S. Ray (1972) discusses the dosage issue in terms of chemical, biologic, and clinical equivalents. Chemically equivalent drugs contain essentially identical amounts of active ingredients in identical dosages. Biologically equivalent drugs, when used in equal dosage, provide the same biologic or physiologic availability of the drug to the body tissues. Clinically equivalent drugs are chemical equivalents that, when given in the same amounts, result in the same therapeutic effect. Controversy over the generic equivalence of drugs recently emerged when the U.S. Food and Drug Administration Commissioner stated that drugs that purport to be equivalent and may be chemically equivalent may not be therapeutically equivalent. The biologic availability of a drug, and thus its therapeutic effectiveness, must be carefully monitored beyond the chemical equivalence.

Relating Drug Dosage to Human Response

Several recent research projects have examined the issue of dosage in antipsychotic-drug administration. Gardos et al. (1973), in an extensive article on dose-response studies, contend that it is pointless to describe clinical effects of antipsychotic drugs unless dose level is specified, and yet little attention is paid to posology in psychopharmacologic literature. Although the literature is replete with articles on the clinical effectiveness of antipsychotic drugs, the vast majority name the drug with no mention of the dose level. Klein and Davis (1969) found that no studies had used dose-response curves in the phenothiazine treatment of schizophrenics. Not only are dose-response studies rarely done in clinical psychopharmacologic research, but also more conventional clinical studies rarely even attempt to relate observed clinical changes to specific dose levels. Most publications note only the mean dose level or the dosage range and advise the practitioner to adjust dosage to the needs of the patient.

Prien and Klett (1972) found that long-term schizophrenic patients receiving the equivalent of 350–600 milligrams per day of chlorpromazine showed no significant change in their clinical condition when their dosage was reduced to 300 milligrams per day. Prien et al. (1969), in a study of 325 chronic hospitalized schizophrenics, also found no significant differences between patients on high (80-milligrams) and low (15-milligrams) dosages of trifluoperazine. Both dosages were, however, significantly superior to a placebo.

Carscallen et al. (1968) conducted a 6-month double-blind study using a high dose (100-milligrams) of trifluoperazine and a usual dose (10-milligrams) and found no significant clinical differences on the Lorr Morbidity Scale. This finding supports the efficacy of low dosage.

Prien and Cole (1968), conducting a study with 838 chronic schizophrenics, concluded that high daily dosages of chlorpromazine (2000 milligrams) were significantly superior to dosages of 300 milligrams for patients under 40 years of age with less than 10 years of psychiatric hospitalization. In older, more chronic patients, there was no advantage to the higher doses, and the elevated doses increased the likelihood of side effects. Clark and Davis (1970) also found that patients under 40 years of age with fewer years of hospitalization responded better to higher doses of chlorpromazine.

Gardos et al. (1973) conclude their review of the dose-response literature by stating that only treatment-resistant schizophrenic groups require high or very high doses of antipsychotic medications. Low-dose therapy for many patients is certainly indicated.

The paucity of dose-response studies indicates the serious methodological difficulties encountered in this type of research. A fixed dose level, while methodologically necessary for the research team, may have harrowing effects on the patient, the clinician, and the staff. If, however, the doses are adjusted, the clarity of the research design is weakened. Thus many researchers prefer the high-dose-versus-low-dose protocol.

Several psychopharmacologists have discussed the problem of individual absorption and metabolism of antipsychotic medications. Oral dosages can be considered only an approximation of the available drug, and a precise determination of the physiologically active level of these drugs is difficult to obtain. (This problem compounds the debate over the equivalencies of antipsychotic drugs; studies that claim to find no significant differences between two drugs are frequently criticized for having inaccurate dose equivalents.)

The most difficult aspect of the dosage is the outcome measure. The efficacy of any drug-treatment regimen is dependent on a precise measuring instrument for success. Wing et al. (1972) discuss the problem of accurate initial diagnosis of schizophrenia. In reporting on the U.S.–U.K. Diagnostic Project, they note several disagreements over the common diagnosis of schizophrenia. A vast amount of empirical evidence has delineated ways in which environment can modify the symptomatic picture of the schizophrenic patient. Both overstimulation and understimulation may severely affect the patient's ability to cope; thus outcome measures for certain antipsychotic drugs must be cautiously examined.

WHO IS TAKING WHAT AND HOW MUCH

Of the 12,430 residents in sheltered care in our study, 88% were taking drugs of some type (either psychiatric or nonpsychiatric) and 76% were taking antipsychotic drugs at the time of the interview. There are 13 antipsychotic drugs, 12 of which were in use by members of the sheltered-care population. Of those on antipsychotic drugs, 38% were on more than one and 99% were taking at least one of the three most frequently prescribed drugs.

The most common antipsychotic drug prescribed for this population is thioridazine (Mellaril®); 38% of the population is taking it. The dosages range from 15 to 900 milligrams, with most patients (7%) taking 200 milligrams per day. Thorazine is the second most prescribed antipsychotic drug; 33% are taking daily dosages ranging from 25 to 4000 milligrams; 4.5% of the group are at the 200-milligram level, which was the modal category. The third most commonly prescribed drug is Stelazine; 28% of the residents are taking daily dosages ranging from 2 to 98 milligrams. (The dosages discussed in this section are actual prescribed dosages; thus, Stelazine, which is a more potent drug than Mellaril milligram for milligram, cannot be compared unless the equivalency is computed. The data in this section are purely descriptive, to give the reader a sense of the scope and variety of drug use among this population.) Of the sample, 9% were taking Prolixin. The other drugs were distributed as follows: Navane®, 5%; Compazine®, 2%; Quide®, 2%; Haldol®, 2%; Serentil®, 0.7%; Taractan®, 0.3%; Trilafon®, 0.1%; and Tindal®, 0.2%.

The number of drugs that a patient is required to take has become a target of controversy recently. Opponents of the psychopharmacologic revolution charge that the new drugs are "merely chemical strait jackets"—bars for the mind rather than the body. Criticism of multiple-drug prescribing as a social-control mechanism is becoming more frequent and widespread (Lennard, 1971; Lennard & Bernstein, 1974). An additional concern is that doctors are prescribing antipsychotic drugs that have known and frequently severe side effects (e.g., tardive dyskinesia, akathisia, dystonia [cramps], and Parkinsonism). Other drugs must be prescribed to offset the effects of the first drug. It has been charged that doctors continue to base prescriptions of drugs on symptoms caused by previous drug prescriptions (Caligari, 1974). In our study, 88% of residents take some type of medication, 65% take two or more drugs, and 13% take four or more drugs daily; 61% take two or more psychiatric drugs and 10% take four or more psychiatric drugs daily.

The frequency with which patients are required to take drugs is important to the patient's degree of independence from the community-care home. The vast majority of patients do not keep their own drugs, taking them only under supervision. We assumed that, the higher the frequency of medications required, the more attached the patient to the house. The data show that, of the residents taking medications, 14% must take their medications four times a day, 32% three times a day; 23% two times a day; and 16% once. Prien and Klett (1972) question the multiple-dose schedules entirely. They contend that requiring a patient to take drugs more than two times a day is unnecessary (inconsistent with the pharmacology of psychotropic drugs) and inconvenient.

The antiparkinsonian drugs are a particularly important category of medications. These drugs are used primarily to suppress the extrapyramidal disorders due to central nervous system drugs such as the phenothiazines; 29% of those taking antipsychotic drugs were taking Tremin (or Artane, the chemical equivalent) and 7% are taking Cogentin.

Individual Characteristics and Medication

Sex. In this study 81% of the women and 72% of the men are taking antipsychotic medication. Of all the residents not taking antipsychotic drugs, 65% are male. The sheltered-care population in California is 54% male and 46% female. The dosage between males and females is fairly evenly distributed.

Age. Of the study group 36% are under 40 years of age; 22% of those under 40 take no antipsychotic drugs and 16% of those over 40 years of age are not prescribed these drugs.

For residents under 40 taking antipsychotic drugs, 36% are on low doses, 33% are on moderate doses, and 31% are on high doses. In contrast 47% of those over 40 taking antipsychotic drugs take low doses, 36% take moderate doses, and 17% take high doses. This indicates that the clinical practice of doctors in California is consistent with current research, which suggests that higher dosages of antipsychotic drugs are more effective with younger patients (Clark & Davis, 1970; Prien & Cole, 1968).

Two or More Years of Continuous Hospitalization. Of the sample, 43% had spent 2 or more years of continuous residency in a psychiatric hospital. Although it would be important to control for the year of first admission, since the changing hospital and legislative policies would strongly influence the length of stay in a hospital, a rough idea of time spent in a hospital and the drug level could be examined. A strong pattern may be seen. Those who have spent 2 or more continuous years in a hospital do indeed take higher amounts of medications. Of those who have spent at least 2 years continuously in a psychiatric institution, 25% are taking high doses and 11% are not taking antipsychotic drugs. For the group without 2 years of institutionalization, 35% are not taking antipsychotic drugs and only 9% are on high doses.

Hospitalized During the Past Year.   Of the sample, 78% had not been hospitalized during the year previous to the interview. The following question emerges in this regard: Are residents on higher dosages of drugs less likely to need hospitalization, owing to the preventive properties of the antipsychotic drugs, and therefore are they more likely to respond "no" to the question about recent hospitalization? Or, alternatively, are residents on the highest dosages indeed the sickest sector of the sample, more likely to need rehospitalization (and therefore likely to report recent hospitalization)? The data offer slight support for the former alternative. Of the recently hospitalized, 68% were taking antipsychotic drugs, compared with 78% of those not hospitalized. Therefore, those taking the drugs were less frequently hospitalized. This lends some support to the theory that the medications are a factor in inhibiting hospitalization; however, dosage level made no difference.

Without a specific assessment of the reasons for rehospitalization, it is difficult to offer any definitive answer to this issue of preventing hospitalization. Certainly patients are rehospitalized to adjust medication levels. Such appropriate clinical action would lead to an inflated percentage needing rehospitalization who are also on antipsychotic drugs. We believe the problem in interpretation lies with the criterion of rehospitalization being viewed as something to be prevented. Hospitalization should be considered as a device to meet specific patient needs, and as such, the assessment of whether or not it should be prevented is meaningful only for a given treatment plan.

Facility Characteristics and Medication

Facility Size.   The facilities in this study ranged from 1 bed to 280 beds. By comparing the size of the facilities with the dosage levels of the residents, we hoped to determine whether patients in larger, hospital-like facilities were receiving higher doses of drugs.

The data indicate that, of the residents taking low doses of medications, 25% live in the large facilities and 38% in the smallest. No clear relation emerges, however, between high dosage levels and facility size.

Supervision and Dispensing of Medications.   The importance of medications in the opinion of facility operators is illustrated in data on procedures used in dispensing drugs: 83% of the operators responded that all their residents are supervised during the dispensing of medications; 14% reported that some were supervised, and 3% reported that none were supervised.

Our goal was to determine whether residents with higher dosages were viewed with more concern by operators and whether supervision was thus seen as more necessary among this group. These data show that, in facilities that do not supervise the taking of drugs, there are no residents on high doses of drugs; on the other hand, 17% of the facilities that supervise medications for all their residents have residents on high doses. Of the facilities that do not supervise medication dispensing, 56% have residents who do not take antipsychotic drugs, compared with 23% of the facilities that do supervise. This finding could imply that appropriate supervision is being offered to highly dosed residents and also supports the hypothesis that cautious operators are more likely to have clients on high doses of antipsychotic drugs. The latter case should be given careful scrutiny in regard to operator-training programs.

To the question "Do residents keep their own medications?" 5% of the operators reported that all residents do; 23% responded that some do; and 72% said that none do. Apparently the process of residents' taking their medication is fairly well regulated. The majority of facilities report that patients do not keep their own medications, are supervised during the dispensing of the medications, and (in 83% of the facilities) are subjected to formal procedures to ensure that the medications are in fact taken.

General Medical Care. At least four-fifths of the residents in the sample reported that it was very easy or easy to arrange for medical care, including medications, at the sheltered home. Only 8% felt it was difficult or very difficult; 52% felt it would be easy or very easy to obtain medical care (including medications) outside the facility or without the operator's help.

At least four-fifths of the operators have made arrangements for a house doctor to service the community-care facility. This doctor presumably is called whenever there is a medical problem for any of the residents and in particular whenever there is a need for a medication renewal or alteration. Many medication changes are conducted over the phone, the operator describing the problem and the doctor suggesting dosage changes.

Physicians do visit the homes when they feel it is necessary; Medicaid allows each patient to select his own physician, but in most cases the doctor is arranged for by the operator and approved by the residents; 9% of the operators reported that the doctor comes more than once a week, 26% said that a doctor comes once a month, and 55% said doctors are on call. Our impression is doctor visits are "for sickness," and phone calls are used for "normal problems with the meds."

Heins (1975), in a study of Canadian community physicians, found that psychiatrists have turned over the responsibility for chronically mentally ill community care to the general practitioner. As a result these patients tend to be maintained on the same drug and dosage as when they left the hospital. Gray (1974) also reports a stable dosage level following hospital release. Heins (1975) assumed that the general practitioner, who is less informed about antipsychotic medications, is reluctant to make any alterations unless a specific problem occurs. Whereas our study did not include the length of time a resident has been on the same medication, several doctors and facility operators in the San Francisco area report a similar pattern of drug maintenance for California. Medical services, in combination with psychiatric drugs, have been considered an important variable in former mental patients' "success" in the community (Davis et al., 1974; Pasamanick et al., 1967). Studies have indicated that, if psychiatric support services (social workers, public-health nurses, etc.) are readily available to former patients, crises may be weathered and a return to a hospital may be avoided.

Of the facility operators surveyed, 78% reported that day-hospital/day-care treatments were available or easily available; 11% considered these services unavailable; and 11% felt these services were available with difficulty. Whereas these statistics generally indicate that the operators feel that psychiatric backup services are available to them when needed, 22% of the sample felt that these services—services that could help an operator provide short-term therapy for the patient or give the operator a rest break—were unavailable or could be used only with difficulty; 15% of the operators have used this type of service "often or very often," but 47% used it rarely or never.

Psychiatric inpatient care was considered to be more easily obtainable by the operators; 85% felt that psychiatric inpatient services were "easily available" or "available," but only 13% of the operators use this service "often" or "very often."

AVERAGE DAILY DOSE RECOMMENDATIONS

In this section we compare the dosage levels of the 76% of the sheltered-care population on antipsychotic medications with dosages recommended by authoritative sources. This comparison has implications for the social control as well as the helping function of antipsychotic medication.

Hollister's chlorpromazine equivalents being used, the dose level of prescriptions for residents ranges from 10 to 3400 milligrams per day. The Meyers' equivalents range from 15 to 2400 milligrams per day. Although the few studies that report dose levels do not agree on what constitutes a high dose, most of the studies we referred to agree that more than 600 milligrams of chlorpromazine (or its equivalent) is a large dose; 300–600 milligrams is generally considered moderate, and less than 300 milligrams is a low dose.

According to the Hollister conversion scales, 17% of our study group take high doses of antipsychotic drugs, 26% take moderate doses, and 33% take low doses; 24% of the total population were not taking any *antipsychotic* medications, and only 12% of the group are completely drug free.

As noted earlier, Prien and Cole (1968) suggest that large doses of drugs are indicated for treatment-resistant schizophrenics and those under 40 years of age with less than 10 years of hospitalization. Although our data did not examine "treatment-resistant patients," our findings regarding "age" and "years of hospitalization" indicate that many residents for whom research does not recommend high doses are in fact receiving high doses. Only 17% of the entire sample are on high dosages of drugs, and yet 27% of the group 40 or older with more than 10 years of hospitalization are on high doses.

As previously noted, the "average daily dose" of a drug is a recommended range within which it is suggested drug prescriptions be confined. Each resident's converted relative-potency dosage (on Hollister's scale) was compared with the "average daily dose." Three sources of recommended dose ranges were used: Hollister, the AMA, and the *PDR*. Because of the disagreement over what constitutes a low or high dose, we analyzed the California sample against the suggestions, respectively, of a psychopharmacologist, physicians, and drug companies.

Compared with Hollister's recommended daily dose levels (50–400 milligrams of Thorazine or equivalent for "outpatient care"), 60% of those in our study taking antipsychotic drugs were doing so at the recommended level; 39% were above this level, and only 1% were below this level.

Compared with the AMA's *Drug Evaluations* (30–1000 milligrams—an extremely broad range), 89% of the residents are within the prescribed range, 10% are above the recommendation, and 0.07% are below it.

The *PDR* had the smallest range of recommended daily doses of all the sources examined: 30–75 milligrams. This is somewhat surprising because the drug manufacturers themselves supply the recommendations for the *PDR* (1974). Compared with this range, only 8% of the California study group are within the recommended dosage range, 91% are above it, and 0.07% are below it.*

These findings illustrate a trend noted by several authors, among them Scheff (1966):

[Most] physicians learn early in their training that it is far more culpable to dismiss a sick patient than to retain a well one (p. 110).

Translated into prescription patterns, the rule is that it is better to offer too much cure than not enough. No matter how one interprets the "average daily dosage" comparisons, the tendency is to err in the direction of more rather than less drugs. (Certainly this prescription pattern might be justified by the needs of the population. In the final section of this chapter we directly address this issue.)

The ranges recommended by our three sources vary considerably:

*More recent editions of the *PDR* have broadened their recommended range.

Hollister's list is from 50–400 milligrams; the AMA's from 30–1000; and the *PDR*'s from 30–75 milligrams. Hollister's statistical range (the difference between the highest and the lowest recommended dosage) is 350; for the AMA it is 970; and for the *PDR* 45. This dispersion illustrates how vastly the concepts of dosage recommendation differ.

Obviously even the best physicians function with very vague guidelines for the use of antipsychotic medications. A good example of these guidelines is the *PDR*'s discussion of chlorpromazine. Thorazine, the patented brand of chlorpromazine, is discussed by its manufacturer Smith Kline Corporation as follows:

Dosage and Administration:

Adjust dosage to individual and the severity of his condition, recognizing that the milligram for milligram potency relationship among all dosage forms has not been precisely established clinically. It is important to increase dosage until symptoms are controlled. Dosage should be increased more gradually in elderly patients. In continuing therapy, gradually reduce dosage to the lowest effective maintenance level after symptoms have been controlled for a reasonable period (1974, p. 1386).

SOCIAL INTEGRATION AND THE ANTIPSYCHOTIC DRUGS

How does the level of prescribed antipsychotic medication affect the internal and external integration of residents? These medications, though known to be successful in preventing readmissions to psychiatric hospitals of patients living in the community, must be examined with a more refined measure (Englehart et al., 1967; Hogarty, 1973). Whereas maintenance of a former patient in the community may be considerably better than maintenance in a back ward of a large hospital (Goffman, 1961), more research is needed on the quality of life and existence a patient in the community is experiencing.

Since 1956, when the phenothiazine chemicals were introduced into state hospitals, studies have repeatedly demonstrated the effectiveness of psychoactive drugs in reducing florid symptomatology among the mentally ill. Later studies describing the negative medical side effects of prolonged use of phenothiazines raise serious ethical questions about this widely used treatment modality (American College of Neuropsychopharmacology Study, 1973).

Little attention has been given to the relationship between medication and the psychological, social, and interactional functioning or behavior patterns of the mentally ill living in the community.

External Integration

An initial examination of study findings reveals little relationship between external-integration scores and antipsychotic medications. The direction of this weak (nonsignificant) relationship is negative—those residents not taking antipsychotic drugs found external integration easier than those taking any dosage. Those on the highest doses found such integration "difficult" or "very difficult." While not significant, this negative trend has two possible interpretations: Either the most ill, who have the most difficulty with social integration, are receiving high levels of antipsychotic medications because they need them, or the use of high levels of antipsychotic drugs actually depresses residents' levels of integration. The latter possibility is supported by the large number of residents taking moderate to high doses of the antipsychotic drug as maintenance.

Controlling for Psychopathology. In an attempt to relate levels of antipsychotic medication to residents' level of external integration, we controlled for individual levels of psychopathology, using a similar approach to that employed in the assessments of the differential effects of psychopathology on the external- and internal-integration models. The Brief Psychiatric Rating Scale (BPRS), based on 16 psychiatric symptoms, was employed as an index of resident psychopathology (Overall & Gorham, 1962). The sum of ratings on all 16 symptoms was divided into three categories, category three characterizing the most disturbed residents and category one, the least disturbed.

When psychopathology was controlled for, drug doses for the most ill portion of the population (category three in the BPRS) were significantly related to external integration in a positive direction ($r = .34$, $p < .05$). Having discovered this significant positive relationship for the most disturbed subgroup, we sought to account for any confounding effects resulting from our methodology, which involved judging level of disturbance at the same time individuals were on medication and on the basis of their assessed symptom scores, which the drugs are supposed to affect. We took account of these effects by obtaining the partial correlation between external-integration scores and drug dosage levels, controlling for BPRS symptomatology ratings within the most disturbed group; we thus obtained an assessment of the relationship between external integration and drug dosage level after current symptom assessments had explained all the variation they could in the latter two variables. The result of this procedure strengthened our results (the partial correlation equaled .39). Thus, for the severely disturbed (16% of the study group), antipsychotic drugs exert a positive influence on external integration. However, no one in this disturbed group found external integration "very easy"—only 6% found it "easy"; 33% of this group not taking antipsychotic drugs and 5% of those taking high dosages, found external integration very difficult. The largest subset of the severely disturbed group consisted of the residents on high dosages of medication who found external integration "difficult" or "not much trouble" (28%). This suggests that, even for the most ill, drugs do not facilitate high levels of external integration, although those on high doses experience less difficulty.

In sharp contrast to this finding is the significant negative association between drugs and external integration for the 29% of the population who scored in the healthiest subgroup (category 1 on the BPRS). With the same methodology as that employed to assess the relationship between external integration and drug dosage in the severe group, the partial correlation between these two variables in the healthiest subgroup, the current level of symptomatology being controlled for, was $-.24$ ($p < .05$). Of crucial importance is that only 25% of those in the subgroup with no medication, compared with 61% of those in the subgroup who were most medicated, found external integration "difficult" or "very difficult." Thus it is clear that, in the healthier group, drugs (especially at high dosages) *hinder* external integration.

Goldstein (1970), in an experimental study of premorbid adjustment and patterns of response to phenothiazines in acute schizophrenia, obtained data in support of our findings:

When the behavioral and psychophysiological measures are used, good and poor premorbid schizophrenics vary in their response to 21-day drug or placebo regimens. Poor premorbid patients respond to drug or placebo treatment according to clinical expectation, but good premorbid patients show a reverse pattern of response (p. 37).

Unfortunately, from our perspective, this type of negative finding is reproduced in our internal-integration data.

Internal Integration

The overall association between antipsychotic dose level and internal integration is slightly negative. The relationship is not significant but is in the anticipated direction. Our assumption was that residents who are more outgoing and able are not likely to be on high doses of drugs, which tend to restrict their ability to negotiate successfully the life of the facility.

Controlling for Psychopathology. In the disturbed group (category 3 on the BPRS) we obtained a positive, though nonsignificant, partial correlation between internal integration and drug dosage, controlling for symptom assessments. Given the general trend of the interaction we observed in the external-integration analysis—that is, the tendency of the relationship between external integration and drug dosage to change from negative to positive with increased resident psychopathology—we divided the disturbed group in two (according to the degree of their disturbance). Looking at the relationship between internal integration and drug dosage and controlling for current symptom assessments for the most severely disturbed subset of the disturbed group (8% of the study population), we found a significant and positive partial correlation equal to .28 ($p < .05$). Thus for the *most* severely ill subset of the disturbed group, drugs assist residents in coping with the facility environment. But drug doses for residents who scored lowest on the BPRS (i.e., the healthiest group) were significantly and *negatively* related to internal-integration scores (the partial correlation between internal integration and drug dosage in the healthiest subgroup, controlled for symptom assessments, being equal to $-.22$ ($p < .05$)). That is, for the healthiest portion of the sample, drugs work *against* the patient's ability to negotiate his or her needs through the operator and the facility.

The positive impact of increased drug dosage on external integration occurs in a group with less overall disturbance than the group in which we find a positive relationship between internal integration and drug dosage. It is the differential impact of psychopathology on external and internal integration that accounts for this finding. Psychopathology has a greater impact on external than on internal activities, the former involving greater social outreach, and therefore the drugs have their impact on those with lesser disturbance.

These findings are quite disturbing in view of the high risk factors associated with taking medications if no benefit can be attributed to their usage. The "no benefit" conclusion is certainly supported by our data, at least with respect to all but the most severely ill residents, if we employ internal and external integration as our outcome criteria.

Given our pattern of results—which suggests a more discriminating use of drugs—it seems necessary to look at the relationship between social integration and drug doses when other important factors in drug treatment are controlled for—for example, resident age and the chronicity of his illness.

AGE, CHRONICITY, AND SOCIAL INTEGRATION

To examine the relation of age and chronicity to social integration and antipsychotic drug use, the population was divided into four categories: under 40 with less than 10 years in a psychiatric institution, under 40 with 10 years or more in a psychiatric institution, and the same categories for those over 40 years of age. Previously cited research studies have demonstrated the general beneficial effect of antipsychotic drugs on those under 40 with fewer years of hospitalization. We wished to determine whether this held true for the California sheltered-care population. Also of interest were the differences between patients, in an era when incentives in the mental-health system clearly tend toward community-based treatment programs.

Our data indicate that young residents with short hospital histories experience a weak negative effect on their external integration when we consider only the relationship between external integration and drug dosage. However, when severity of symptomatology is controlled for, this relationship becomes a weak positive one. This change is due to the fact that, for the young with only short periods of hospitalization, there is significant and strong positive relationship between drug dosage and severity of symptomatology ($r =$ .38, $p < .01$). Thus prescribing for the young with brief hospitalization is related to symptomatology. This latter relationship decreases and becomes slightly negative as one gets older and accumulates hospital time—for those over 40 with more than 10 years of hospitalization it is $r = -.11$. It thus seems that prescribing for those who are older and have more hospital time is done as a matter of course or with reference to some underlying disorder as opposed to being related to the more specific criterion of symptomatology.

The older, more chronic subset (those over 40 with more than 10 years of hospitalization) experience a very strong, highly significant negative effect of antipsychotic medications on internal integration (the partial correlation between internal integration and drug dosage, when symptomatology is controlled for, being $-.36$, $p < .01$) and a small negative effect on external integration.

There were no other significant associations between internal or external integration and antipsychotic drug dosage within age and chronicity subgroups.

If the antipsychotic drugs are effective only for a small subset of the mentally ill population, but 76% of the population are taking these powerful medications, are the drugs really therapeutic, or are they merely a mechanism of social control? If the drugs are therapeutic, why is the prescribing pattern so extensive when research has demonstrated the selective effectiveness of the antipsychotic medications (Clark & Davis, 1970; Prien & Cole, 1968)?

We do not question the prescribing of high doses of antipsychotic drugs for groups where such dosing procedures have proved effective for promoting their social integration, for example, the most severely disturbed. However, because of the disabling side effects of these powerful drugs, we question the wisdom of such broad prescription of these drugs to a population known to be less likely to benefit from them. Furthermore maintaining a patient on the same drug and dosage without modification "unless there is a problem" impedes the patient's chances of being successful on lower doses or even of getting off the drugs for rest periods. Certainly the population over 40, for whom the drugs are not as effective and who comprise almost two-thirds of the population in sheltered care in California, might benefit from some dosage reductions or drug "holidays"—especially that portion of this group evidencing no severe psychiatric symptomatology.

REFERENCES

American College of Neuropsychopharmacology, FDA Task Force. "Neurologic Syndromes Associated with Antipsychotic Drug Use." *New Engl. J. Med.* **289**(1), 20–23 (1973).

The American Medical Association. *Drug Evaluations,* 1st ed. Chicago: AMA, 1971.

Dr. Caligari (pseudonym). "Pursuing Spychiatric Pill Pushers," in Sherry Hirsch et al. (Eds.). *Madness Network News Reader.* San Francisco: Glide Publications, 1974, pp. 98–121.

Carscallen, H. B., H. Rochman, and T. D. Lovegrove. "High Dose Trifluoperazine in Schizophrenia." *Canad. Psychiat. J.* **13**, 459–461 (1968).

Claridge, G. *Drugs and Human Behavior.* London: Penguin Press, 1970.

Clark, M. L. and J. M. Davis. "Chlorpromazine in Chronic Schizophrenia: Behavioral Dose Response Relationships." *Psychopharmacologia* (Berlin), **18**, 260–270 (1970).

Davis, A., et al. *Schizophrenics in the New Custodial Community: Five Years after the Experiment.* Columbus: Ohio State University Press, 1974.

Englehart, D., et al. "Phenothiazines in Prevention of Psychiatric Hospitalization." *Arch. Gen. Psychiat.* **16**(1), 98–117 (1967).

Gardos, G., J. Cole, and M. Orzack. "The Importance of Dosage in Antipsychotic Drug Administration: A Review of Dose Response Studies." *Psychopharmacol.* **29**, 221–230 (1973).

Goffman, E. *Asylums.* Garden City, New York: Doubleday and Company, Inc., 1961.

Goldstein, M. "Premorbid Adjustment, Paranoid Status, and Patterns of Response to Phenothizaine in Acute Schizophrenia." *Schizophrenia Bulletin,* National Clearing House for Mental Health Information, No. 3, pp. 24–37, Winter, 1970.

Gray, J. "Psychotropic Medication and the Approved Home Resident." Unpublished memo. North Battleford, Saskatchewan, Canada, 1974.

Heins, T. J. "Prescription Audit in the Evaluation of Community Physicians Care of Chronic Psychiatric Patients in Foster Care." *Ann. Royal Coll. Phys. and Surg. Canada,* **8**, 1–5 (1975).

Hogarty, G. "Drug and Sociotherapy in the Aftercare of Schizophrenic Patients." *Arch. Gen. Psychiat.* **28**(1), 54–64 (1973).

Hollister, L. *Clinical Uses of Psychotherapeutic Drugs.* Springfield, Illinois: Charles C. Thomas, 1973.

Klein, D. F., and J. M. Davis. *Diagnosis and Drug Treatment of Psychiatric Disorders.* Baltimore: Williams and Wilkins Co., 1969.

Lennard, H. *Mystification and Drug Misuse: Hazards in Using Psychoactive Drugs.* San Francisco: Jossey-Bass, Inc., 1971.

Lennard, H. and A. Bernstein. "Perspectives on the New Psychoactive Drug Technology," in Ruth Coperstock (Ed.). *Social Aspects of the Medical Use of Psychotropic Drugs.* Toronto, Canada: Addiction Research Foundation, 1974.

Meyers, F., et al. *Review of Medical Pharmacology,* 4th ed. Los Altos, California: Lange Medical Publications, 1974.

Overall, J. and D. Gorham. "The Brief Psychiatric Rating Scale." *Psychologic. Rep.* **10**, 779–812 (1962).

Pasamanick, B., et al. *Schizophrenics in the Community.* New York: Appleton, 1967.

The *Physicians' Desk Reference,* 28th ed. Oradell, New Jersey: Charles E. Baker, Jr., Publisher, Medical Economics Company, 1974.

Prien, R. and J. Cole. "High Dose Chlorpromazine Therapy in Chronic Schizophrenia." *Arch. Gen. Psychiat.* **18**, 482–495 (1968).

Prien, R. and C. J. Klett. "An Appraisal of the Long-term Use of Tranquilizing Medication with Hospitalized Chronic Schizophrenics." *Schizophrenia Bull.*, National Clearing House for Mental Health Information, No. 5, Spring, 1972.

Prien, R., J. Levine, and J. Cole. "High Dose Trifluoperazine Therapy in Chronic Schizophrenia." *Am. J. Psychiat.* **126,** 53–61 (1969).

Ray, O. *Drugs, Society and Human Behavior.* St. Louis: C. V. Mosby Company, 1972.

Scheff, T. *Being Mentally Ill: A Sociological Theory.* Chicago: Aldine Publishing Company, 1966.

Wing, J., et al. "Preventive Treatment of Schizophrenia: Some Theoretical and Methodological Issues, in J. Cole et al. (Eds.). *Psychopathology and Psychopharmacology.* Baltimore: John Hopkins Press, 1972.

FIFTEEN

Consumer or Commodity?

I feel that I have lost too much time in my life, that I didn't realize my true potential. Oh, that I wasn't in this unfortunate situation! Most of my life I've always made my own decisions and now someone else is telling me something I feel is completely wrong, but these are people you can't argue with (sheltered-care resident).

In most human-service organizations the distinction between consumer and commodity is blurred. The individual participant is viewed to some extent as both a consumer and a commodity. The factor in a particular service that determines whether he is more the former than the latter is the extent to which he exercises control over and participates in major decisions in the service process that affect his life circumstances.

To a greater or lesser extent, all participants in the sheltered-care controversy have assumed the role of patient helper. They are all doing something for the residents of the sheltered-care home that they assume these individuals are incapable of doing for themselves. Even grassroots organizations involved in the situation do not have a clear understanding of what the residents' role should be in the system. Little clarity exists about the question of whether the resident is to be a commodity of, or a consumer in, the system;

whether he is to be an object of "people-processing" and "people-changing" organizations or a person who uses a service.

SHELTERED CARE AS A COMMODITY MARKET

When the sheltered-care system is viewed as a commodity market, two factors conflict with the goals of external and internal integration:

1. An empty facility bed represents an operating loss to the facility in terms of revenue and increased overhead per resident (though it may represent more choice for the consumer).
2. The state lacks a system of quality control by which to determine whether sheltered-care facilities achieve social-integration goals.

In considering the first factor, we should realize that residents who achieve complete economic independence and move to independent living arrangements represent empty beds to facility operators. No matter how good the intentions of operators, in most cases they are in business to make a living, and an empty bed is an economic burden. However, the small portion of the population who will achieve this level of independence does not pose a serious financial threat to most operators. In fact many operators—especially in small facilities—showed pride and encouragment at the outreach efforts of able residents.

The empty bed is, in terms of its negative effects on internal and external integration, more of a problem from the perspective of the placement system than when it is considered a factor in blocking individuals from leaving the system. Werner (1974) cites four placement channels in the system: private mental-health professionals, county inpatient services, the Public Guardian's Office, and the local Community Care Services Section of the Department of Health (CCSS). She correctly points out (pp. 45–46):

The most commonly alleged criticism against placement agencies is probably most applicable to the non-CCSS inputs into the board and care system. Improper matching to the most suitable type of facility, non-contact with ex-patients, and lack of evaluation of residents' progress and conditions appears more likely given that proper mental health aftercare referral is not the principal function of these agencies.

In addition at least 20% of the residents are placed by operators and other informal participants who have neither organizational nor professional accountability. Competition to fill empty beds has led operators to develop their own referral sources and to press politically for a referral system based on equity between facilities rather than resident need. In areas where there are not enough residents to fill available beds, the effect on development of a placement system based on resident need is even more acute. One area, situated near a closed state hospital, lacks sufficient mentally ill to keep facility beds filled, and operators advocate bringing in out-of-county residents to fill the void.

The system is currently unable to ensure supervised placement in accordance with individual needs, and it is questionable that such a referral system can even be developed; therefore, the active participation of informed consumers is essential to supplement and expand the supervisory potential of the professional placement personnel. Continuation of the current system of placement, which functions in many areas of the state primarily to fill empty facility beds, can lead only to an increased number of "involuntary residents," who develop feelings of helplessness and resentment that block their external and internal integration.

The second factor that brings the commodity-market perspective into conflict with the goals of social integration is the lack of a means by which to ensure high-quality care for residents. As a commodity the resident is barter for $270 a month. This is the legal maximum payment allowed to operators for board and care under state regulations effective June 1, 1975, and applies primarily to Supplemental Security Income (SSI) recipients, who comprise 81% of the sheltered-care population. This amount is determined by the Director of the Department of Health, Department of Benefit Payments. On the basis of California State Bill AB853, which set the legal board-and-care minimum at $225 per month, the Department of Benefit Payments makes a yearly budget adjustment to the maximum rate determined by average cost-of-living increases in Los Angeles and San Francisco. No reasonable cost analysis of sheltered care has been completed, and the possibility of doing such a study, given the problems of obtaining valid data, is in serious question (Charles, 1973). Yet the achievement of high quality in the facilities' "people-changing effort" requires financial and manpower inputs in excess of the fees currently allowed on the basis of cost of care. Program grants, private fund raising, payment of private fees to compensate for low SSI fees, and undervaluation of the operator's labor are some of the methods used by concerned operators to maintain quality of care.

At the opposite end of the spectrum are low-quality, large institutions that may get $810 a month for three women occupying a single bedroom that would rent for no more than $175 per month without the supervisory component. It is hardly conceivable that these facilities are offering a $635 differential in food and programs (Werner, 1974, p. 30). Interviewers' impressions confirm that a service differential of this magnitude is not evident: "the thing that stands out . . . as a generalization is that . . . most residents are totally confined to the facilities and do nothing. They're not even interested in watching TV anymore. . . . Most of them just lay down in their beds, sit in their rooms, or sit on the porch and watch the people walk by."

With no understanding of the cost of the components of high-quality care—many of which are so diffuse as to defy cost accounting—it seems reasonable to give credence to the claims of operators of high-quality facilities that fees for service are too low. Yet for the state to put more money into sheltered care, it must be assured that the experience of the state hospital's back wards will not be repeated. High-quality care was not maintained in the small number of state hospitals with a monitoring system based solely on professional manpower. Can it be hoped that the quality of care in hundreds of sheltered-care facilities can be adequately assessed, especially without the aid of an active consumer? Unless changes are made to determine how consumers may best work with professionals to supplement their efforts, we might expect to see the development of operations similar to the Public Guardian's Office in Los Angeles. Twenty deputy guardians make placements for the entire county; because of the small staff further evaluation is limited to investigating residents' complaints. Such a situation assumes consumerism without encouraging it and without assessing residents' capabilities to perform such a role (particularly important in this example because of the residents' need for public guardianship).

SHELTERED CARE AS A CONSUMER MARKET

In regarding the sheltered-care system as a consumer market, it is appropriate to consider five questions posed by Karno and Schwartz (1974):

1. Who are the participants?
2. How are decisions to be made?
3. What are the constraints on participation?
4. Who is accountable for the consequences of joint decisions?
5. What happens in case of irreconcilable conflicts?

Who are the Participants?

At a minimum the participants in any consumer action are the consumer and the provider of the service. In sheltered care they are the resident and an operator, CCSS social worker, welfare worker, physician, or other service providers. Other parties may be involved in four capacities: (1) as facilitators, (2) as participant observers, (3) as advocates, and (4) as mediators. These participant roles are discussed in greater detail later. We have already noted, however, that service providers in the sheltered-care situation see themselves, to a greater or lesser degree, as fulfilling some of the third-party roles in addition to their primary service functions. This factor may make it difficult for them to be confronted by residents with consumer demands. But it also makes them more amenable to accepting consumer-proposed alternatives.

How are Decisions to Be Made?

Many of the most basic decisions in the sheltered-care environment are made in direct negotiations between the resident and the service provider. In one small facility a resident had arranged for his own room with an outside entrance. He has his own keys and is more of an independent boarder than other house residents who live under a family atmosphere. Most residents in sheltered care are, however, more passive and engage in consumer actions only with the supportive efforts of third-party participants. The most consumer-oriented role these participants assume is that of facilitator. In this role the participant provides the resident with education and consultation and, at the most active level, may attempt to raise the consciousness of the consumer group to promote independent action. Ideally, when facilitators function in this way, the consumers themselves bring their demand to the service providers.

The success of New Opportunities Through Voluntary Action (NOVA), a Los Angeles organization that has attempted during the past 4½ years to promote an activist orientation among sheltered-care residents, provides a good example of the use of this third-party role. Acting in an educative capacity, this group "convinced some individuals to stand up, assert themselves, and advocate their own principles. . . . One woman who internalized the teachings of survival in a complex world, . . . questioned the relevance of past mental illness to driving ability, . . . by herself. [She] fought the Department of Motor Vehicles for three years to get a driver's license" (Werner, 1974, p. 101).

In the following situation NOVA acted in a consciousness-raising capacity: A chain of board-and-care home operators had food prepared in a central kitchen, and it arrived cold to the facilities. A "food survey" among the residents was taken. The effect of the survey was to demonstrate residents' discontent with the service, and this led the owners to install separate kitchens.

This type of third-party role is in accordance with Alinsky's observations on helping relationships.

It is impossible to over-estimate the enormous importance of people doing things themselves. It is the most common reaction that successful attainment of objectives is much more meaningful to people who have achieved the objectives through their own efforts (Alinsky, 1946, p. 12).

In light of Alinsky's thoughts, compare the following statement of a NOVA member with the statement of the sheltered-care resident quoted at the beginning of this chapter:

I have found NOVA to be a very helpful organization that has substantially benefited my life. Participating in the organization has stimulated me to take new interest in my physical and social environment and to make greater efforts to control my own life. In my experience as a resident for 13 years at Fredmarc Manor, NOVA has represented the only opportunity for residents to engage in the type of meaningful self-help activities which would enable them to exert greater control over their own lives. It is only through NOVA that the residents will change from passive "patients" to active and functioning members of the community (Werner, 1974, p. 105).

Amos Fried, NOVA's director, states that the agency's role is to help residents learn "that they are responsible for their own lives and we are teaching them to use that responsibility "(Minnehan, 1974, p. 9). To achieve this goal, NOVA organizes the residents in a facility, helps them elect a chairman and officers, and then withdraws into the background, leaving leadership to the group itself.

And NOVA, like other service organizations, has frequently lapsed into other third-party roles in the consumer process. At times they have become the "participant observer." In this role the third party joins the consumer in his negotiation efforts and by his presence bolsters those efforts. The following example of this type of activity was given by a NOVA organizer:

One NOVA member failed to receive his ATD grant for several months until the organizers and members contacted his caseworker at the Department of Public Social Services. According to the NOVA newspaper, the worker "put things off and distorted the truth in her statements." After a meeting, an attempt was made to meet with the District Director—but the secretary refused to make an appointment. Finally a group of 18 members of NOVA and a NOVA staff person stormed the welfare office and interrupted the Director in a meeting. As a result, the member received his grant, which amounted to more than $1000 (F.N.).*

This type of help for clients in challenging the welfare process and violations of their rights is a role more commonly assumed by social-service organizations than by facilitators. It represents a social prosthesis (i.e., the addition of support to a person's interaction) rather than a purchase of services to supplement an individual's abilities (e.g., hiring a lawyer).

The "advocate" as a third party in consumer negotiation has a more encompassing role in the support offered than the participant observer has. In this arrangement of roles it is the advocate who takes the action, usually, but not necessarily, at the request of the consumer. In one situation NOVA organizers, noting that a facility cleaned its windows only once a year, threatened to call the health inspectors; the operator cleaned the windows. In

---

*F.N. refers to field notes taken at the time of a structured or open-ended interview.

another instance NOVA staff persons (not resident members) attempted to influence a CCSS worker to change the wording of a form that informed residents of their right to refuse services and that in effect required the client to acknowledge by his signature that he was "mentally ill." Here NOVA's efforts were directed at eliminating the stigma-producing effects of the process.

Another illustration of the advocate role is legal action taken on behalf of 100 residents who attended the Thunderseed Social Rehabilitation Program in San Francisco. San Francisco Neighborhood Legal Assistance Foundation filed a suit against the City and County of San Francisco and several other city and state employees to prevent the closure of the social rehabilitation program. Although it is not clear that the suit itself led to the discovery of funds for the continuation of this program, Thunderseed is now operating and continuing its work.

The final third-party role in consumer negotiation is the mediator. This role is perhaps more common for service organizations other than NOVA in the sheltered-care situation and is characteristically assumed by the person who arranges placement for released mental patients. We found, for example, that 33% of the residents who stated that they chose to come to their facility did not see it beforehand but had trusted the opinion of the person who recommended it to them. Even more than the advocate, the mediator is actually required to make the decisions. And NOVA's avoidance of this role is the major difference between its client-centered efforts and the efforts of other service organizations. Yet even NOVA views the professional organizer as an indispensable person in consumer efforts involving former mental patients. For this reason, and because of NOVA's deemphasis of third-party roles other than that of facilitator, this organization, though it is the most effective client-centered organization in the state, has only begun to give credibility to consumerism among former mental patients. A step-by-step withdrawal of professionals from a well-organized resident group, always with the assurance that the support will be there if necessary, is the next stage. This pattern would also allow for optimum use of available professional manpower. Such a process assumes that residents have the capacity for running a well-organized consumer group. Evidence for this is not clear, though some of our data reported later indicate they at least have the capacity to assess their situations adequately. We must support the highest degree of autonomy possible and will find what the highest degree is only if we are first willing to experiment with granting such autonomy.

What Are the Constraints on Participation?

There are four constraints to the participation of sheltered-care residents from the consumer perspective:

1. Psychological disability and learned social passivity.
2. Geographic dispersion and residents' unwillingness to participate in group action.
3. Conflict of interest between service provision and the promotion of consumerism.
4. Resources for influence.

Psychological Disability and Learned Social Passivity. The major assumption about the mentally ill with regard to consumerism is that they are too psychologically disturbed and socially passive to provide an adequate assessment of their environment. Further, it is assumed that this disturbance is a significant constraint on their ability to act as informed consumers. Yet only 17% of the population we studied actually had conservators. Therefore the validity of this "psychological handicap" assumption must be questioned.

To evaluate the environment in which the resident lives, a 20-item consumer-response scale was developed, the items of which were concerned primarily with the characteristics of the facility. (The complete consumer-response questionnaire is contained in Appendix E.) The total score of respondents summed over all 20 items in the consumer-response scale was significantly related to the degree of their external and internal integration. That is, the better the resident's report of the environment, the more likely he was to have a higher level of external and internal integration. The correlation of the consumer-response scale with internal integration was, however, much greater than its correlation with external integration.

The finding that consumer response is predictive of internal and external integration leads one to ask what the best predictors of consumer response scores are. Are these predictors valid in the sense of reflecting an adequate assessment of the environment, or are they related to a person's mental handicap and social passivity and thus indicative of a poor and inaccurate assessment of the environment?

To test the validity of the stereotype of the mentally ill as unable to assess their environment accurately, a consumer-response model was developed by using three types of variables as predictors of the consumer-response score: (1) facility environment descriptions, (2) measures of psychological disorder and social passivity, and (3) resident's desire to remain at his current residence (see Figure 15.1).

Four variables describing the social-psychological environment of the facility that showed the strongest positive relations to the consumer response score were included in the model: program involvement, order and organization, support, and spontaneity. These four variables are subscales of the Community Oriented Program Environment Scale (COPES). With the exception of "order and organization," which refers to system-maintenance characteristics of the facility, these subscales describe social relationships within the facility.

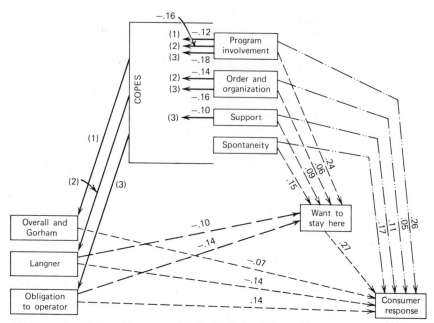

Figure 15.1. Consumer model. The values associated with each path refer to the value of the model's partial standardized regression coefficients. The size of these regression coefficients indicates their relative importance in the model. Nonsignificant paths, evaluated at the .05 level, have been eliminated.

Three measures of psychological disturbance and social passivity were included in the model. The first was the resident score on the Overall and Gorham Brief Psychiatric Rating Scale (BPRS). This score, as noted in previous chapters, represents ratings on 16 psychiatric symptoms: somatic concern, anxiety, emotional withdrawal, conceptual disorganization, guilt feelings, tension, mannerisms and posturing, grandiosity, depressive mood, hostility, suspiciousness, hallucinatory behavior, motor retardation, uncooperativeness, unusual thought content, and blunted affect. The second measure of psychological disturbance was the Langner Scale, which consists primarily of residents' self-reports of psychophysiologic disturbance and has been found to be predictive of psychiatric ratings of psychological disturbance (Srole et al., 1962). The third measure was a scale developed to assess residents' feelings of obligation toward the operator. Such feelings of obligation were viewed as a measure of social passivity, though it would also seem logical to interpret them as a measure of gratitude toward the operator for a good service.

Finally a validation variable was included in the model. Based on the belief that an individual who felt he was in a good program would wish to remain there, resident response to the question, "How would you view the prospect of staying on in this facility for a long period of time?" was included in the model.

We found that the environmental variable with the greatest impact on reducing levels of psychopathology and social passivity was program involvement (See Figure 15.1). Program involvement requires the participation of the individual in the social situation and thus reduces his concentration on psychological problems. Whereas a high level of "order and organization" in the facility was associated with a reduction in the self-report of psychophysiological symptomatology (i.e., reduction in Langner scores) and also tended to contribute to a reduction in the resident's obligation to the operator, it was not related to psychiatric-symptom ratings as measured by the Overall and Gorham Scale.

The "supportive" environment tended to reduce the resident's feelings of obligation to the operator, perhaps by virtue of his ability to gain needed support from other individuals in the facility. This variable had no impact on psychopathology.

The fourth facility characteristic, "spontaneity," had no impact on psychological disturbance or social passivity.

In looking at the consumer-response score as the major dependent variable in the model, the validational concept "want to stay here" had the strongest positive relationship (measured by the partial standardized regression weight) in the anticipated direction. But the size of the positive standardized regression coefficient describing the impact of a unit change in "want to stay" on the individual's consumer-response score (given the influence of the other variables in the system) leads us to the conclusion that "wanting to stay" is only one component of consumer response and not necessarily a measure of criterion validity. Thus individuals who thought the facility was good were *more likely* to want to remain.

The second most powerful set of predictors were the facility-environment factors. All four of these variables were related to consumer response in the same way—that is, the more program involvement, order and organization, support, and spontaneity in an environment, the more residents were likely to assess it positively. This was true even after psychological disturbance and social passivity had been taken into account. This does not, however, imply that these factors do not influence consumer response. The Overall and Gorham, Langner, and Obligation-to-the-Operator scales were all significantly related to consumer-response scores. We found that, the higher the level of disturbance and the lower the feelings of obligation to the operator, the more negative the evaluation of the facility.

Thus psychological disturbance and social dependency do add a degree of ambiguity to consumer ratings and therefore pose some obstacle to the interpretation of these consumer ratings; however, the more powerful and independent components of consumer ratings are facility characteristics.

Geographic Dispersion and Residents' Unwillingness to Participate in Group Action.
The tendency of residents to avoid being identified with other residents was
already discussed when we looked at the influence of isolation on internal
integration. To some extent identification with the resident group means
acceptance of society's definition that one is mentally ill. This is a definition
of self that many residents strongly resist, and their resistance is a significant
constraint on group participation in a resident-consumer organization. Their
unwillingness to be identified with an organized group is reflected in the fact
that most people would find the following cartoon funny:

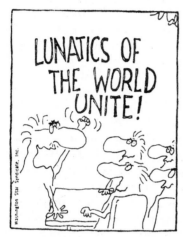

It is easiest to organize residents where they are highly concentrated, such
as in large facilities and in the residential ghetto. It is here that consumer
organizations have functioned best, as witnessed by the success of NOVA in
organizing residents in Los Angeles and the attempt at resident organization
in San Jose. In these environments it is more difficult to resist identification
because residents are more publicly visible, whereas small, geographically
dispersed facilities make group identification less likely and organization of
residents more difficult. Thus greater effort is required to facilitate resident
organization among dispersed populations than in more impacted areas.

*Conflict of Interest Between Service Provision and Promotion of Consumer Service Assess-
ments.* To the extent the resident is dependent on service providers, he may
be "biting the hand that feeds him" when he promotes his own self-interests.
The dependence of the resident upon the operator far exceeds the dependence of a tenant upon his landlord. The resident may be a consumer in
name only if the operator receives and deposits his support check and doles
out his spending money. Priscilla Allen (1974a), a resident advocate currently
living in sheltered care, notes that:

When I moved into the board and care home where I live, my first ATD check was presented to me, face down, ready for signature. Its envelope had, of course, been opened and the check removed by the operator. Before the rent came due again, I opened a bank account and presented the operator with a check for the approaching month's rent. I continued to follow this policy, and she has not, to my knowledge, opened any more of my mail (p. 13).

Fully 53% of the residents in sheltered care who do not have a legal conservator report that, when their checks arrive, the operator opens their mail and has them sign the full amount of the check over to him.

Also contributing to residents' dependence on the operator is the fact that the resident does not have the legal safeguards of eviction proceedings such as the 30-day notice. Sometimes operators even have reciprocal arrangements with other operators so that a recalcitrant resident can be transferred to another facility at a moment's notice. Viewed in this context, resident fear of consumer activism is understandable.

Another illustration of the fear of becoming involved in consumer activitism is reported in the experiences of one resident activist. This man attempted to involve the residents of his board-and-care facility in complaining to state licensing about possible violations by the facility operator. The residents told him "Stop, because you are going to make it worse for us." Ultimately this man praised the wisdom of his fellow residents, for when licensing ultimately did come in to inspect the facility, the lot of the residents was in fact worsened. Residents who formerly had been living in attractive attic rooms were forced, because of fire hazard, to move down to much less attractive basement facilities.

Operators and other service providers see their roles in the life of the residents as ongoing and essential. Many operators went into the business because the former mental patient was expected to be a "compliant resident"—one who would not raise objections about living facilities or service and who would remain a long time. Encouraging independence may change this population characteristic and confront the operator with a more difficult and expensive service task. The idea of phasing out service supports to promote independence has been given only limited expression in the development of satellite housing programs (i.e., programs that emphasize less supervision and more independent living in a subsidized apartment). In our view there should be increasing efforts in this direction in light of the stated goals of resident independence. The lack of development in this area may indicate a conflict of interest between residents and operators.

Resources for Influence.   As effective consumers former patients must be able not only to organize themselves for action but also to exert influence so that their demands will be heeded. In both these activities they are handicapped by a lack of resources with which to promote organization and with which to engage in effective bargaining. The cost of transportation to meetings might itself be an obstacle, let alone the finances necessary to promote their aims. This forces residents to be dependent on outside groups to support their efforts. In addition the nature of their common bond—mental illness and social dependency—detracts from their credibility in the eyes of policymakers. They are truly a powerless group. Even the threat of disruption used by other powerless groups is hardly a viable one for this population: Mental patients do not engage in group riots—they act as isolated individuals.

Who Is Accountable for the Consequences of Joint Decisions?

Ideally one would expect that the service provider, if he plays a major role in making decisions, would also share responsibility with the resident for their consequences. In fact, though, it is usually the resident who is held accountable—regardless of how the decision is made. For example, whether or not a resident participates in choosing his facility, he alone must live with that choice and pay for failure by returning to the hospital. Although the Lanterman-Petris-Short (LPS) Act has restored the right of self-determination to the released mental patient (to participate in the market), it has provided few of the resources necessary (e.g., professional facilitators to educate, consult, and help develop consumer action or functional support) for this vulnerable and highly disaffiliated population to exercise such a right.

What Happens in Case of Irreconcilable Conflict?

If the current system is to be taken as an indication, nothing happens in the instance of irreconcilable conflict. The system enters a state of limbo in which the primary losers are the residents. This is illustrated by the lack of a solution to the zoning problem after several years of controversy. In a political standoff residents are powerless to initiate change that is in their interest. Whether the encouragement of effective consumer action could bring about change at a significant level is questionable. However, success in the smaller issues (as demonstrated by the NOVA experience) will provide the confidence and initiative needed to take on more significant controversies.

RESIDENTS AS CONSUMERS: PLACEMENT CHOICE

Which residents choose their own facility, what organization brokered their placement, and which facilities did they choose?

We asked residents whether or not they chose their current living arrangement. Overall 64% of the residents said they had. The resident who chose a facility could be any age, sex, or marital status but is likely to be from a higher socioeconomic status and have his or her own spending money. This money is available on a predictable, regular basis. These residents are more internally and externally integrated.

When we looked to see how residents' choice varied by placement broker, we found that 75% of the facilities brokered by the CCSS scored in the "choice" range when the responses of their residents to the question were aggregated. Likewise 73% of the facilities brokered through family, friends, and residents scored in this range. Facilities serviced by public-welfare and county mental-health services had only 50% in the "choice" range when the responses of their residents were aggregated and averaged. Thus CCSS as the major placement broker seems to be giving the residents it places as much or more choice of living situation than other placement brokers.

Concerning the validity of this choice differential by placement broker, we considered current residents' satisfaction with the facility and the qualitative reasons given for their choice. Residents of facilities brokered by CCSS and "self, family, friends" are more likely to say they are satisfied with their facility. When asked for qualitative reasons for choosing the facility (e.g., they liked the operator, the residents, the area, or the living arrangement), in contrast to some nonchoice reason (e.g., trusting the recommender or liking everything about the facility), both the "self, family, friends"-brokered residents and the CCSS-brokered residents had a higher percentage (37% and 28% as compared to 12% and 4% respectively, cite specific qualities of the facility) than groups referred by other brokers.*

While there was little clear-cut relationship between resident's choice of facility and the facility's program, residents who chose looked for either quiet (farm) areas or mixed business and residential areas. Residents are also likely to choose a facility in an upper class area.

Choice was related to the resident population of the facility. Those facilities with all mentally ill or no mentally ill residents were less likely to have residents who felt they chose the facility. Facilities with residents who could be characterized as extreme are less likely to have been chosen; that is, all or none of their residents were abandoned by their families, all or none of their residents can work, and all or none of their residents have been in a state hospital for more than 5 years. Thus residents seem to look for a mix of other residents and for situations wherein they will be neither the worst off nor the best off. The exception to this rule is, however, those facilities where the operator said all the residents had been hospitalized within the year. These facilities had a very high probability of choice, perhaps indicative of changing policies in placement giving residents more choice. Finally facilities with residents having a full-age range of characteristics are the most likely to be chosen.

---

*Such findings, besides indicating the validity of resident choice, could be viewed as efforts to reduce cognitive dissonance resulting from having made a choice.

Given this information, we assume that residents are exercising very reasonable criteria in their selection of facilities and perhaps could benefit from additional information on available facilities to enhance their consumer efforts.

CONSUMER RIGHTS OR ADVOCATE PREROGATIVES?

Current actions on behalf of residents emphasize the need to clarify or at least focus attention on the distinction between consumers' rights and the prerogatives of their adovcates to act on their behalf. Whereas the consumer and his advocate often have complementary interests, there is much room for conflict between them.

Conflict between the rights of residents and the prerogatives of their advocates can spring from two basic facts:

1. Sheltered-care residents are often deprived of their rights as free-living citizens—that is, they are a vulnerable population in need of protection.
2. Extending protection to residents in the community limits their rights as free-living citizens.

A Vulnerable yet Free-Living Population

Priscilla Allen (1974b) has recently written a Bill of Consumer Tenant, and Civil Rights for Citizens Using Mental Health Services. In her statement of intent relating to the bill, Allen writes that:

Unless they are subject to specific legal limitations, persons living in the community utilizing mental health services are entitled to all the rights and privileges that ordinarily accompany citizenship. In fact, however, they are denied many of these rights. This bill has been formulated in order to bring into sharper focus some of the areas where the greatest deficiencies in true citizenship are most frequently encountered.

In offering this "bill of rights," Allen raises the reality of a very vulnerable, yet legally free-living population. Seven basic rights are detailed in this proposed bill: (1) the right to treatment, (2) the right to refuse treatment, (3) the right to confidentiality of personal records, (4) the right to use fully the economic rights and benefits to which a client is entitled, (5) the right to a humane psychological and physical environment, (6) the right to conduct life with maximum freedom and independence suitable to each free-living person, (7) the right to information.

The most important facts about these rights are that (1) a majority of them have already been guaranteed to involuntarily confined individuals in state institutions,* and yet no such recognition has been granted to residents in

---

*The provisions of Article 7 of the LPS Act relating to legal and civil rights of persons confined in mental institutions note:

facilities that have taken over many of the previous functions of the state hospital system, and (2) the basis for entitlement for the right to treatment—loss of due process rights—conflicts with the others.

It is the contention of many mental-health professionals (Shadoan, 1975, among others) and some resident advocates such as Allen, that these rights should now be extended to individuals living in residential-care facilities for the mentally ill. There is no doubt that the rights of this vulnerable population in sheltered care are in need of protection. Yet we must consider, from the consumers' point of view, the implications of extending these rights, previously granted involuntarily committed patients in mental hospitals, into the community.

Protection Limits Residents' Rights

It is our contention that, without significant consumer input into the determination of which rights should be extended into the community and how the extension should be made, the result will be an extension of the prerogatives of the advocates of the mentally ill to impose treatment or other services as opposed to an extension of the rights of the mentally ill themselves. This contention can best be substantiated by a look at the "right-to-treatment" issue.

The "right-to-treatment" argument has been generated primarily from a series of legal decisions, the most important cases being *Wyatt* v. *Stickney*, F.2d (1972) and *Donaldson* v. *O'Connor*, 493 F.2d (1974) and F.2d (1975). In both

---

"5325. Each person involuntarily detained for evaluation or treatment under provisions of this part shall have the following rights, a list of which shall be prominently posted in English and Spanish in all facilities providing such services and otherwise brought to his attention by such additional means as the Director of Mental Hygiene may designate by regulation:

(a) To wear his own clothes, to keep and use his own personal possessions including his toilet articles; and to keep and be allowed to spend a reasonable sum of his own money for canteen expenses and small purchases.

(b) To have access to individual storage space for his private use.

(c) To see visitors each day.

(d) To have reasonable access to telephones, both to make and to receive confidential calls.

(e) To have ready access to letter writing materials, including stamps, and to mail and receive unopened correspondence.

(f) To refuse shock treatment.

(g) To refuse psycho surgery.

5328. All information and records obtained in the course of providing services to either voluntary or involuntary recipients of services shall be confidential (Cal. Welf. & Inst. Code., §5325, §5328)."

In addition, the "right to treatment" has been guaranteed by the courts to the involuntarily confined.

the *Wyatt* case and in the first *Donaldson* decision, Judge Wisdom of the U.S. Fifth Circuit Court of Appeals handed down an opinion stating that:

To deprive any citizen of his or her liberty upon the altruistic theory that the confinement is for humane therapeutic reasons and then fail to provide adequate treatment violates the very fundamentals of due process (493 F.2d, at 521).

Using this line of reasoning and noting that these two decisions related primarily to involuntary inpatients in state hospitals, a recent suit filed in the Superior Court in the State of California—*Williams et al.* v. *the City and County of San Francisco et al.*—attempted to expand the notion of involuntary commitment to include community care, and to establish that, although people released from state hospitals to community-sheltered facilities are legally free to leave whenever they choose, they are in fact held in an involuntary capacity in the facilities in which they live. The attorneys for plaintiffs (residents in these facilities) noted in the complaint that:

Plaintiffs are informed and believe and thereon allege that as a result of their mental disorders they did not knowingly participate in the preparation of the aftercare plan prepared prior to their release from the State mental hospital; that State employees prepared said plan in order to obtain the release of plaintiffs from such institutions as mandated by the Lanterman-Petris-Short and Short-Doyle Acts; that State employees made all arrangements for the placement of plaintiffs in their respective board and care facilities; that State employees in State-owned vehicles transported plaintiffs to their board and care homes and that State employees arranged for plaintiffs to receive welfare assistance to support and maintain plaintiffs in said homes. Plaintiffs are further informed and believe and allege each of said homes is licensed and regulated by the State of California, Department of Health. Plaintiffs are further informed and believe and thereon allege that had any of plaintiffs objected to these activities, state and county officials would have applied for and obtained an involuntary Lanterman-Petris-Short Act conservator for such plaintiffs and that said conservator would have effected such placement for plaintiffs. . . .

As a result of the foregoing, defendants had as much control over plaintiffs as had been present when plaintiffs were "committed" to the State mental institutions.

Thus, as a matter of law, defendants are infringing plaintiffs' liberty. Therefore, defendants have a duty of providing plaintiffs with treatment designed to assist plaintiffs in overcoming their mental disabilities (Lenvin & Gesmer, 1975, pp. 10-11).

Given this line of reasoning, attorneys Lenvin and Gesmer have tried to show that in reality the vast majority of the plaintiffs were in no position, because of their mental illness and previous hospital experience, to raise objections to their placement. Thus Lenvin and Gesmer would argue that these residents of sheltered-care facilities are de facto involuntarily housed and due the "right to treatment."

The importance of the "right to treatment" should not be underemphasized, but let us look at the concurring arguments of Mr. Chief Justice Berger in the Supreme Court decision in *Donaldson* v. *O'Connor*, June 24, 1975. Although the Court did not address the controversial "right-to-treatment" issue in the *Donaldson* decision, Chief Justice Berger's concurring opinion with his colleagues did. Berger clearly disagrees with Justice Wisdom's "right-to-treatment" arguments in the latter's circuit-court decision.

Justice Wisdom's decision in the "right-to-treatment" cases largely rests on a *quid pro quo* theory of civil commitment. He notes that "there must be a *quid pro quo* extended by government to justify confinement and the *quid pro quo* most commonly recognized is the provision of rehabilitative treatment" (493 F.2d at 522). Justice Berger responds to this argument by noting that:

Rather than inquiring whether strict standards of proof or periodic redetermination of a patient's condition are required in a civil commitment, the *quid pro quo* theory accepts the absence of safeguards but insists that the State provide benefits which, in view of a court, are adequate "compensation" for confinement. . . . Given the present state of medical knowledge regarding abnormal behavior and its treatment, few things could be more fraught with peril than to irrevocably condition a State's power to protect the mentally ill upon the providing of "such treatment as will give [them] a realistic opportunity to be cured." Nor can I accept the theory that a State may lawfully confine an individual thought to need treatment and justify that deprivation of liberty solely by providing some treatment. Our concepts of due process do not tolerate such a "tradeoff." Because the Court of Appeals analysis could be read as authorizing these results, it should not be followed (43 LW 49367).

What is apparent in this argument is that the right to treatment is a double-edged sword that can itself lead to the deprivation of one's due-process rights. For example, the "right-to-treatment" issue is currently the basis for a lawsuit challenging the patient's right to refuse shock treatment. That is, the treatment institution is arguing that because electroshock treatment is the treatment of choice, it is obligated to provide such treatment, as the patient's right, even though that patient may refuse it. Thus the right of the patient becomes the right of the servicer to ensure service delivery.

If a person were to refuse medication in a community-care home, would the extending of the "right-to-treatment" to that environment mean that the operator of the facility (as a patient's advocate) could force the individual to take the medications against the resident's wishes? Once we move into the realm of community care, it is not clear whether such rights guarantees are really in the best interest of the resident or whether they create a situation open to more abuse than the benefits produced by the guarantee.

Without the significant input of the consumer in the planning of such treatment efforts the "right-to-treatment" simply ensures the prerogatives of the advocate to provide such treatment to a passive patient population. This in part is what Meisel (1975) alludes to when he notes that the implementation of such rights is contingent upon the benevolence of mental-health professionals.

Meisel (1975) also alludes to the vulnerability and powerlessness of the population. Let us look at the less controversial ruling of *Souder v. Brennan* (1973)—a case relating to the protection of mental patients from institutional peonage. The ruling in this case guaranteed that patient workers should be covered by the provisions of the Federal Fair Labor Standards Act, which entitled them to minimum wages and overtime compensation. This ruling also indicated that the "economic reality" is the test of employment: "So long as the institution derived any consequential benefit the economic reality test would indicate an employment relationship rather than a mere therapeutic exercise" (42 U.S.L.W. 2271, D.D.C., Nov. 14, 1973). Meisel (1975) indicates that the court in *Souder v. Brennan* gave the Department of Labor 1 year to begin to apply the Fair Labor Standards Act for patient workers. He notes further, however, that, as of the December 1974 deadline, the department had not yet published the regulations governing the application of the law to mental institutions. As a member of a Pennsylvania survey team, Meisel (1975) found that, whereas almost all patient labor in institutions had been abolished, a few patients who were still permitted to work received no pay as late as January 1975. Similarly, Meisel points out, the right of patients to refuse treatment provided by the 1972 *Wyatt* decision has not been totally protected in good faith; at least four patients at Alabama's Brice Hospital have received electric shock therapy (ECT) without their consent. The hospital's written policy on the use of ECT, issued after the 1972 *Wyatt* decision, appears to be directly contrary to the court order; it permits ECT to be administered over the patient's protest as long as consent has been obtained from the family or someone else he had designated to act for him. Meisel notes that in early 1975 court proceedings were initiated against several medical staff members and against the Brice Hospital's administration for these violations. The conclusion from these facts seems to be that without strong consumer input the rights of the sheltered-care population are contingent upon the beneficence of their mental-health advocates.

A CONSUMER'S VIEW OF THE SYSTEM

With all its drawbacks the sheltered-care system is more consumer oriented than its state-hospital predecessor, and, in a real sense, it offers significant advantages as a long-term placement. The consumer's situation is expressed in an interviewer's report:

Jane is in her mid 40s. She was hospitalized for two years. She will have lived in this board-and-care home two years this February. She likes it better than the hospital as one is free to come and go as one pleases. She feels the residents get good food and care from the operator. She didn't like the state hospital, and feels freer now. When asked about what she does, it seems TV is a major activity. She sometimes goes to a nearby coffee shop, a lot of board-and-care residents frequent, as one can get as much coffee as one wants for 20¢—some stay there a good part of the day. She also goes to a pizza parlor. Sometimes, she walks in the neighborhood and occasionally goes out to the big shopping center. When asked about wanting to move to an independent living situation, she said she couldn't afford it with rent, food, utilities, and probably needing a car to get around. She seemed to feel living in the community was fine, except it got "boring" sometimes (F.N.).

When asked about their lives in sheltered care, 48% of the California residents indicated that they were "satisfied" with their current living arrangement, 31% said they were "somewhat satisfied," and 21% were dissatisfied.

When asked how they would view different living arrangements, 84% of the residents said they would object to returning to a mental hospital; 55% thought it would be at least all right to stay in their current board-and-care home for a long period of time. This in itself is testimony to the improvement over hospitalization that community residence represents, though it is far from perfect.

Given the desirability of community care, should we extend special rights to former mental patients in the community? If one assumes that former hospital patients are capable of self-determination, then there is no need to extend special rights—they are "free-living" individuals with the same rights as anyone else. If one assumes that they are not capable, the rights extended are not always residents' but in special situations their advocates'. Since the issue becomes a problem for those situations where there is considerable ambiguity regarding the ability of the former patient, we offer the following suggestions regarding sheltered-care residents:

1. Assume that the formerly hospitalized sheltered-care resident is vulnerable (more so than the general public) but capable (assuming he/she is not under conservatorship) in that they can say what they want or do not want.
2. Since the "right to treatment" relating to mental illness has implications leading to the conclusion that people may be forced to participate in the treatment they do not want "for their own good," do not extend this right to former hospital patients in community care. These individuals, unless adjudicated to be in need of conservatorship or to be dangerous to themselves or others or gravely disabled, are capable of choosing, as are members of the general population, what type of service would best suit them.

3. Confine the "right to treatment," especially as it relates to forced participation to situations where extensive due-process safeguards can be guaranteed (as they have been under LPS for the involuntary mental-hospital
admission).

4. Guarantee, in the community-care system, the right to access to quality
environmental conditions (such as those specified under Section 5325 [a]
through [e] in the LPS Act), legal, treatment and social services, as well as
the right to refuse such services.

In extending special rights to the former mental-hospital patient in community-based sheltered care, a distinction must be embedded in these rights
between access and participation. For the "free-living" individual, we can
ensure only access. Proverbially we should be able to ensure that they get to
the water, but be unable to force them to drink. Such guarantees would
create a situation of operator accountability that we believe would lead to a
higher quality of care. Access to legal, treatment, and social services should
be guaranteed, since in supervised living arrangements the individual is vulnerable to exploitation. These access rights must be implemented with the
help of consumer-action organizations, state licensing and certification agencies, mental-health and social-service personnel, and legal-assistance agencies. Participation of residents in such activities would take them more into
the consumer role and make them less likely to be the system's commodity.

REFERENCES

Alinsky, S. D. *Reveille for Radicals*. Chicago: University of Chicago Press, 1946.

Allen, P. "Background and Reference Material for Outpatient Bill of Rights." Unpublished
memo. Sacramento, California: Citizens Advisory Council, March 1974 (a).

Allen, P. "A Bill of Rights for Users of Outpatient Mental Health Services." Unpublished
memo. Sacramento, California: Citizens Advisory Council, November 1974 (b).

Charles, M. "Analysis and Recommendations Relating to Rate Structure for Residential Care
Homes." Unpublished memo. San Jose, California: Santa Clara County Department of Social
Services, July 6, 1973.

Karno, M. and D. A. Schwartz. *Community Mental Health: Reflections and Explorations*. Flushing,
New York: Spectrum, 1974.

Lenvin, N. C. and G. M. Gesmer. "Complaint for Declaratory and Injunctive Relief." Superior
Court of the State of California in and for the City and County of San Francisco, Williams et al.
v. City and County of San Francisco et al., June 1975.

Meisel, A. "Rights of the Mentally Ill: The Gulf Between Theory and Reality." *Hosp. and
Community Psychiat.* 26(6), 349–353 (1975).

Minnehan, C. "Project NOVA Unites Residents to Solve Common Problems." *Health News*,
1(11), 9, 1974.

Shadoan, R. A. "Right to Treatment in Community Residential Facilities." Unpublished
memo. San Francisco, California, 1975.

Souder v. Brennan, 42 U.S.L.W. 2271 (D.D.C., November 14, 1973); 367 F. Supplement 808 (D.D.C. 1973).

Srole, L., T. S. Langner, S. T. Michael, P. Kirkpatrick, M. K. Opler, and T. A. C. Rennie. *Mental Health in the Metropolis: The Midtown Manhattan Study.* New York: Harper Torchbooks, 1962.

Werner, G. D. S. "Observations on the Board and Care System of Los Angeles." Unpublished paper. Los Angeles: University of California, School of Law, December, 1974.

Williams et al. v. the City and County of San Francisco et al. Superior Court in and for the City and County of San Francisco, State of California, June 20, 1975.

Wyatt v. Stickney, 493 F. Supplement 521, 522 (1972).

SEVEN
CONCLUSION

SIXTEEN

Toward A Better System of Sheltered Care

The development of a community-based sheltered-care system in California is the first major social experiment in the care of former mental patients in the past 100 years. As so often happens with major social experiments, great hopes, fears, and disappointments are reflected in the controversies that emerge around the changes they produce. One thing for sure, those involved in the controversy around the development of community-based sheltered care have realized that problems of mental illness and issues related to the delivery of proper care and rehabilitation of the mentally ill cannot be simply solved by the act of moving the mentally ill from the state hospitals to community-based sheltered-care facilities.

We have considered the history of the return to community care for the mentally ill. We saw how the basic social functions of public policy relating to the care of the mentally ill were influenced by various social trends. We saw how these trends brought about a complete change in the care and treatment of the mentally ill—from community to hospital and back to the community.

We have looked at the pattern of change in California in the organization of community-care services. We have also discussed the influx of former mental patients into local communities and the unanticipated consequences of the return of the mentally ill to the community.

Various community groups have tried to establish measures to bar the mentally ill from certain neighborhoods and put them into ghetto areas. Other groups, for a variety of reasons, have been trying to open the gates of many communities to accept the mentally ill. The reform in the mental-health system in California created the opportunity for the former hospitalized mental patient to assume the role of service consumer rather than the status of a system's commodity. We have seen, however, that the degree of psychopathology of some former psychiatric patients, combined with environmental forces, limited their ability to exercise their new potential status. Market conditions alone were not sufficient to ensure the civil rights of, as well as the quality of services provided to, the mentally ill in the community. The state has reacted to the situation by moving toward regulations. But the effect of regulations and other efforts to improve the lot of the mentally ill in the community is limited because of the basic lack of accurate knowledge and the prevalence of misconceptions about the population and the system that the regulations are aimed at.

The purpose of our study was to describe accurately the people in sheltered care, the facilities in which they reside, the people who operate those facilities, and the placement and services that have emerged around the sheltered-care system.

In an effort to enhance the quality of life of formerly hospitalized patients in the community, we concentrated our research on illuminating factors that facilitate and hinder the social integration of sheltered care residents. We specified factors related to integration both within the facility and in the external community. Finally, as another means of understanding those devices that might enhance the quality of life of residents, we considered the relationship between the helper and the person who is being helped in the sheltered-care situation.

MAJOR FACTORS IN RESIDENTS' QUALITY OF LIFE

The ultimate success or failure of the California experiment in community-based sheltered care must hinge upon its consequences for the individuals who reside in its system. Thus, in looking to future improvements of the system, let us review four major factors relating to the nature of sheltered care and the character of its residents—let us also discuss the program and policy implications of these four factors that seem to have the most significant impact on residents' quality of life as measured by their levels of internal and external integration. These four factors are (1) the impact of psychological disturbance, (2) the impact of the community, (3) the helper-client relationship, and (4) the impact of the resident's current level of social integration (in the sense we would consider the impact of a country's current level of economic development on its potential for future economic development).

The Impact of Psychological Disturbance

The level of psychological disturbance, as measured by the severity of symptom manifestations, is a key factor in determining the differential impact of factors facilitating and hindering internal and external integration of the sheltered-care resident. These impact differentials have implications for three program and policy issues in the development of a better system. These issues are:

1. The type of services that should be offered and who should receive them.
2. The type of residential facilities necessary to ensure an effective system.
3. The level and type of skill or professional competence needed by service givers.

The Type of Services Offered and Who Should Receive Them. Two types of services should be offered in the sheltered-care system. First are clinical services primarily related to the formerly hospitalized patient's illness. Second are social-support services relating to attempts to enhance social functioning by providing rehabilitative and community resources to the resident. The crucial elements in determining who should get clinical and social-support services are the ability of residents to use such services to enhance their social and psychological functioning and the assurance that offering these services will not lead to a reduction in social or psychological functioning.

Our findings indicate that people with different levels of psychopathology use services and help in different ways. It therefore seems reasonable to employ level of psychopathology as an aid in determining the type of services that should best be offered to differential subgroups in this population. Looking first at the most disturbed subgroup, we find a group of people in whom psychological disturbance is so great that it predominates in their social interactions. The level of external and internal integration of these people is very low, and few factors will work to enhance these types of integration. This is, however, one group for which the level of internal and external integration is enhanced with increasing levels of antipsychotic medication. The internal integration of this population is also enhanced by the ideal psychiatric environment (one emphasizing higher levels of resident social involvement, support, spontaneity and autonomy; one encouraging a practical orientation to problems and the expression of personal problems and anger and aggression; and one stressing program clarity, order, organization, and minimal staff control). Few other factors contribute to the social benefit or quality of life of this severely disturbed group. We must conclude that a clinical or therapeutic approach seems most appropriate to employ with this population.

Looking at the group having very minimal psychological disturbance, we found a large number of factors related to their ability to enhance their internal and external integration. These included community environment and facility characteristics, as well as individual characteristics. In viewing this population, which has very little psychological disturbance, we also observe what might be considered an overuse of clinical resources. Although this group benefited substantially from the ideal psychiatric environment, their level of social integration was depressed significantly by the higher doses of antipsychotic medication.

Those with moderate degrees of psychological disturbance are more like their less disturbed fellows in being more capable of using social supports to enhance their social integration than the severely disturbed are. These supports involve not only direct rehabilitative-type services but also placement services that put individuals in environments that will enhance social functioning—for example, those close to community resources.

Given the limited resources allotted to the mental-health industry, it is essential that these resources be used differentially, based on the needs of the group, the availability of alternative resources, and their potential benefit. The most efficient use of limited clinical services would therefore involve a concentrated effort with the most severely symptomatically disturbed, since few alternatives are open to them. Social supports and social-support services should be concentrated on groups with lesser degrees of symptomatic disturbance.

Type of Residential Services Necessary. In accord with our notions regarding the type of service and who should get what type of service, we see the need for two basic types of facilities in the sheltered-care arena. First is that facility geared to be an ideal psychiatric environment and organized to deal with high levels of psychological disturbance. The second type would be a board-and-care home with primarily socially oriented programs. Individuals going to such board-and-care homes would be less overtly disturbed and more capable of using the social benefits of their environment. They would not be in the position of having to rely almost solely upon facility-based clinical resources to enhance their social integration. This does not imply that the less disturbed individuals in the population could not benefit from being in an ideal psychiatric environment. Our data show that they certainly would benefit greatly. Unfortunately there are not enough ideal psychiatric environments to go around. Moreover, these environments often involve the use of other clinical resources, such as high doses of medications, which are contraindicated for those with little psychological disturbance. If we consider the halfway house as an indicator of the number of ideal psychiatric environments available, we find that this facility serves only 3% of the sheltered-care population. The severely psychologically disturbed, on the other hand, constitute 16% at minimum, of this population. If, as a way of maximizing the efficiency of use of available clinical or therapeutic resources, we took the most disturbed subset of the population in sheltered care and moved them into halfway houses, we would still have a large number of clinically oriented psychiatric environments to develop in the community before we could begin to say we are serving the needs of this population subset. In addition the differential between the number of halfway houses available and the estimated need for them is exacerbated by the fact that halfway houses are less likely to be serving those who are most severely psychologically disturbed.

Level of Skill or Professional Competence Needed by Service Givers in Sheltered Care. It is difficult to tell people who make policy that the primary factor in distinguishing the needs of the sheltered-care population or subsets of this population is the level of psychological disturbance or psychopathology. This is particularly true because of the difficulty of assessing psychopathology. Yet we are in a situation where we do not have a simple answer and where we have found that levels of pathology measured by symptom assessments are most capable of distinguishing subsets of this population with differential service needs. We have also found that one does not need a psychiatrist to make this distinction, but that with brief training individuals with experience such as social workers can make such assessments. It seems that at minimum, service to this population must be offered by individuals with training at distinguishing levels of psychopathology that characterize their clients. This is particularly necessary for those individuals responsible for the prescription of antipsychotic medications, since the overprescription of such medications is most likely to lead to the occurrence of iatrogenic effects—specifically the reduction of individual levels of social functioning.

Service givers who staff the clinically oriented facilities must in fact have the skills to deal with the severely psychologically disturbed. They must be aware of what psychopathology is and how it develops and have an understanding of growth and development concepts and of how to treat psychopathology. On the other hand those individuals who staff the board-and-care facilities can contribute to enhancing the social integration of residents with less disturbance, with little education in this area. The focus of any training efforts for this latter group should be on the social situation and on how to better that situation. Such training should deemphasize psychopathology. In these socially oriented facilities, where it is possible with a less disturbed population to substitute social supports for clinical supports, this effort should be a primary focus of service.

The Impact of the Community

The impact of the community on both the external and internal integration of sheltered-care residents is experienced both directly and indirectly by residents. Direct community outreach to individuals in these facilities has enhanced their external and internal integration. Adverse community reaction to residents as a group of mentally ill people, for example, a large number of complaints, has the effect of reducing individual levels of external integration. Not only the social but also the physical characteristics of a community have an important influence on the external integration of residents—most particularly, distance from community resources. Those closer to resources have enhanced levels of social functioning.

The impact of community upon sheltered care is most pertinent with respect to two issues: (1) the development of a placement system and how much difference it will make and (2) the protection of the civil rights of formerly hospitalized mental patients.

Placement: Its Organization and How Much Difference It Will Make.   To achieve the most beneficial arrangement of resources or a more efficient investment of therapeutic resources, we are in need of more efficient placements to bring the overtly symptomatic to a more therapeutic environment. It is also important that we have a more selectively oriented service system than one that simply responds to the principle of the "squeaky wheel." To achieve this goal, we need skilled professional placement personnel who are aware of the needs of this population, have dealt with it over a period of time, and are able to make decisions regarding placements that maximize the use of factors outside the normally thought of therapeutic realm—factors relating to community acceptance, distance from resources, and the provision of resources to the individual client.

The crucial argument regarding placement revolves around an assessment of how much difference it will make—or more specifically, how strong are factors in our models that can be taken into account in making placements. As a whole, community factors are the most important predictors of both external and internal integration, especially for those individuals with less psychological disturbance. Whereas our models admittedly explain a little less than a third of the differences in levels of social integration in the population, we are inclined to believe that the relationships summarized in these models are important and stable. We would consider them as representing the strongest relationships in the system—where their strength is indicated by the fact that they consistently predict external and internal integration. Perhaps the best analogy is to the signal picked up by a crystal set radio in a situation with a good deal of interference. Such a signal is the strongest signal in the system but may appear to come through weakly because of the relatively primitive instrumentation. Currently social-science measures are at a primitive stage in their development, and we believe that only the strongest relationships will come through clearly, though often weakly. Given this perspective, it can be concluded from our data that effective placement would greatly enhance the efficiency of the sheltered-care system in that it would permit the most effective use of clinical resources with those individuals who could maximally benefit from them and, in addition, would enable us to substitute the necessary social supports to maintain the level of social integration of the less disturbed population.

Our data indicate that it will be extremely difficult to rationalize the placement system totally. Yet the goal of the system should be to add to its discriminating ability. This goal might best be achieved with a maximum effort to centralize placement decisions within the community in a single organization—such as the Community Care Services Section (CCSS). Such centralization will give this agency considerable leverage in the placement negotiation process to encourage the development of facilities having needed social and clinical resources. If operators cannot get outside placements, they will be more willing to make resource modifications to get placements from this single agency. Such centralization of the placement function might also have the consequence of reinstituting the higher level of continuous care available before mental-health reform. It would also, as indicated by our data, ensure that the placement worker has a greater level of competence.

Civil Rights of Former Mental Patients.   Our broadly focused analysis of the political situation relating to the development of sheltered-care facilities in the community has demonstrated the use by communities of such exclusionary tactics as zoning ordinances and bureaucratic maneuvering to keep out these facilities. Such action raises the need for countermeasures in terms of legal and social action. There can be no justification of the violation of state law by communities in excluding small residential facilities from residential neighborhoods. The case against these exclusionary tactics must be won in the courts.

Whether or not individuals are placed in such exclusionary neighborhoods should, however, be determined on the basis of the social supports these neighborhoods offer them with respect to enhancing their social integration. Neighborhoods at a distance from community resources and demonstrating exclusionary attitudes toward former mental patients are not the best places to put them. On the other hand some neighborhoods, such as San Jose, California, which we have spoken about previously as a mental-patient ghetto, offer compensatory or complementary benefits and drawbacks relating to community social support. On the one hand the San Jose community offers access to resources to the former mental patients. It offers them access to each other in terms of developing their own consumer awareness and developing friendship groups, albeit, groups that relate these patients to other former mental patients. At the negative end of the scale such a community demonstrated a severe negative reaction to their large concentration of these patients. Given these conflicting situations, a professional service role should be developed to maximize the benefits that such a community might offer to these residents. Such a task is being achieved in San Jose and is focused around the involvement of the community with former mental patients in a way geared to modify negative attitudes. To the extent that attitude change is successful, areas like San Jose become potentially useful placement resources. They offer the social setting that by virtue of easy access to community resources and a lack of the serious social problems of a large downtown urban area, provide the social supports for the less disturbed that they so need to maintain their external and internal social integration.

The Helper-Client Relationship

Our findings emphasize the need of residents to participate in decisions relating to their life situation and indicate their ability to assess the quality of their environments. Thus they point to two significant issues in the system: (1) consumer organization and activism and (2) licensing and/or certification.

Consumer Organization and Activism. Perhaps the most beneficial way to approach serving this population is on a basis of encouragement of consumer organization and activism. But how does one do this? Undoubtedly a more competitive market in sheltered care can enhance self-determination. Our findings indicate, however, that it is not enough. This population is vulnerable and has a significant amount of social handicap. We need the authoritative intervention of a regulatory agency and the sensitivity and competence of the professionally trained worker to avoid making decisions for the client he is capable of making for himself and to act as a significant force to ensure quality of care. In any population, however, there will be a variance in ability and there will be a small group most interested and capable of consumer-oriented action. Such action by virtue of its very existence constitutes a force that makes for maximum independence on the part of many more than just those clients involved. Such groups can be funded to deal specifically with issues that residents are most capable of dealing with, such as helping in evaluation of facilities (in an anonymous way to protect residents from reprisal) and helping in finding prospective residents placements that would be most desirable.

One might envision a consumer group's having a desk or place at the inpatient facility and being involved in facilitating placements along with placement workers. Social workers of CCSS of the Department of Health were most effective in allowing the resident a maximum amount of self-determination in choosing his placement. This is perhaps one of the key skills of social-work practice, the ability not to "take over" for a client.

We would not recommend, at least initially, the attempt to involve consumers at all levels in the system, for example, with all decision-making bodies. Such involvements should develop from the specific request of a consumer group for representation. It seems that there is a tendency to involve consumers just for the sake of having them. Such situations often lead to consumer frustration and unwillingness to participate. Involvement at the care-giving level, at the everyday level of enhancing the social functioning of other residents, offers many opportunities to help in the development of a better service system and to enhance and supplement the activities of the mental-health professionals serving residents in sheltered care.

Licensing and/or Certification. The ability of residents to assess the quality of their social environment leads to some significant conclusions or raises some issues about how licensing and/or certification should proceed in the system. To date, the limited number of personnel involved in the licensing of facilities has made it impossible to do anything but respond to complaints. In addition we do not foresee a change in this situation given the availability of future resources. We would therefore suggest that licensing activities be confined to those characteristics of facilities—such as the physical environment and its social amenities (e.g., the character and nature of the food, physical plant, availability of personal space and of toilet access). We would further suggest that a certification system be developed that would involve the interaction of resident groups and placement workers around the certifying of facilities with respect to the quality of their social environment. Such assessment requires a more judgmental approach to the problem and by virtue of his position it is already a part of the placement worker's job. It requires an approach to the problem for which there is often little hard evidence other than the assessment of a professional in the system and the additional input of the residents. In such a situation we would have two criteria for assessing facilities: The first would be a set of physical characteristics that reside with the facility and that can be licensed. In this type of situation the facility has the right to operate a business and is licensed as such; the power to operate is the facility's under state license. In the certification system the certification belongs to the agency that grants it, and it is easy for them, or relatively easy, to remove it. In no case can clients be forced in and out of the facility, since we are talking simply about access to information with respect to the quality of the facility. Initially a large proportion of residents would be in noncertified facilities, but as resident consumer groups become more active and involved in the certification process along with mental-health professionals, we believe the result would allow a greater potential for the development of higher quality of care within the system. Without the joint cooperation of the client and the helper, the assurance of quality of care in such a broadly based system would be extremely difficult.

The Impact of Social Integration

Our findings with regard to the level of social integration of this population, aside from their immediate level of participation, lead us to believe that this group was never integrated into the mainstream of society. The issue this finding addresses is that of evaluations of outcome in the system. If the expectation is community reintegration, it will not be fulfilled on a broad scale and will be achieved in a very marginal way by only a small proportion of the population currently living in sheltered care. If the expectation is external and internal integration, that is, enhanced involvement in the outside world independent of the facility and enhanced involvement within the facility in which a person is currently living, there is significant opportunity to achieve such goals. The outcome of community care then must not be assessed in terms of the number of people, the head count, returning to independent economic productive activity but must be assessed in terms of the number of people maintaining an adequate level of functioning who, given our past experience, might deteriorate to a less than adequate level of social functioning if they were confined to large institutional settings.

The 1975 ammendments to the Community Mental Health Centers Act have added to the definition of a comprehensive community mental health center the need to provide halfway-house services on a transitional basis and residential care to those who will need longer term living arrangements. The emphasis in the future will, given their numbers, have to be on those needing longer-term living arrangements. There will be a continuing need for involvement in a social supportive role on the part of the community mental-health center with the long-term sheltered-care resident. The community mental-health center responsible for a given catchment area will have to develop a service team with highly skilled placement personnel, direct-service personnel, and resident consumer-oriented or consumer-action development personnel. It is only in this way that we can expect the optimum use of sheltered care in achieving the goal of maximum social integration. In addition formal evaluative systems of community mental-health services will have to be augmented with new measures of success, measures related to the prevention of social deterioration as opposed to the achievement of rehabilitation.

Toward a Better System of Sheltered Care

It is our firm belief that, with all the drawbacks the community-based sheltered-care system has, and it has many, it offers an opportunity to explore a new and untried mode of caring for the chronic mentally ill. Change never occurs without suffering, and many residents whom we read about in the newspapers daily are suffering. If our study had been an evaluation, we might have painted a bleaker picture of the sheltered-care environment. Instead, we looked at this environment in a way that seeks to maximize our understanding of the benefits it offers or can offer to the formerly hospitalized mental patient. It is our view, as it is the view of many of the residents we have spoken to, that at least this environment is a place where there is more freedom to determine one's personal life than there was in the hospital. What has emerged from our study to date, and what we have attempted to outline in our book, are the crucially important factors involved in optimizing the chances of individuals to enhance their functioning in the community. In considering the impact of such factors in future sheltered-care programming, we will be making use of a unique opportunity to create a better system of care for the mentally ill in the community.

Survey Methodology

The methodology employed in the survey involved three primary tasks: (1) the development of the sample survey design, (2) data gathering, and (3) the data analysis. With regard to data analysis two methods were employed: (1) analysis of the resident's response data and the characteristics of the environment of each resident (here the resident was the unit of analysis) and (2) analysis of the characteristics of facilities and their operators.

SURVEY SAMPLE PLAN

The sample is a self-weighting, representative sample of all individuals between 18 and 65 years of age with a past history of mental illness, currently living in sheltered-care facilities (i.e., family-care homes, board-and-care homes, and halfway houses) for the mentally ill in California (Kish, 1965).

To obtain the sample, the state was divided into three master strata:

1. Los Angeles County.
2. The Bay Area—that is, Alameda, Contra Costa, Marin, Napa, San Francisco, San Mateo, Santa Clara, Solano, and Sonoma Counties.
3. All other counties in the state.

In the Los Angeles and Bay Area strata, the sample was drawn from the total population. In each of these areas a two-stage cluster sample was designed with sheltered-care facilities as the primary sampling units, and individuals within facilities as the second sampling stage.

Facilities were stratified by size in both Los Angeles and the Bay Area, and a sample was drawn of paired facilities (primary selection units) taken probability proportionate to size. Individuals within facilities were sampled by using systematic random sampling from specially prepared field listings. Individuals were sampled in clusters of three in those facilities with four or more residents. In facilities with three or fewer residents one interview was completed.

In the third stratum, comprising "all other counties," a three-stage cluster sample was designed by using counties as primary selection units, facilities as the second stage, and individuals within facilities as the third stage. All counties within this stratum with 20 or fewer facilities were arbitrarily excluded from the sample. This procedure eliminated only 3% of the estimated population (618 residents) from consideration and allowed us to draw conclusions with respect to the other 97%. The remaining counties were further divided into two substrata, north and south. Two counties were picked as paired primary sampling units from the north (Mendocino and Sacramento) and two from the south (San Diego and Ventura). The facility and individual samples in this stratum were taken within each of the selected counties by using systematic random sampling for the latter and selections probability proportionate to size for the former.

Given our expectations about the degree of relationship necessary to detect as significant, anticipated losses due to refusals and illness, and available resources, our sampling fraction was set at 1/36.

Unanticipated Problems

The major unanticipated problems with the design resulted from the inaccuracy of sheltered-care facility lists at the time we drew our sample. In the Los Angeles area we used a list of facilities compiled by the County Department of Mental Health, and for the rest of the state we used a list put together by the Community Care Services Section (CCSS) of the State Department of Health for fire-clearance purposes. In the Los Angeles area, despite an initial telephone survey, several facilities had closed before we could interview in them. Further, the fact that the aged, physically disabled, mentally retarded, mentally ill, alcoholics, and drug abusers were often housed in the same facility reduced the number of interviews we had expected in many facilities (i.e., since the estimated number of eligible residents was initially based on facility's bed capacity). In the Bay Area pretest the loss due to ineligibility was much less than that in Los Angeles. Despite the fact that the Los Angeles Mental Health Department's listing indicated, and the operator confirmed, that a facility served the mentally ill, interviewers frequently arrived at the facility only to find that there were no eligible residents. After 2 weeks of interviewing, it was determined that only half of the expected interviews in Los Angeles were actually available. For this reason we increased the sample size to obtain a sample population of reasonable size. In the Los Angeles area a supplemental list of new facilities, opened after the development of the County Mental Health list, was compiled. The sampling fraction in Los Angeles was doubled so that we would interview 1 out of every 18 residents instead of 1 out of every 36 as originally planned. Although we anticipated that the procedure employed in Los Angeles would be necessary in the other sampled areas, in fact the supplemental list developed in these areas increased the anticipated number of beds by 100% in each location. Owing to this increase, the sampling fraction in other areas was maintained at $\frac{1}{36}$.

Design Effect

The design effect in the study was relatively high, averaging about two when estimated for proportions. The large design effect is primarily the result of two study characteristics. The first is the fact that only two pairs of counties were chosen in the "all other county" stratum, owing to budget limitations. The second is the large number of losses because of ineligibility.

Because of the exploratory nature of the study, significance tests were carried out by using the standard formulas for simple random sampling. Reduction of the number of degrees of freedom used in statistical tests to one-fourth of those available was employed throughout most of the analysis to compensate for the large design effect.

DATA GATHERING

In spite of the unanticipated problems experienced during the data-gathering phase of the project, all data-gathering tasks were completed by September 1973; 499 resident interviews were attempted with a loss (due to refusal and inaccessibility) of 12%; 10% of the 234 operators contacted refused to participate in the study.

Contacting Facilities

Every facility was initially contacted by telephone to determine whether it had residents appropriate for the study. The study's purpose and procedures were explained to the operators, and permission was obtained from the operator for researchers to enter the facility. A specific interview time was arranged. If an operator refused to allow researchers into his or her facility, the central research office in Berkeley sent a letter to the resistant operator, and contact was reinitiated by telephone. If a refusal was obtained following the letter, the contact was terminated.

Resident Interviews

Upon entering a facility, interviewers obtained a list of names of eligible residents from the facility operator. The names were arranged alphabetically and numbered from one to "n" (the last name on the list). Interviewers then chose their prospective interviewees on the basis of preselected numbers made available to them in their sampling instructions for the facility.

No interview was conducted with a resident until he had signed a consent form, which also gave the interviewer permission to ask the facility operator about the type and dosage of the resident's medication. Once the form was signed, it was detached from the interview schedule, and thus any reference to the resident by name on the form was eliminated and his identity protected. Medication information was usually obtained at the time the list of eligible residents was made and was checked before the interviewer left the facility, when the list of names was destroyed (along with medication information obtained about residents who did not wish to be interviewed).

Language Barriers

We encountered a small but significant number of residents who spoke only Spanish. To avoid losing their participation in the study, the interview schedule was translated into Spanish and used throughout the state whenever necessary. On these occasions our Spanish-speaking interviewer was flown to the area to conduct the interview. The only other resident who did not speak English spoke Cantonese and was lost to the sample, since we could not find on short notice an affordable Cantonese-speaking interviewer.

Interviewers and Interview Training

The 10 study interviewers were all social-work graduate students or professional social workers with at least 1 year of graduate work and 1 year of experience in working with a sheltered-care or state-mental-hospital population. They received intensive training focused on study procedures and on the use of our survey instruments—especially those relating to the assessment of residents' psychopathology. The training sessions involved interviewers in role plays of resident and operator interviews wherein they were given feedback from senior staff on their performances. The sessions also involved practice in assessing psychopathology with the aid of filmed interviews of mental-hospital patients and feedback from our staff psychiatrist.

DATA ANALYSIS

The project data analysis is focused on two units of analysis—the resident and the facility or the facility operator. For the resident analysis four primary tasks have been completed: (1) a simple demographic description of the population through cross-tabulation techniques; (2) development of two dependent variables, that is, measures of external and internal integration; (3) delineation of a series of predictors of social integration; (4) consideration of the interrelationships between these predictors and social integration.

The sheltered-care operator being taken as a unit of analysis, two major efforts have been undertaken: (1) a simple demographic description of the facilities and operators through cross-tabulation techniques and (2) determination of the relationship between the characteristics of facilities and their use of social, medical, and rehabilitative services. The first task in both the resident and the facility analyses is rather straightforward: to describe the two populations by using cross-tabulation. This section of our methods appendix focuses on the remaining tasks in the resident and facility analyses. Each of these tasks used more complex statistical procedures and relied on the construction of composite indices.

Developing the Social-Integration Scales

Initially all those items included as part of the original conception of social integration that were skewed more than 90% were eliminated from consideration as possible scale items. All items originally thought to belong in the external-integration scale and internal-integration scale respectively were separately intercorrelated to produce two matrices of approximately 80 items per matrix. These matrices were initially cluster analyzed by hand to determine what major clusters could be distinguished within the internal- and external-content areas and whether these clusters would correspond to our initial conception of social integration. (A component analysis was used to facilitate this cluster analysis.) Once the best clusters had been derived, the cluster items selected from the two original correlation matrices were put into one large correlation matrix containing both internal-integration and external-integration clusters. This large correlation matrix was then factor analyzed by using the principal factor solution with a varimax rotation to simple structure. These procedures produced the 12 subscales that now comprise the social-integration scale scores, 7 comprising an external-integration score and 5 an internal-integration score. There was little overlap between items loading on the external factors and those loading on the internal factors. This seems to be a practical validation of the original conceptual distinction between the items.

The conceptual distinction between external- and internal-integration items having been established, two smaller correlation matrices including the items of the external and internal subscales *weighted* by the sample weights were then generated and factor analyzed by using a principal-factor procedure with a varimax rotation. We returned to using the smaller matrices in the weighted analysis because it was more economical. No substantial differences in the scales derived were found in the weighted versus the unweighted analysis.

Once these cluster-analytic procedures had been completed, the internal consistencies (as measured by Alpha) of the subscales derived in the weighted analysis making up the internal- and the external-integration scores were computed. Also computed was the average item-to-subscale correlation for each subscale and the average item-to-other-subscale correlation for each subscale. The major criterion used for retaining a subscale was a high average item-to-subscale correlation versus a low average item-to-other-subscale correlation. All 12 subscales met this criterion (see Table A.1), and so all the scales were retained for analysis with the predictor variables (Lord and Novick, 1968).

Factors Used as the Basis for External- and Internal-Integration Subscales

A detailed outline of the interaction patterns described by the social-integration scales is included in Chapter 9. In this section we focus on how the scales were constructed.

The seven factor analytically derived external-integration subscales are:

1. Attending to oneself.
2. Access to community resources.
3. Access to basic and personal resources.
4. Familial access and participation.
5. Friendship access and participation.
6. Social interaction through community groups.
7. Use of community facilities.

Each subscale score was constructed by adding the normalized values of the items that loaded on the derived factor. In constructing the subscale score, unit weighting was used, and the mean item score was substituted for nonresponse in situations where at least half the items in a subscale were answered. No factor accounting for less than 5% of the total communality was included.

Throughout the analysis of the external-integration subscales, we attempted to employ a general criterion of rejecting items for a subscale if their factor loadings fell below .4. Whereas we managed to stay within this criterion for the internal-integration analysis that follows, we violated it five times in de-

Table A.1   Internal Consistencies and Average Item-to-Subscale and Other Subscale
Correlations for External- and Internal-Integration Subscales.

	Alpha	Average Item-Subscale Correlation	Average Item-Other Subscale Correlation
External-Integration Subscales			
Attending to oneself	.70	.65	.26
Access to community resouces	.91	.71	.30
Access to basic and personal resources	.86	.76	.32
Familial access and participation	.83	.73	.27
Friendship access and participation	.87	.78	.39
Social interaction through community groups	.70	.73	.29
Use of community facilities	.65	.71	.27
Internal-Integration Subscales			
OP to community resources	.91	.74	.22
OP facilitates activity	.73	.69	.18
OP provides necessities	.66	.71	.21
Socializing in house	.73	.71	.17
Supplies in house	.62	.69	.11

veloping the external-integration subscales. In each of these cases the items with lower loadings were included when they seemed to enhance the substantive meaning of the factor and when no items with a higher loading (but a loading less than .4) would have to be eliminated to maintain substantive clarity. The addition of these items produced minimal change in the internal consistency of the subscales they were added to (e.g., for the "attending to oneself" subscale, the addition of the item relating to time spent in the evening reduced the Alpha coefficient from .72 to .70). These items often would have reached the acceptable criterion of a .4 loading for inclusion in the scale if a different extraction or rotation procedure had been used.

Table A.2 shows the relationship of the subscales of the external-integration scale to each other and to the external-integration-scale score. Given the positive significant relationship of all the subscales to each other, the decision was made to add the normalized scores from each subscale to generate the external-integration-scale score. This procedure gave equal weight to each

Table A.2   Intercorrelations of External-Integration Subscale Scores

		1	2	3	4	5	6	7	8[a]
Attending to oneself	1	—	.45	.41	.30	.39	.38	.42	.68
Access to community resources	2		—	.69	.31	.46	.25	.34	.71
Access to basic or personal resources	3			—	.38	.48	.22	.33	.71
Familial access and participation	4				—	.50	.36	.29	.64
Friendship access and participation	5					—	.68	.42	.80
Social interaction through community groups	6						—	.46	.69
Use of community facilities	7							—	.67
External-integration score	8								—

[a] The total external-integration score includes each respective subscale score.

subscale in the total score. While there is the problem that such total scores may mask relationships between facilitating and hindering factors and individual subscale scores, the procedure does greatly facilitate the initial data analysis. The limited time of our project, the need to provide early feedback to the community who favorably supported the study, and the wish to provide at least basic understanding of the predictive factors in the social integration of the sheltered-care resident have led us to take this approach to the data.

The five factor analytically derived internal-integration subscales are:

1. Operator will transport residents to community resources.
2. Operator facilitates activity through the facility.
3. Operator provides basic necessities.
4. Socializing with other residents and the operator.
5. Supplies purchased by the house.

The internal-integration subscales are distinguished from the external-integration subscales by virtue of the former's emphasis on involvement within the facility or involvements with the outside community that are mediated by the facility. The internal-integration subscales were developed in the same manner as the external-integration subscales and were likewise significantly related to each other in a positive direction (see Table A.3). Thus the same procedure used to develop the external-integration score was used for the internal-integration score.

Relating external and internal integration to each other proved quite interesting. It was originally thought that internal integration might be negatively correlated with external integration, given the concept of the hospital as a total institution and the notion that the sheltered-care facility is simply a "back ward" of the hospital transferred to the community. This did not, however, prove to be the case. In fact, internal integration and external

Table A.3   Intercorrelations of Internal-Integration-Subscale Scores

		1	2	3	4	5	6
Op to community resources	1	—	.45	.32	.31	.12	.66
Op facilitates activity	2		—	.30	.19	.09	.64
Op provides necessities	3			—	.30	.27	.70
Socializing in house	4				—	.14	.59
Supplies in house	5					—	.53
Internal integration	6						—

[a] The total internal-integration score includes each respective subscale score.

integration, as scores of a group of subscales under each rubric, are significantly correlated at a positive level of $r = .35, p < .01$.

To illustrate this relationship further, the external- and internal-integration scores were dichotomized at their means and cross-tabulated.

Table A.4 gives the joint distribution of these dichotomized variables. This procedure was used only for illustrative purposes because the categorization of data in this fashion generally tends to reduce the strength of relationships in the data.

Finally, in considering the development of the social integration scales, we have listed the original items by subscale in Table A.5.

PREDICTORS OF SOCIAL INTEGRATION

In the process of developing predictors of social integration, 650 variables were organized by content areas. When the variables were arranged in content areas—that is, resident demographic characteristics, resident psychological and social perceptions, resident psychological characteristics, facility environment characteristics, operator characteristics, and characteristics of the resident's neighborhood—the variables in each content area were intercorrelated with themselves in individual correlation matrices. Included in each one of the content-area correlation matrices were all the social-integration

Table A.4   Relating External and Internal Integration Scores

		Internal Integration		
		High	Low	
External Integration	High	3,520 (28.5)	2,680 (21.6)	6,200
	Low	2,620 (21.2)	3,540 (28.6)	6,160
		6,140	6,220	N = 12,360

Table A.5 Social Integration Scales

The social-integration scales are composed of two major scales: external and internal integration. The external-integration scale has seven subscales. The internal-integration scale has five subscales.

External-Integration Scale

I. Attending to Oneself Subscale

	Scoring				
	Very Often	Often	Sometimes	Rarely	Never
1. On a typical day do you go to a coffee shop or restaurant?	5	4	3	2	1
2. On a typical day do you go to the shopping center or local shopping areas?	5	4	3	2	1
3. How often in a typical week do you order food from outside or eat out at a local restaurant?	5	4	3	2	1
4. How often in a typical week do you make a purchase at a local store?	5	4	3	2	1

	None	A Little	Half/ Half	Most	All
5. On a typical day how much of your time between 8:00 a.m. and 5:00 p.m. is spent at the house?	5	4	3	2	1
6. On a typical day how much of your time between 5:00 p.m. and 11:00 p.m. do you spend at home?	5	4	3	2	1

II. Access to Community Resources Subscale

	Scoring				
	Very Easy	Easy	Not Much Trouble	Difficult	Very Difficult
If you have to arrange your own transportation, without the aid of (operator's name), or walk how easy would it be to:					
1. Go to a shopping center or a large shopping area	5	4	3	2	1

Table A.5 *(Continued)*

		Very Easy	Easy	Not Much Trouble	Difficult	Very Difficult
2.	Go to a park	5	4	3	2	1
3.	Go to a library	5	4	3	2	1
4.	Go to a movie	5	4	3	2	1
5.	Go to a community center	5	4	3	2	1
6.	Go to a restaurant or coffee shop	5	4	3	2	1
7.	Go to a bar	5	4	3	2	1
8.	Go to a public transportation	5	4	3	2	1
9.	Go to the place of worship you prefer	5	4	3	2	1
10.	Go to an organization that offers individuals an opportunity to do volunteer work	5	4	3	2	1
11.	Go to a barber shop or beauty parlor	5	4	3	2	1
12.	Take a walk in a pleasant area	5	4	3	2	1

III. Access to Basic or Personal-Resources Subscale

	Scoring				
	Very Easy	Easy	Not Much Trouble	Difficult	Very Difficult
If you wanted, how easy would it be to obtain, outside this house or without the aid of (operator's name) the following things:					
1. Meals	5	4	3	2	1
2. Medical care	5	4	3	2	1
3. Laundry services	5	4	3	2	1
4. Clothing	5	4	3	2	1
5. Toilet supplies and incidentals	5	4	3	2	1
6. A telephone	5	4	3	2	1

Table A.5 *(Continued)*

IV. Familial-Access and Participation Subscale

	Scoring				
	Very Easy	Easy	Not Much Trouble	Difficult	Very Difficult
How easy would it be, if you want to:					
1. Telephone and just talk to a member of your immediate family	5	4	3	2	1
2. Telephone and just talk to a more distant relative	5	4	3	2	1
3. Get together with a member of your immediate family	5	4	3	2	1
4. Get together with a more distant relative	5	4	3	2	1

	Very Often	Often	Sometimes	Rarely	Never
On a typical day how often do you visit with:					
5. Members of your immediate family	5	4	3	2	1
6. More distant relatives	5	4	3	2	1

V. Friendship-Access and Participation Subscale

	Scoring				
	Very Easy	Easy	Not Much Trouble	Difficult	Very Difficult
How easy would it be, if you want to:					
1. Telephone and just talk to a close friend outside the house	5	4	3	2	1
2. Telephone and just talk to an acquaintance outside the house	5	4	3	2	1
3. Get together with a close friend not in this facility or another like it	5	4	3	2	1
4. Get together with an acquaintance not in this facility or another like it	5	4	3	2	1

Table A.5 *(Continued)*

On a typical day, how often do you:	Very Often	Often	Sometimes	Rarely	Never
5. Visit with close friends not in this house	5	4	3	2	1
6. Visit with acquaintances not in this house	5	4	3	2	1

VI. Social Integration Through Community Groups Subscale

Scoring

On a typical day, how often do you:	Very Often	Often	Sometimes	Rarely	Never
1. Visit with close friends not in this house	5	4	3	2	1
2. Visit with acquaintances not in this house	5	4	3	2	1
3. Do volunteer work	5	4	3	2	1
4. Join in the activities of social or political groups outside the house for people who are not considered former patients	5	4	3	2	1

VII. Use of Community Facilities Subscale

Scoring

On a typical day how often do you:	Very Often	Often	Sometimes	Rarely	Never
1. Go to the park	5	4	3	2	1
2. Go to the library	5	4	3	2	1
3. Participate in some outside sports activity	5	4	3	2	1
4. Go to special sports or entertainment events	5	4	3	2	1

Internal-Integration Scale

I. Operator Will Transport Residents to Community Resources Subscale

			Scoring		
How easy would it be for you to get the operator, a staff member, or a member of the operator's family to take you to a:	Very Easy	Easy	Not Much Trouble	Difficult	Very Difficult
1. Supermarket or large shopping center	5	4	3	2	1
2. Park	5	4	3	2	1
3. Library	5	4	3	2	1
4. Movie theater	5	4	3	2	1
5. Community center	5	4	3	2	1
6. Public school, high school, or college providing adult education	5	4	3	2	1
7. Restaurant or coffee shop	5	4	3	2	1
8. Public transportation	5	4	3	2	1
9. The place of worship you prefer	5	4	3	2	1
10. Organization that offers an individual an opportunity to do volunteer work	5	4	3	2	1
11. Barber shop or beauty parlor	5	4	3	2	1

II. Operator Facilitates Activity Through the Facility Subscale

			Scoring		
How easy would it be for you to arrange the following:	Very Easy	Easy	Not Much Trouble	Difficult	Very Difficult
1. Trips to sports events with other house residents	5	4	3	2	1
2. Social activities at the house	5	4	3	2	1
3. Vocational training at the house	5	4	3	2	1
4. Religious services at the house	5	4	3	2	1
5. Individual or group therapy at the house	5	4	3	2	1

Table A.5 *(Continued)*

III. Operator Provides Basic Necessities Subscale

	Scoring				
	Very Easy	Easy	Not Much Trouble	Difficult	Very Difficult
How easy is it for you to get or arrange the following:					
1. Laundry service at the house	5	4	3	2	1
2. Help from (operator's name) in getting clothing	5	4	3	2	1
3. Toilet supplies and incidentals from (operator's name) or in a vending machine here	5	4	3	2	1
4. Use of the telephone in the house	5	4	3	2	1

IV. Socializing with Other Residents and the Operator Subscale

	Scoring				
	Very Often	Often	Sometimes	Rarely	Never
On a typical day, do you:					
1. Join with other residents in the house to play cards, games, or some other activity	5	4	3	2	1
2. Try to make friends with other residents in the house	5	4	3	2	1
3. Sit and talk with other residents	5	4	3	2	1
4. Talk to (operator's name) or other house visitors (and staff)	5	4	3	2	1

V. Supplies Purchased by the House Subscale

	Scoring				
	Very Often	Often	Sometimes	Rarely	Never
How often do you purchase the following things at the house from the operator of the house:					
1. Laundry services	5	4	3	2	1
2. Clothing	5	4	3	2	1
3. Toilet items or other incidentals	5	4	3	2	1
4. Grooming services—for example, prepaid beauty shop or barber shop appointments	5	4	3	2	1

subscales and the external- and internal-integration scores. This enabled us to select significant predictors within each content area.

It is realized that this procedure tended to violate several measurement assumptions; however, the benefit of using a parametric approach to facilitate data reduction outweighed a purist approach to the data. We have continued to check our findings through cross-tabulation procedures to ensure their validity.

Exploratory stepwise regressions were run to determine the independent contribution to predicting social integration of each of the selected predictor variables or scales, because many predictors were scores of established scales (e.g., Overall & Gorham Brief Psychiatric Rating Scale [BPRS], 1962). Having obtained some idea of the relative importance of particular variables, and of their relative independent contribution to predicting social integration, we were able to construct models that formed the basis of our concluding which factors facilitate or hinder an individual's integration into the community.

We used 26 significant predictors ($p < .10$) in the analysis. These predictors were included in a causal model on the basis of two criteria: (1) they were policy relevant—that is, they were modifiable by policy action or represented individual characteristics that had to be controlled for in the analysis to interpret the effects of more modifiable variables on the criterion measures; and (2) they added a reasonable amount of additional independently explained variance to the model.

All path-analytic causal models were tested by using standard multiple-regression procedures where the model's path coefficients are equal to the standardized partial-regression coefficients in the equation. To control for individual factors such as "degree of psychological disturbance" and "individual ability," each model's input variables were residualized by the predictors most accurately approximating these characteristics: For example, the variance explained in the scale measuring "ideal psychiatric environment" by the five predictors "distress," "chronic," "single," "high-class father," and "autonomous" was subtracted out of this predictor variable, creating a new residualized input measure.

Thus if

Y_1 = ideal psychiatric environment
X_1 = distress and symptomatology
X_2 = chronic
X_3 = single
X_4 = high-class father
X_5 = autonomous

and $\hat{Y}_1$ equals the linear prediction of Y_1 given X_1 through X_5, so that
$$\hat{Y}_1 = a + bx_2 + bx_3 + bx_4 + bx_5$$
then the residualized input variable "ideal psychiatric environment" may be defined as Y_R, where

$$Y_R = Y_1 - \hat{Y}_1$$
or $\quad Y_R = Y_1 - (a + bx_1 + bx_2 + bx_3 + bx_4 + bx_5).$

Model input variables were residualized by factors requiring control in the analysis, given our understanding of the sheltered-care system. In the example just cited the "distress/symptoms" and "chronic" variables were used in the controlling procedures as indicators of psychological disturbance; the "single," "high-class father," and "autonomous" variables were used as indicators of individual ability. All model inputs were residualized by these indicators of psychological disturbance and individual ability unless the input variable was itself one of the controls. This was true only for "distress" in the internal-integration model. In the internal-integration model the input "distress" was residualized only by individual ability.

Following the development of causal models to predict external and internal-integration scores, a step backward was taken and models were developed to predict each of the predictors of the major criterion. The causal models were also run within dichotomomized or trichotomized categories of major intervening variables such as resident level of psychopathology, assessed by the scores on the BPRS (Overall & Gorham, 1962).

Analysis of Facility Characteristics

In addition to the descriptive analysis of facility characteristics, we sought the variables significant in predicting the use of services by a facility. In conducting an analysis of predictors of service usage, a scale was developed to demonstrate how often facilities use 11 types of social, medical, and rehabilitative services. Each operator was asked how often his residents use a service. An operator indicated whether they used it very often, often, sometimes, rarely, or never (scored 1 to 5 respectively). The total of the 11 normalized item scores is our indicator of "service usage." The procedure for constructing this service-use scale gives equal weight to each type of service in making the assessment of how much service is used by a facility. While this may improperly place emphasis on certain types of services, it was difficult to offer more meaningful weights, given our current limited understanding of the sheltered-care environment. We therefore chose the unit-weighting procedure as a means of obtaining a rough indication of overall service usage by facilities.

THE STRENGTH OF OUR FINDINGS AND CONCLUSIONS FOR POLICY ACTION

In considering the results of this study, especially as they relate to inferences that can be drawn regarding policy decisions relating to factors that facilitate and hinder social integration, the magnitude of significant correlations are in the range of .2. This means that a given factor may account for only 4% of the behavior differences in the population on a given criterion. Some will argue that making policy decisions or even recommendations regarding such decisions based on such small relationships is inappropriate. We would argue, however, that the robustness of these observed relationships and their strength allow them to be detected despite the considerable measurement error involved in survey research methodologies.

COMMENTS ON METHODOLOGY

In conducting the data analysis and designing the survey sample for the study, we employed the most powerful set of procedures possible to obtain the best indication of what it is like to live in sheltered care and what can be done to better this living situation. In many instances, we pushed the robustness assumption in our models very far. By no means could it be said that we adopted the purist approach in our analysis. Yet we believe that, when all is said and done, the results reported justify the approach we have taken.

REFERENCES

Kish, L. *Survey Sampling*. New York: John Wiley and Sons, Inc., 1965.

Lord, F. and M. Novick. *Statistical Theories of Mental Test Scores*. Menlo Park, California: Addison-Wesley Publishing Co., 1968.

Overall, J. E. and D. R. Gorham. "The Brief Psychiatric Rating Scale." *Psychological Rep.* **10**, 799–812 (1962).

APPENDIX B

Harmon House Weekly Schedule

Residents agree to be in structured program/activities between 4:00 p.m. and 10:00 p.m., Monday through Friday

Monday	4:00 — 5:00	Harmon Folk Group rehearsal (Last Monday of each month singing at various community convalescent hospitals)
	5:00 — 6:00	Monday night therapy (community welcome)
	7:00 — 9:00	Work jobs
Tuesday	6:00 — 7:15	Minority awareness (community welcome)
	8:00 — 10:00	Women's Consciousness-Raising Group (community women welcome)
Wednesday	1:00 — 4:30	Potential clients' final screenings
	4:30 — 6:00	Staff meeting
	7:00 — 9:00	Residents' mandatory house meeting
Thursday	4:00 — 10:00	Work jobs
	5:00 — 6:00	Men's Consciousness-Raising Group (community men welcome)
	7:00 — 9:00	Thursday night activity
	7:00 — 10:00	Basketball game (Jones Jr. High School)
Friday	6:00 — 7:30	Grocery shopping
	9:00 — 1:00	Night Club Group
Sunday	9:00 a.m. to 12 noon	Transportation to church facilities and basketball practice
	1:00 — 5:00	Sunday outing

Creative Arts Center: see monthly schedule
Photography Darkroom: see monthly schedule

APPENDIX C

Harmon House Rules

1. No alcohol or illegal drugs permitted in the house.
2. Attendance at house meeting is mandatory.
3. Everyone is to do his or her housekeeping duty.
4. Everyone is to shop and cook when it is their time unless prior okay is received.
5. There is to be no rough-housing, excessive noise, or fighting in the house.
6. No one is allowed in anyone else's room without their permission.
7. Everyone is to be responsible for their own medication.
8. Everyone is to keep an orderly room.
9. Each resident is to be responsible for their personal hygiene.
10. Everyone is to be in an ongoing therapeutic process (i.e., therapy group or therapist).
11. Everyone is expected to be at their daytime activity.
12. Two weeks' written notice is required if leaving house.

APPENDIX D

Resident/House Contract

_____ House is a residential care home licensed by the State Department of Health. We provide a homelike atmosphere and a program for the residents. We do not discriminate regarding race, creed, color, religion, national origin or ancestry in our admission policy or in service offered to residents.

For the stipulated monthly rate of _____ the house will provide:

1. Safe and healthful accommodations.
2. Ample food for three nutritious meals per day (to be prepared by the residents).
3. Laundry facilities available for personal use.
4. Planning and arranging of transportation to local services in case of emergency or when public transportation is not available.
5. A program of recreational activity.
6. Development of a personal rehabilitation plan with each resident which includes arrangements for all necessary community services.
7. Assistance with obtaining a doctor's services as needed.
8. Assistance, as needed, with taking prescribed medications in accordance with physician's instructions.
9. Bedside care for temporary illness.

The rate set forth above is the monthly fee for room, board, and services. Rooms are arranged for double occupancy. Rates will not be changed without thirty (30) days' notice to the residents. The house staff has the right to consult with the resident's physician regarding medications. The house is not licensed for, and will not provide, nursing or medical care.

I understand what is expected of me while I am living at _____ House.

1. I have read the house rules and agree to cooperate with the house regulations.
2. I understand that I am to see an outside therapist on a regular basis, take my own medications and participate in an outside daytime activity and in all required phases of the house program.
3. I also agree to pay my rent of _____ before the tenth (10th) of the month, and if I leave the house I will give at least two weeks' notice before leaving. If I do not do this, I will forfeit the entire month's rent. After giving notice, I am responsible to pay the pro-rated amount for each day until I leave the house.

If I do not cooperate with the aforementioned rules and with what is expected of me in the house, I will jeopardize my opportunity to be a house resident.

_____ Date

_____ Signature of resident and/or conservator

_____ Signature of house representative

APPENDIX E

Consumer-Response Scale Items[a]

Please give us your opinion on the following items. (Circle one)

	1	2	3
1. Do you find the living arrangements here to be:	Good	Adequate	Poor
2. For what you get, the amount you pay to live here is:	A bargain	A fair amount	Too much
3. If you knew of someone looking for a residential care home, would you recommend this place:	Highly	With reservations	Not at all
4. Living here is:	Very comfortable	Comfortable enough	Uncomfortable
5. The food here is:	Good	Adequate	Poor
6. Are you bored here:	Almost never	Occasionally	Usually
7. The rules here are:	Good	Adequate	Poor
8. Do you feel that the appearance and cleanliness of the house is:	Good	Adequate	Poor
9. The amount of privacy here is:	Good	Adequate	Poor
10. Do you feel that living here is:	Very safe	Somewhat safe	Definitely unsafe
11. Do you feel that living here is:	Very helpful to me	Somewhat helpful to me	Not helpful to me
12. How satisfied are you with the amount of influence you have in what goes on in the house:	Very satisfied	Somewhat satisfied	Dissatisfied

APPENDIX E *(Continued)*

	1	2	3
13. How satisfied are you with how much you are expected to participate in house activities and chores:	Very satisfied	Somewhat satisfied	Dissatisfied
14. How satisfied are you with the amount of therapy or treatment you get:	Very satisfied	Somewhat satisfied	Dissatisfied
15. Do you feel that the amount of recreational facilities and activities here are:	Good	Adequate	Poor
16. How satisfied are you with the number of close friends you have here:	Satisfied	Somewhat satisfied	Dissatisfied
17. About how often do you feel as though you want to move from here:	Often	Occasionally	Almost never
18. Do you feel that your needs are taken care of here:	Well	Okay	Poorly
19. As far as doing what *you* want to do or say around here, do you feel that you are:	Very satisfied	Somewhat satisfied	Dissatisfied
20. Do you feel safe on the street:	Almost always	During the day but not at night	Almost never

---

[a]We wish to thank Dr. Edward Oakland and Dr. Thomas Powers for their participation in developing this scale.

AUTHOR INDEX

SUBJECT INDEX

Abshire Act, 35
Access and social integration, 145, 146, 149-
150, 157, 159
as a measure of integration, 55-56
Access to basic or personal resources, 149
Access to community resources, 149
Accommodations, provider involvement in
sheltered care, 64-65, 68
Action for Mental Health, 28
Activity structuring, 221-222
Admissions to mental hospitals, 136
control of, 41
first, 140
number of, 140
rates after LPS, 70, 140, 257-258
Advocacy, 257-258 definition of quality
care and, 75
external social service, 228
interest groups, 73-75
Aftercare, see Services
Age, aged in hospitals, 4-7

control of medications and, 195
drugs and, 238, 240, 244, 248-249
female operator and, 195
ideal psychiatric environment and, 191
neighbor response and, 189
operator perceives services as helpful and,
192
residence club and, 193
resident, see Residents of sheltered care
rurality and, 189
social isolation and, 193
subgroup analysis, 169, 172, 173, 181,
182-183, 187, 195
Aid to the Totally Disabled, 64. See also
Public assistance; Supplemental
Security Income (SSI)
Antipsychotic drugs, see Drugs
Appropriations, 33. See also Community
Care Movement, economics of
Arrests, rates of mentally ill, 67
resident, 142

317